T0226827

Pediatric Liver Disease

Editor

PHILIP ROSENTHAL

CLINICS IN LIVER DISEASE

www.liver.theclinics.com

Consulting Editor
NORMAN GITLIN

November 2018 • Volume 22 • Number 4

ELSEVIER

1600 John F. Kennedy Boulevard • Suite 1800 • Philadelphia, Pennsylvania, 19103-2899

http://www.theclinics.com

CLINICS IN LIVER DISEASE Volume 22, Number 4
November 2018 ISSN 1089-3261, ISBN-13: 978-0-323-64333-7

Editor: Kerry Holland
Developmental Editor: Meredith Madeira

Clinics in Liver Disease (ISSN 1089-3261) is published quarterly by Elsevier Inc., 360 Park Avenue South, New York, NY 10010-1710. Months of issue are February, May, August, and November. Business and Editorial Offices: 1600 John F. Kennedy Blvd., Ste. 1800, Philadelphia, PA 19103-2899. Customer Service Office: 3251 Riverport Lane, Maryland Heights, MO 63043. Periodicals postage paid at New York, NY and additional mailing offices. Subscription prices are $292.00 per year (U.S. individuals), $100.00 per year (U.S. student/resident), $509.00 per year (U.S. institutions), $403.00 per year (international individuals), $200.00 per year (international student/resident), $631.00 per year (international institutions), $338.00 per year (Canadian individuals), $200.00 per year (Canadian student/resident), and $631.00 per year (Canadian institutions). Foreign air speed delivery is included in all *Clinics* subscription prices. All prices are subject to change without notice. **POSTMASTER:** Send address changes to *Clinics in Liver Disease*, Elsevier Health Sciences Division, Subscription Customer Service, 3251 Riverport Lane, Maryland Heights, MO 63043. **Customer Service: Telephone: 1-800-654-2452 (U.S. and Canada); 314-447-8871 (outside U.S. and Canada). Fax: 314-447-8029. E-mail: journalscustomer service-usa@elsevier.com (for print support); journalsonlinesupport-usa@elsevier.com (for online support).**

Reprints. For copies of 100 or more of articles in this publication, please contact the Commercial Reprints Department, Elsevier Inc., 360 Park Avenue South, New York, NY 10010-1710. Tel.: 212-633-3874; Fax: 212-633-3820; E-mail: reprints@elsevier.com.

Clinics in Liver Disease is covered in *MEDLINE/PubMed (Index Medicus)*, Science Citation Index Expanded, Journal Citation Reports/Science Edition, and Current Contents/Clinical Medicine.

Contributors

CONSULTING EDITOR

NORMAN GITLIN, MD, FRCP (LONDON), FRCPE (EDINBURGH), FAASLD, FACP, FACG
Head of Hepatology, Southern California Liver Centers, San Clemente, California, USA

EDITOR

PHILIP ROSENTHAL, MD
Director, Pediatric Clinical Research, Director, Pediatric Hepatology and Liver Transplant Research, Director, Pediatric Hepatology, Professor, Departments of Pediatrics and Surgery, University of California, San Francisco, USA

AUTHORS

LEE M. BASS, MD
Associate Professor of Pediatrics, Division of Pediatric Gastroenterology, Hepatology and Nutrition, Ann & Robert H. Lurie Children's Hospital of Chicago, Northwestern University Feinberg School of Medicine, Chicago, Illinois, USA

KEVIN E. BOVE, MD
Professor of Pediatrics and Pathology, Divisions of Pediatric Gastroenterology, Hepatology and Nutrition, and Pathology, Cincinnati Children's Hospital Medical Center, University of Cincinnati College of Medicine, Cincinnati, Ohio, USA

LAURA N. BULL, PhD
Professor, Department of Medicine and Institute for Human Genetics, University of California, San Francisco, UCSF Liver Center Laboratory, Zuckerberg San Francisco General, San Francisco, California, USA

ALBERT CHAN, MD
Division of Gastroenterology, Hepatology and Nutrition, Golisano Children's Hospital, University of Rochester Medical Center, Rochester, New York; Division of Pediatric Gastroenterology, Hepatology and Nutrition, University of Florida, Gainesville, Florida, USA

CATHERINE A. CHAPIN, MD
Instructor of Pediatrics, Division of Pediatric Gastroenterology, Hepatology and Nutrition, Ann & Robert H. Lurie Children's Hospital of Chicago, Northwestern University Feinberg School of Medicine, Chicago, Illinois, USA

MELISSA GILBERT, PhD
Fellow, Division of Genomic Diagnostics, Department of Pathology and Laboratory Medicine, The Children's Hospital of Philadelphia, Perelman School of Medicine, University of Pennsylvania, Philadelphia, Pennsylvania, USA

JAMES E. HEUBI, MD
Professor of Pediatrics, Associate Dean, Clinical and Translational Research, Divisions of Pediatric Gastroenterology, Hepatology and Nutrition, and Pathology, Cincinnati Children's Hospital Medical Center, University of Cincinnati College of Medicine, Cincinnati, Ohio, USA

NANDA KERKAR, MD, FAASLD
Professor of Pediatrics, Director, Pediatric Liver Disease and Liver Transplant Program, Division of Gastroenterology, Hepatology and Nutrition, Golisano Children's Hospital, University of Rochester Medical Center, Rochester, New York, USA

DANIEL H. LEUNG, MD
Associate Professor, Department of Pediatrics, Baylor College of Medicine, Director of Viral Hepatitis Program, Division of Gastroenterology, Hepatology, and Nutrition, Texas Children's Hospital, Houston, Texas, USA

KATHLEEN M. LOOMES, MD
Division of Pediatric Gastroenterology, Hepatology and Nutrition, The Children's Hospital of Philadelphia, Professor, Department of Pediatrics, Perelman School of Medicine, University of Pennsylvania, Philadelphia, Pennsylvania, USA

PATRICK McKIERNAN, MD
Professor of Pediatrics, Department of Pediatric Gastroenterology and Hepatology, University of Pittsburgh School of Medicine, Children's Hospital of Pittsburgh, Pittsburgh, Pennsylvania, USA

TAMIR MILOH, MD
Associate Professor, Pediatric Gastroenterology, Hepatology, and Nutrition, Baylor College of Medicine, Director of Pediatric Hepatology and Liver Transplant Medicine, Texas Children's Hospital, Houston, Texas, USA

ELLEN MITCHELL, MD
Fellow, Division of Pediatric Gastroenterology, Hepatology and Nutrition, Children's Hospital of Pittsburgh, University of Pittsburgh Medical Center, Pittsburgh, Pennsylvania, USA

DOUGLAS B. MOGUL, MD, MPH
Assistant Professor, Department of Pediatrics, Johns Hopkins School of Medicine, Baltimore, Maryland, USA

KRUPA R. MYSORE, MD, MS
Associate Professor, Department of Pediatrics, Baylor College of Medicine, Director of Viral Hepatitis Program, Division of Gastroenterology, Hepatology, and Nutrition, Texas Children's Hospital, Houston, Texas, USA

KENNETH NG, DO
Assistant Professor, Department of Pediatrics, Johns Hopkins School of Medicine, Baltimore, Maryland, USA

DHIREN PATEL, MD
Assistant Professor, Department of Pediatrics, Division of Gastroenterology, Hepatology and Nutrition, Saint Louis University School of Medicine, St Louis, Missouri, USA

EMILY R. PERITO, MD
Assistant Professor of Pediatrics, Department of Pediatric Gastroenterology, Hepatology, and Nutrition, University of California, San Francisco, San Francisco, California, USA

YEN H. PHAM, MD
Assistant Professor of Pediatrics, Pediatric Gastroenterology, Hepatology, and Nutrition, Baylor College of Medicine, Texas Children's Hospital, Houston, Texas, USA

KENNETH D.R. SETCHELL, PhD
Professor of Pediatrics and Pathology, Divisions of Pediatric Gastroenterology, Hepatology and Nutrition, and Pathology, Cincinnati Children's Hospital Medical Center, University of Cincinnati College of Medicine, Cincinnati, Ohio, USA

SARA KATHRYN SMITH, MD
Assistant Professor of Pediatrics, Department of Pediatric Gastroenterology, Hepatology, and Nutrition, University of California, San Francisco, San Francisco, California, USA

JAMES E. SQUIRES, MD, MS
Assistant Professor of Pediatrics, Department of Pediatric Gastroenterology and Hepatology, University of Pittsburgh School of Medicine, Children's Hospital of Pittsburgh, Pittsburgh, Pennsylvania, USA

ROBERT H. SQUIRES, MD
Professor of Pediatrics, Department of Pediatric Gastroenterology and Hepatology, University of Pittsburgh School of Medicine, Children's Hospital of Pittsburgh, Pittsburgh, Pennsylvania, USA

JEFFREY H. TECKMAN, MD
Professor, Departments of Pediatrics, Biochemistry and Molecular Biology, Division of Gastroenterology, Hepatology and Nutrition, Saint Louis University School of Medicine, St Louis, Missouri, USA

RICHARD J. THOMPSON, MD, PhD
Professor of Molecular Hepatology, Institute of Liver Studies, King's College London, King's College Hospital, London, United Kingdom

Contents

> Alagille syndrome is a complex multisystem autosomal dominant disorder with a wide variability in penetrance of clinical features. Most patients have pathogenic mutations in either the *JAG1* gene, encoding a Notch pathway ligand, or the receptor *NOTCH2.* No genotype-phenotype correlations have been found in any organ system. Liver disease is a major cause of morbidity in this population, whereas cardiac and vascular involvement accounts for most of the mortality. Current therapies are supportive, but the future is promising for the development of targeted interventions to augment Notch pathway signaling in involved tissues.

> In homozygous ZZ alpha-1-antitrypsin (AAT) deficiency, the liver synthesizes large quantities of AAT mutant Z, which folds improperly during biogenesis and is retained within the hepatocytes and directed into intracellular proteolysis pathways. These intracellular polymers trigger an injury cascade, which can lead to liver injury. This process is highly variable, and not all patients develop liver disease. Although the injury cascade is not fully described, there is likely a strong influence of genetic and environmental modifiers of the injury cascade and of the fibrotic response. With improved understanding of liver injury mechanisms, new strategies for treatment are now being explored.

> Genetic cholestasis has been dissected through genetic investigation. The major PFIC genes are now described. *ATP8B1* encodes FIC1, *ABCB11* encodes BSEP, *ABCB4* encodes MDR3, *TJP2* encodes TJP2, *NR1H4* encodes FXR, and *MYO5B* encodes MYO5B. The full spectra of phenotypes associated with mutations in each gene are discussed, along with our understanding of the disease mechanisms. Differences in treatment response and targets for future treatment are emerging.

> Inborn errors of bile acid metabolism are rare causes of neonatal cholestasis and liver disease in older children and adults. The diagnosis should be considered in the context of hyperbilirubinemia with normal serum bile

acids and made by urinary liquid secondary ionization mass spectrometry or DNA testing. Cholic acid is an effective treatment of most single-enzyme defects and patients with Zellweger spectrum disorder with liver disease.

Autoimmune hepatitis (AIH) is characterized by elevated serum aminotransferases, immunoglobulin G, autoantibodies, and interface hepatitis, in the absence of a known diagnosis. Presentation is varied. Therapy is with immunosuppression. There is inflammation of the intrahepatic and/or extrahepatic bile ducts in sclerosing cholangitis (SC), and when associated with inflammatory bowel disease, it is known as primary SC (PSC), with ursodeoxycholic acid used for therapy. The overlap of clinical, biochemical, and histologic features of AIH and PSC is known as autoimmune sclerosing cholangitis (ASC) or overlap syndrome. Liver transplant is performed when medical treatment fails, and both AIH and PSC may recur posttransplant.

Hepatitis B virus (HBV) and hepatitis C virus (HCV) infections represent a major global public health and economic burden, with an estimated 257 million and 71 million people, respectively, having chronic infection worldwide. The natural history of HBV and HCV in children depends on the age at time of infection, mode of acquisition, ethnicity, and genotype. Most children infected perinatally or vertically remain asymptomatic but are at a uniquely higher risk of developing chronic viral hepatitis, progressing to liver cirrhosis and hepatocellular carcinoma, hence classifying HBV and HCV as oncoviruses. This article discusses the epidemiology, virology, immunobiology, prevention, clinical manifestations, evaluation, and advances in treatment of hepatitis B and C in children.

Pediatric nonalcoholic fatty liver disease (NAFLD) is the most common cause of liver disease in children. The spectrum of NAFLD ranges from steatosis to nonalcoholic steatohepatitis (NASH) to fibrosis. Obesity rates in children continue to increase and, as a result, NAFLD in children is becoming more prevalent. The pathophysiology, natural history, and progression of disease are still being elucidated, but NAFLD/NASH in children may represent a more severe phenotype that will benefit from early identification and management.

Cirrhosis is a complex process in which the architecture of the liver is replaced by structurally abnormal nodules due to cirrhosis. Cirrhosis frequently leads to the development of portal hypertension. In children, portal hypertension may have a wide range of causes, including extrahepatic portal vein obstruction, biliary atresia, alpha 1 antitrypsin deficiency, and autoimmune hepatitis. Gastroesophageal varices and ascites are two of the complications of portal hypertension likely to cause morbidity and mortality. This article also discusses extrahepatic manifestations of portal hypertension and treatment options.

Although liver tumors are rare in the pediatric population, they are common in the setting of children with specific risk factors requiring increased awareness and, in some instances, screening. The evaluation of a liver mass in children is largely driven by the age at diagnosis, the presence of any medical comorbidities, and initial testing with alpha fetoprotein and imaging. Specific guidelines for the management of different tumors have been implemented in recent years such that a multidisciplinary approach is ideal and care should be provided by centers with experience in their management.

Pediatric acute liver failure (PALF) is a dynamic, life-threatening condition of disparate etiology. Management of PALF is dependent on intensive collaborative clinical care and support. Proper recognition and treatment of common complications of liver failure are critical to optimizing outcomes. In parallel, investigations to identify the underlying cause and the implementation of timely, appropriate treatment can be lifesaving. Predicting patient outcome in the era of liver transplantation has been unfulfilling, and better predictive models must be developed for proper stewardship of the limited resource of organ availability.

Liver transplant (LT) for children has excellent short- and long-term patient and graft survival. LT is a lifesaving procedure in children with acute or chronic liver disease, hepatic tumors, and a few genetic metabolic diseases in which it can significantly improve quality of life. In this article, the authors discuss the unique aspects of pediatric LT, including the indications, patient selection and evaluation, allocation, transplant surgery and organ selection, posttransplant care, prognosis, adherence, and transition of care.

CLINICS IN LIVER DISEASE

THE CLINICS ARE AVAILABLE ONLINE!
Access your subscription at:
www.theclinics.com

Preface

Advances in Pediatric Hepatology

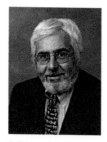

Philip Rosenthal, MD
Editor

The field of Pediatric Hepatology has seen tremendous advances in the past decade with the advent of molecular techniques. These methods have allowed for a better understanding of the cause, natural history, diagnosis, and treatment of childhood liver disease. This issue devoted specifically to pediatric liver disease is both timely and relevant. For pediatric hepatologists, it is an update on the current state-of-the-art. For adult hepatologists who are caring for more and more children who have survived to adulthood with childhood liver disorders, it is a quick and easy reference guide to inform them of the disorders that they will be seeing in their practices. For all medical personnel who care for these patients, it is a useful resource to familiarize themselves with these liver disorders that present in childhood.

Philip Rosenthal, MD
Division of Pediatric Gastroenterology
Hepatology, and Nutrition
University of California, San Francisco
550 16th Street, Mailcode 0136
San Francisco, CA 94143, USA

E-mail address:
prosenth@ucsf.edu

Clin Liver Dis 22 (2018) xi
https://doi.org/10.1016/j.cld.2018.08.001
1089-3261/18/© 2018 Published by Elsevier Inc.

Alagille Syndrome

Ellen Mitchell, MD[a], Melissa Gilbert, PhD[b],
Kathleen M. Loomes, MD[c,d,*]

KEYWORDS

- *JAG1* • *NOTCH2* • Pediatric • Cholestasis • Liver transplant

KEY POINTS

- Alagille syndrome (ALGS) is a multisystem disorder with variable phenotypic penetrance caused by heterozygous mutations in 1 of 2 genes that are fundamental components of the Notch signaling pathway, *JAGGED1 (JAG1)* and *NOTCH2*.
- Features of the syndrome include characteristic facies, bile duct paucity, chronic cholestasis, and abnormalities in cardiac, renal, vascular, skeletal, and ocular systems.
- Indications for transplantation include severe pruritus, liver synthetic dysfunction, portal hypertension, bone fractures, and growth failure.
- Genotype-phenotype correlation studies have not shown a link between mutation type and clinical manifestation or severity, leading to the hypothesis that a second gene could function to modify the effects of a *JAG1* or *NOTCH2* mutation. Several candidate genetic modifiers have been identified in animal and human studies.
- Current therapies for ALGS patients are supportive and focus on clinical manifestations. In the future, new therapeutic approaches may involve modulation of Notch pathway signaling, cell-based therapies, or correction of specific mutations in vitro or in vivo.

INTRODUCTION

Alagille syndrome (ALGS) is an autosomal dominant, multisystem disorder with variable phenotypic penetrance that was first described in 1969 by Daniel Alagille. Initial diagnosis was based on the presence of intrahepatic bile duct paucity and at least 3 other clinical features: chronic cholestasis, cardiac disease, ocular abnormalities, skeletal abnormalities, and characteristic facial features. Although not currently included in the diagnostic criteria, patients also have a high prevalence of renal and

Disclosure Statement: No disclosures to report.
[a] Division of Pediatric Gastroenterology, Hepatology and Nutrition, Children's Hospital of Pittsburgh, University of Pittsburgh Medical Center, 4401 Penn Avenue, Pittsburgh, PA 15224, USA; [b] Division of Genomic Diagnostics, Department of Pathology and Laboratory Medicine, Children's Hospital of Philadelphia, Perelman School of Medicine, University of Pennsylvania, 3615 Civic Center Boulevard, Philadelphia, PA 19104, USA; [c] Division of Pediatric Gastroenterology, Hepatology and Nutrition, Children's Hospital of Philadelphia, 3401 Civic Center Boulevard, Philadelphia, PA 19104, USA; [d] Department of Pediatrics, Perelman School of Medicine, University of Pennsylvania, 3400 Civic Center Boulevard, Philadelphia, PA 19104, USA
* Corresponding author. 3401 Civic Center Boulevard, Philadelphia, PA 19104.
E-mail address: LOOMES@email.chop.edu

Clin Liver Dis 22 (2018) 625–641
https://doi.org/10.1016/j.cld.2018.06.001
1089-3261/18/© 2018 Elsevier Inc. All rights reserved.

liver.theclinics.com

vascular disease. Early approximations based on the diagnosis of cholestasis in infants estimated the frequency as 1 in 70,000 live births. Molecular diagnosis, however, has increased the number of cases detected and the true incidence is probably closer to 1 in 30,000.[1]

ALGS is caused by various mutations in JAGGED1 (*JAG1*), which encodes the ligand Jagged1 in the Notch signaling pathway.[2,3] A majority of patients have a detectable mutation in JAG1 (more than 90%), but there is also a smaller percentage with mutations in *NOTCH2*.[4,5] The same genetic mutation often has different phenotypic characteristics within the same family. There is ongoing investigation into the genetic modifiers of this disease to further elucidate the relationship between genotype and phenotype.

CLINICAL FEATURES
Hepatic

Initial reports of ALGS identified patients based on bile duct paucity. As more has been learned about the disease, it has been shown that although hepatic involvement is common, it is not always present. More recent reports found cholestasis in only 89% of patients and bile duct paucity in 75%.[6] Cholestasis can vary from mild to severe. Hepatitis, if present, is usually mild and synthetic dysfunction is rare. Bile salt levels can be elevated even with normal bilirubin. Bile ducts are also damaged with elevations in alkaline phosphatase and gamma glutamyltransferase. If a patient has liver disease, it typically develops in the neonatal period and presents with direct hyperbilirubinemia. Liver disease does not develop outside of early childhood, and mild disease often improves during this time period.[7,8] Because the mechanism for resolution is poorly understood, it can be difficult to predict which children will improve and which will go on to develop cirrhosis. Total bilirubin above 6.5 mg/dL, conjugated bilirubin above 4.5 mg/dL, and cholesterol above 520 mg/dL under the age of 5 are predictors for sustained and more severe liver disease.[9]

In a recent prospective study of liver disease outcomes in ALGS, the morbidity was much higher than previously reported.[7,10] The cohort was limited to those patients presenting with cholestasis, but 50% had ascites, 25% had at least 1 episode of variceal bleeding, and only 20% survived childhood with their native liver.[11]

There are many complications of chronic cholestasis and some of the most bothersome to children include pruritus and xanthomas. Pruritus also develops early and is often more severe than the degree of cholestasis as measured by laboratory indicators. Intractable itching can be 1 of the most debilitating symptoms of this disease. Patients with impaired bile secretion also have reduced secretion of cholesterol. Cholesterol levels can be more than 1000 mg/dL to 2000 mg/dL, often resulting in the formation of xanthomas. These lesions typically develop over the first few years of life and resolve as cholestasis improves.

Histopathology

Bile duct paucity is the most consistent feature of ALGS (**Fig. 1**C). The normal bile duct to portal space ratio ranges from 0.9 to 1.8. Alagille based his original definition of bile duct paucity as a bile duct to portal tract ratio less than 0.5. It is recommended to examine at least 6 portal tracts to make an accurate diagnosis, but many pathologists require 10 to 20 portal tracts.[12] In 1 large clinical study, bile duct paucity was present in only 60% of liver biopsies done prior to 6 months of age and in 95% of those done after 6 months of age.[7] Ductular proliferation and giant cell hepatitis can also been seen in infancy and have led to misdiagnosis of biliary atresia (**Fig. 1**A, B). The mechanism for the progression of bile duct paucity over the first months of life is unknown but may be

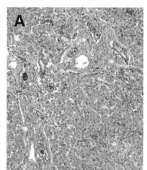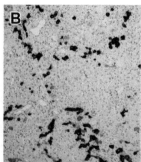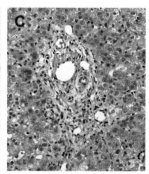

Fig. 1. Variability in histologic features in ALGS. (A) Liver biopsy from a 3-month-old infant with ALGS shows features consistent with biliary obstruction, including bile duct proliferation, bile plugs, and portal tract expansion (hematoxylin-eosin, original magnification ×100). (B) Cytokeratin 7 staining in a 2-month-old infant with ALGS highlights ductular reaction and some aberrant staining in hepatocytes but no interlobular bile ducts (hematoxylin-eosin, original magnification ×100). (C) Hematoxylin-eosin staining of the biopsy (B) presents a portal tract with a branch of the portal vein and hepatic artery but no bile duct, indicative of bile duct paucity (hematoxylin-eosin, original magnification ×200).

related to continued bile duct development and branching of the peripheral biliary tree postnatally. If bile duct paucity is not established at birth, this may provide a window of opportunity for therapeutic intervention (discussed later).

Cardiovascular

Congenital cardiac disease is another common feature of ALGS, with structural abnormalities found in up to 94% of patients. Stenosis/hypoplasia of the branch pulmonary arteries was the most common and found in 76% of subjects, followed by tetralogy of Fallot. Other anomalies are listed in **Table 1**.[13] Patients with ALGS do not get invasive cardiac imaging routinely so it is likely pulmonary artery disease is underestimated in this population. Cardiac involvement significantly increases mortality. Survival to 6 years is decreased to 40% compared with 95% in patients without intracardiac disease.[7]

Although both mouse and human embryo studies have demonstrated the crucial role of *JAG1* in the development of cardiac and vascular systems, the exact mechanism of disease remains unknown and there is no correlation between the genetic mutation in *JAG1* and the presence or type of cardiovascular disease.[13,14]

Vascular

The initial name for ALGS was arteriohepatic dysplasia due to the high prevalence of vascular anomalies. A wide variety of abnormalities have been reported and often lead to significant morbidity and mortality. Noncardiac vascular anomalies accounted for 34% of mortality in patients with ALGS.[15] Epidural, subdural, subarachnoid, and intraparenchymal bleeds have been reported in up to 25% of patients and the vast majority of those patients were found to have no other risk factors.[7,16] There have been several reported cases of moyamoya, a progressive intracranial arterial occlusive disease.[17] Systemic vascular anomalies of the aorta (both aneurysm and coarctation), renal, celiac, superior mesenteric, and subclavian arteries have all been reported.[15] Screening brain MRIs have detected vascular abnormalities in more than 30% of patients, most of whom were asymptomatic.[18,19] Both arterial and venous abnormalities have been found, and many were detected during the first decade of life.[19] Currently, it is recommended that all patients have a screening MRI/magnetic resonance angiogram when they reach

Table 1
Primary cardiovascular anomalies among 200 subjects with a *JAG1* mutation

Primary Cardiovascular Anomaly	Total (%) (n = 200)	JAG1 Mutation (%) (n = 154)	Alagille Syndrome Without a JAG1 Mutation (%) (n = 46)
Cardiovascular anomalies as defined by imaging modalities	150 (75)	119 (77)	31 (67)
Right-sided anomalies	110 (55)	93 (60)	17 (37)
Tetralogy of Fallot	23 (12)	20 (13)	3 (7)
Valvar pulmonary stenosis	15 (8)	11 (7)	4 (9)
Branch PA stenosis	70 (35)	60 (39)	10 (22)
Pulmonary atresia, intact ventricular septum	1 (1)	1 (1)	0 (0)
Truncus arteriosus	1 (1)	1 (1)	0 (0)
Left-sided anomalies	13 (7)	9 (6)	4 (9)
Valvar AS	4 (2)	4 (3)	0 (0)
Bileaflet aortic valve without stenosis	2 (1)	1 (1)	1 (2)
Supravalvar AS	2 (1)	1 (1)	1 (2)
Coarctation of the aorta	4 (2)	2 (1)	2 (4)
Sinus of Valsalva aneurysm	1 (1)	1 (1)	0 (0)
Other anomalies	27 (14)	17 (10)	10 (22)
Ventricular septal defect	10 (5)	6 (4)	4 (9)
Atrial septal defect	10 (5)	7 (5)	3 (7)
Unbalanced atrioventricular septal defect	1 (1)	0 (0)	1 (2)
Patent ductus arteriosus	2 (1)	1 (1)	1 (2)
Left SVC, absent right SVC	1 (1)	1 (1)	0 (0)
Right aortic arch	1 (1)	1 (1)	0 (0)
Anomalous left coronary artery from the PA	1 (1)	1 (1)	0 (0)
Pulmonary vein stenosis	1 (1)	0 (0)	1 (2)
Normal or no cardiovascular imaging	50 (25)	35 (23)	15 (33)
PPS murmur without documented anomalies	37 (19)	27 (18)	10 (22)
Normal echocardiogram	26 (13)	19 (12)	7 (15)
No cardiovascular imaging	11 (6)	8 (5)	3 (7)
No PPS murmur with normal or no imaging	13 (7)	8 (5)	5 (11)

Abbreviations: AS, aortic stenosis; PA, pulmonary artery; PPS, peripheral pulmonic stenosis; SVC, superior vena cava.

From McElhinney DB, Krantz ID, Bason L, et al. Analysis of cardiovascular phenotype and genotype-phenotype correlation in individuals with a JAG1 mutation and/or Alagille syndrome. Circulation 2002;106(20):2568; with permission.

an age where they do not require sedation for the examination and for physicians to have a low threshold to repeat imaging in the case of trauma or neurologic symptoms.

There is no genotype-phenotype correlation, so the exact mechanism of the development of these vascular abnormalities remains unknown/ The expression of *JAG1* in all major arteries, however, has been established in studies of human embryos.[20] It has been proposed that vasculopathy is the primary abnormality in ALGS and causes bile duct paucity as the development of intrahepatic bile ducts is dependent on intrahepatic arterial branch formation.

Renal

Although the initial study by Alagille reported renal features in up to 73.9% of patients, these reports were not confirmed by a nephrologist.[21] A more recent report found renal involvement in 39% of cases with the most common manifestation being renal dysplasia (58.9%) followed by renal tubular acidosis (9.5%), vesicular ureteric reflux (8.2%), and urinary obstruction (8.2%) (**Table 2**).[22] Based on these findings, it has been proposed that renal anomalies be considered a disease-defining criterion in ALGS. Although Notch is known to play a role in glomerular development, there was no association between genetic mutation and renal disease.[2,22]

Although renal insufficiency, including the need for renal replacement therapy or renal transplant, is rare, all patients should have a full functional and structural evaluation at the time of diagnosis. This evaluation should also be repeated if the patient is considered for hepatic transplantation. Renal disease is not a contraindication, and preliminary data indicate that transplant does not have an impact on renal function in patients with ALGS. Knowing about underlying renal disease, however, can help the transplant team adjust the medication regimen to limit nephrotoxic therapies.

Skeletal Abnormalities

There is a wide range of vertebral anomalies described in patients with ALGS. The most common are butterfly vertebrae, which are vertebral bodies where the anterior arches fail to fuse and the vertebra is split sagittally into hemivertebrae. Patients are asymptomatic and there is no structural significance to the finding, but it can aid in

Table 2
Distribution of renal anomalies in Alagille syndrome study cohort

Categories of Renal Anomalies	Number of Patients with Each Renal Anomaly
Dysplasia	43 (58.9%)
Generalized	28
Focal	8
With vesicoureteric reflux	5
With renal insufficiency	2
Renal tubular acidosis	7 (9.5%)
Vesicoureteric reflux	6 (8.2%)
With hydronephrosis	1
Obstruction	6 (8.2%)
Ureteropelvic junction	2
With hydronephrosis	4
Chronic renal failure	4 (5.4%)
End-stage renal disease	3 (4.1%)
Requiring kidney transplant	1
Acute kidney injury	2 (2.7%)
Renal lipidosis	2 (2.7%)
Renal artery stenosis (bilateral)	2 (2.7%)
Focal segmental glomerulosclerosis	2 (2.7%)
Duplex collecting system	2 (2.7%)
Other	3 (4.1%)

From Kamath BM, Podkameni G, Hutchinson AL, et al. Renal anomalies in Alagille syndrome: a disease-defining feature. Am J Med Genet A 2012;158A(1):87; with permission.

diagnosis as it is found in 33% to 66% of patients.[7,23–25] The wide range of frequency reported is likely due in part in discrepancies in detection. Vertebral anomalies have been misreported in 54% of cases so imaging should always be reviewed with a radiologist familiar with these cases.[23] The presence of butterfly vertebrae does not confirm the diagnosis because it can be found in normal children or associated with other diseases, such as VATER association (vertebral anomalies, imperforate anus, tracheo-esophageal fistula and renal anomalies) and 22q deletion syndrome. Additional skeletal abnormalities include square shape to the proximal finger with tapering of the distal phalanges and extradigital flexion creases, ulna shortening, aseptic necrosis of the femoral or humeral head, and temporal bone abnormalities that increase the risk of chronic otitis media.[25–28]

ALGS patients also have an increased fracture risk and lower bone density beyond what would be explained by deficiencies in vitamin D.[29] Fractures in ALGS patients are more likely to be in the lower extremity, with little or no trauma, and occur at an earlier age compared with peers.[25,30] A genome-wide association study of osteoporosis identified a single nucleotide polymorphism in the *JAG1* gene as associated with higher bone mineral density and decreased risk of osteoporotic fractures.[31] There is also evidence in animal models that *JAG1* and the Notch signaling pathway have an important role in skeletal development.[32] It is likely that increased fracture risk in ALGS is multifactorial and related to clinical factors, such as chronic cholestasis, malabsorption, and fat-soluble vitamin deficiencies as well as underlying genetic etiology of the disease with intrinsic abnormalities of bone development and structure. There is a need for further studies to characterize the bone deficits in these patients because fractures are a significant cause of morbidity and can even be an indication for transplantation.

Facial Features

Patients with ALGS have typical facial features that are often described as triangular and can include a prominent forehead, deeply set eyes, moderate hypertelorism, pointed chin, and bulbous tip of the nose (**Fig. 2**). The use of facial features in diagnosed criteria is controversial because of the subjective nature and there is interobserver variation. When dysmorphologists were presented with patients with ALGS

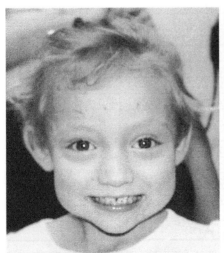 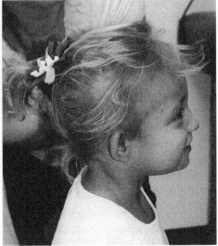

Fig. 2. Typical facial features in ALGS. Front view (*left*) and side view (*right*).

and compared with other early-onset liver disease, they were able to identify patients with a *JAG1* mutation 79% of the time.[26] Although these features typically become more pronounced with age, the adult facial features were most difficult to evaluate successfully. Although the mechanism of the formation of the characteristic facial features remains unknown, the role of *Jag1* in Notch signaling pathway of cranial neural crest cells has been established in mice.[33]

Ocular Abnormalities

Ocular abnormalities do not typically affect vision but can be helpful for diagnostic purposes. There is a wide range of findings but posterior embryotoxon is most common. The term posterior embryotoxon describes a prominent, centrally positioned ring or line at the Schwalbe ring, which is the point when the corneal endothelium and the uveal trabecular meshwork join. Although posterior embryotoxon is found in 56% to 95% of patients with ALGS, it was also detected in 22% of children evaluated in general ophthalmology clinic.[34] A screening ophthalmic ultrasound to look for optic disc drusen may be a more specific way to diagnose ALGS because it was found in up to 95% of children with the disease but only 0.3% to 2% of the general population.[35] Other common findings include retinal pigment granularity, microcornea, anomalous discs and retinal vasculature, mesodermal dysgenesis, lens opacity, and corneal arcus.[36] Although patients with ALGS are often deficient in vitamins A and E, there is no correlation between ocular findings and vitamin levels. A correlation cannot be completely ruled out, however, because current levels do not reflect the levels at time of development.[36] There is also no association between genotype and phenotype.[37]

Growth and Nutrition

Patients with ALGS are known to be significantly smaller in height and weight compared with age-matched peers, with more than half the patients falling below the 5th percentile for height and/or weight.[38] These growth and nutrition deficiencies are likely multifactorial. There is a dietary component because only 20% of children were found to consume adequate calories, fat, and other nutrients.[38] Chronic disease and fat malabsorption from cholestasis are other contributing factors. Growth deficiencies are more significant in children with ALGS, however, compared with other chronic liver diseases, indicating a possible role for *JAG1*.[39] Although any further details on the possible mechanism remain unknown, there is no relationship between height and vertebral anomalies.[40]

Many patients also have steatorrhea and there has been concern for pancreatic insufficiency. Initial studies evaluating pancreatic function included patients only based on paucity of bile ducts. Within that population, children with diarrhea and poor growth had decreased response to pancreatic stimulation and improved growth with pancreatic enzyme supplementation.[41] Later studies, however, showed no difference in fecal elastase or fecal lipase in children with ALGS and so routine screening for pancreatic insufficiency is not recommended.[42,43]

Neurodevelopment

The earliest description of ALGS raised concern for intellectual impairment with 30% of children having an IQ less than 80.[44] Further studies indicated that the number may be lower (16% in a larger cohort) but almost half of ALGS patients have some neurologic deficits and do receive special education.[21,45] Poor nutritional status and severe cholestasis are contributing factors and can also be targets to improve outcomes. The neurologic deficits are greater, however, than those seen in other chronic liver disease patients.[46,47] This indicates a role for *JAG1* in neurodevelopment, and mice with decreased NOTCH1 function had learning deficits.[48]

Children with ALGS are also at risk for mental health issues. In addition to having a chronic disease, children also often suffer from intractable pruritus and xanthomas, which can lead to poor sleep, restrictions in activities, and poor self-image.[45]

GENETICS
JAG1 and NOTCH2

ALGS is an autosomal dominant disorder that is caused by heterozygous mutations in 1 of 2 genes that are fundamental components of the Notch signaling pathway, *JAG-GED1* (*JAG1*) and *NOTCH2*.[2,3,5,49–51] The Notch signaling pathway is a highly conserved system involving 5 transmembrane ligands (*JAG1*, *JAG2*, and *DLL1*, *DLL3*, and *DLL4*) that function to bind 1 of 4 Notch receptors (*NOTCH1*, *NOTCH2*, *NOTCH3*, and *NOTCH4*), expressed on an adjacent cell. In response to this interaction, the Notch receptor undergoes a proteolytic cleavage event that releases an intracellular peptide, which translocates to the nucleus and regulates gene transcription.[52–54] The importance of this signaling pathway in the proper development of multiple organ systems likely explains the pleiotropic nature of ALGS.

Mutations in *JAG1* were first identified in patients with ALGS in 1997 by several groups, and since then more than 500 mutations in this gene have been reported[2,3,50,55] (**Table 3**). These mutations are all found in the extracellular domain of JAG1, which is the portion of the protein that directly binds to NOTCH2 and which contains multiple functional motifs that are crucial for this interaction, including a delta-serate-lag2 domain, 16 epidermal growth factor (EGF)-like repeats, and a cysteine-rich domain.[56] Protein-truncating mutations, which encompass nucleotide-level deletions and duplications, nonsense mutations, large deletions that can span single exons or the entire gene, and nucleotide-level insertion-deletions (indels), are found most frequently in patients with a *JAG1* mutation (75%); however, missense mutations, splice site mutations, large duplications, and translocations have also been reported[49,55,57] (see **Table 3**). Ultimately, mutations in *JAG1* are identified in 94% to 96% of individuals with a clinical diagnosis of ALGS.

Conversely, mutations in *NOTCH2* are found far less frequently and are typically seen in 2% to 3% of individuals with ALGS. A causative link between *NOTCH2* and

Table 3
Type and frequency of *JAG1* mutations found in Alagille syndrome

	Mutation Type	Reported (n)	Frequency (%)
Protein truncating	Small deletions	150	28.4
	Small duplications/insertions	102	19.4
	Nonsense	85	16.1
	Gross deletions	47	8.9
	Indels	12	2.3
Non–protein truncating	Missense	81	15.4
	Splice site	47	8.9
	Gross duplications/insertions	2	0.4
	Translocations	1	0.2
Total		527	100

Data from Stenson PD, Mort M, Ball EV, et al. The human gene mutation database: toward a comprehensive repository of inherited mutation data for medical research, genetic diagnosis and next-generation sequencing studies. Hum Genet 2017;136(6):665–77.

ALGS was first identified in 2006 based on evidence from a mouse model that exhibited ALGS-like symptoms, which prompted screening of *NOTCH2* in patients that did not have a *JAG1* mutation.[5,58] Far fewer mutations have been identified in *NOTCH2*, and unlike *JAG1*, a majority of these mutations tend to be missense (77%), although nonsense, splice site, and nucleotide-level deletion mutations have all been reported[4,5,55,59] (**Table 4**). As seen with *JAG1*, these mutations are clustered in functional motifs that are important in either the JAG1-NOTCH2 interaction (extracellular EGF-like repeats) or required for NOTCH2 to interact with transcription factors and regulate gene expression (intracellular ankyrin repeats).[52,60]

Genetic Diagnosis

A molecular diagnosis is confirmed in up to 96% of individuals with clinically diagnosed ALGS. A majority of *JAG1* and *NOTCH2* mutations can be identified by sequencing all exons, and the immediately adjacent intronic regions to identify splice site mutations, of each gene. Because mutations in *JAG1* are predominant, sequencing of this gene occurs first followed by deletion or duplication analysis via multiplex ligation-dependent probe amplification, chromosomal microarray, or fluorescence in situ hybridization. Sequencing of *JAG1* identifies approximately 85% of ALGS mutations, and deletion/duplication analysis yields an additional approximately 9% of molecular diagnoses. In the absence of an identified mutation in *JAG1*, sequencing of *NOTCH2* identifies another 2% to 3% of mutations in ALGS. There have been no reported large deletion or duplication mutations in *NOTCH2*. A causative mutation for the remaining 2% to 4% of clinically diagnosed ALGS patients has not yet been identified, and the application of various next-generation sequencing techniques could help identify a molecular origin in this population.

Variable Expressivity and Genetic Modifiers

Although the genetics of ALGS is well defined, a lingering question in disease presentation and pathogenesis has centered on the observed variable expressivity of the disease. Individuals with the same mutations, including people in who are in the same family, have been reported to display discordance in both the overall phenotype and/or the severity of the phenotype(s).[1,7,61–65] In support of these numerous observations, genotype-phenotype correlation studies have not identified a link between mutation type and clinical manifestation or severity.[49,66] This inconsistency between mutation and disease presentation has clinical repercussions, with doctors not able to identify at an early age how the disease will progress in a child and how best to tailor therapies, although clinicians are working to identify biomarkers to help with these predictions.[9,67]

Table 4
Type and frequency of *NOTCH2* mutations found in Alagille syndrome

Mutation Type	Reported (n)	Frequency (%)
Missense	10	76.9
Nonsense	1	7.7
Splice site	1	7.7
Small deletions	1	7.7
Total	13	100.0

Data from Stenson PD, Mort M, Ball EV, et al. The Human gene mutation database: toward a comprehensive repository of inherited mutation data for medical research, genetic diagnosis and next-generation sequencing studies. Hum Genet 2017;136(6):665–77.

In the absence of an identified environmental factor that influences disease severity or presentation, scientists have hypothesized that a second gene could function to modify the effects of a *JAG1* or *NOTCH2* mutation to either worsen or alleviate disease features. Through different approaches, several studies have identified putative genetic modifiers to help explain the variable expressivity of this disease.

Two groups have focused on the post-translational modification of both JAG1 and NOTCH2. Both of these proteins contain numerous EGF-like repeats that can be modified through the addition of sugar moieties, a process that is regulated by an enzyme called a glycosyltransferase, which helps with receptor-ligand affinity.[68–75] In 1 study, the glycosyltransferase family of fringe genes, including lunatic fringe (*Lfng*), radical fringe (*Rfng*), and manic fringe (*Mfng*), was studied to determine whether mice with a heterozygous mutation in *Jag1* were further affected when they also had a heterozygous mutation for each fringe gene.[73] The investigators found that double heterozygous mice had increased bile duct proliferation and remodeling compared with mice with only a heterozygous *Jag1* mutation, suggesting a possible modifying effect.[73] Using a similar approach, the second study analyzed mice with heterozygous mutations in both *Jag1* and the liver-specific glycosyltransferase, *Rumi*, and found that these double heterozygotes had a decrease in bile duct paucity compared with mice with a single heterozygous *Jag1* mutation.[75] This suggests that overexpression of *Rumi* in a background of reduced *Jag1* expression may worsen liver disease. Neither of these studies has yet to be translated to humans; however, the biology of each is supportive of a possible, or even likely, functional role.

Finally, a third study aimed to identify genetic modifiers of ALGS through a genome-wide association study that stratified patients with a *JAG1* mutation based on whether they had mild or severe liver disease.[76] Here, an association was found between a single nucleotide polymorphism located upstream of the *THROMBOSPONDIN2* (*THBS2*) gene and severe liver disease. Subsequent protein expression studies and analysis of THBS2/NOTCH2/JAG1 interactions were all supportive of a functional role for THBS2, and the investigators concluded that individuals with increased THBS2, in the background of a *JAG1* mutation, could be at an elevated risk of developing severe liver disease.[76]

MANAGEMENT
Diagnostic Testing

In patients with a suspected diagnosis of ALGS, initial evaluation should include

- Liver function tests, including γ-glutamyl transferase, serum cholesterol and triglycerides, bile acids, complete blood cell count, coagulation studies, and liver ultrasound. Liver biopsy may be done depending on clinical scenario.
- Cardiology evaluation, including echocardiogram
- Renal ultrasound and renal function tests
- Anteroposterior spine radiograph
- Ophthalmic evaluation
- Nutritional assessment, including fat-soluble vitamins
- Genetic testing (discussed previously)

In the era of genomic diagnostics, a diagnosis of ALGS may be determined in patients who do not meet all of the classic clinical criteria, especially in the presence of a positive family history. As time goes on, additional understanding will be gained of the true prevalence of clinical features in individuals with documented mutations in *JAG1* or *NOTCH2*.

Medical Management

It is important to manage a child's pruritus because it can have a significant impact on quality of life. Skin emollients, cutting nails short, and avoiding bathing in hot water can all help minimize itching and excoriations. Ursodiol is a choleretic and stimulates bile flow, making it the first-line treatment of cholestasis.[77] Cholestyramine is a bile acid–binding resin but has to be given 2 hours apart from other medications. Although naltrexone has not been specifically studied in ALGS, it is an opioid antagonist and has been effective in other pediatric cholestatic diseases.[78] The mechanism for which rifampin treats pruritus remains unknown; however, it has been helpful in many children who have not responded to other therapies.[78] Antihistamines should not be the exclusive therapy but can be dosed at night when pruritus interferes with sleep. Children often require a combination of these therapies and they should be added in a stepwise fashion. Patients who fail medical therapy can be referred for a biliary diversion or ileal resection prior to transplantation.[79–81] Recently, clinical studies have been conducted using an ileal bile acid transport inhibitor to interrupt the enterohepatic circulation of bile acids for the treatment of refractory pruritus in ALGS. Results of 1 placebo-controlled study showed that the drug was safe and may reduce pruritus in ALGS.[82] Further studies are required to determine whether this treatment can be effective in this population.

Xanthomas can form on elbows, ankles, knees, and other areas with high friction when cholesterol levels are greater than 500 mg/dL. Although these lesions are not painful, they can be cosmetically disfiguring and bothersome to patients. Xanthomas do not require treatment and typically resolve as cholestasis improves.

Fat-soluble vitamins should be checked routinely and replaced as needed. Each of the vitamins should be dosed individually because a multivitamin contains a fixed ratio and may result in excessive intake of some vitamins to treat insufficient of others. As discussed previously, patients are at risk of malnutrition and growth failure. Therefore, oral nutrition should be optimized with high calorie supplements as needed. Some patients may require nasogastric feeds or placement of a gastrostomy tube to reach caloric intake goals.

Liver Transplantation

Historically, approximately 21% to 31% of ALGS patients require a liver transplant.[82] In 1 recent study of a cholestatic population, however, as many as 70% of patients required a liver transplant during childhood.[11] Indications for transplant include severe pruritus, synthetic dysfunction, portal hypertension, bone fractures, and growth failure. The pretransplant evaluation must include an assessment of cardiac and renal function. Rarely, patients require a cardiac transplant at the time of liver transplant. It is important to ensure the heart can handle the demands of transplant and to repair cardiac disease, when possible, prior to transplant. Renal disease must be evaluated prior to transplant because it can be exacerbated by many of the immunosuppressive medications. Head and abdominal imaging should be completed to identify vascular anomalies because patients are at risk for hemorrhagic bleed and abnormalities in abdominal vasculature could impact the technical aspects of the procedure. Patients who receive a transplant generally do well with improvements in nutrition and growth. One-year patient survival is 80%.[83] Similar survival rates were seen in patients that received a graft from a living related donor.[84] There were no reported cases of complications due to using a family member in these cases. Potential live donors, however, should undergo genetic testing and any individual with a *JAG1* mutation, even in the absence of overt liver disease, should be eliminated from consideration.

FUTURE DIRECTIONS—DEVELOPMENT OF NOVEL THERAPEUTICS FOR ALAGILLE SYNDROME

At present, available therapies for ALGS patients are supportive and focus on clinical manifestations involving each organ system. In the future, new therapeutic approaches may involve modulation of Notch pathway signaling, cell-based therapies, or correction of specific mutations in vitro or in vivo. Although structural cardiac defects occur in early development and are present at birth, involvement of other organs may be more amenable to postnatal interventions. For example, bile duct paucity evolves after birth and there may be a window of time during which a therapeutic intervention could augment bile duct development and branching.

There are several different approaches that could be taken to modulate Notch signaling in vivo.[85] Several pharmacologic compounds are available that can directly promote Notch signaling. Another approach is to increase expression levels of the normal *JAG1* allele or, specifically for the 15% of ALGS patients with nonsense mutations, use a drug that would promote read-through and translation of the mutated *JAG1* allele.[86] Studies are ongoing in other inherited liver diseases using CRISPR/Cas9 technology in human induced pluripotent stem cells to correct mutations in vitro.[87] To date, these studies have focused on hepatocellular rather than biliary defects, but there is potential for future cell-based therapies directed to the bile ducts. In 1 recent study, the mouse extrahepatic biliary tree was successfully reconstructed using human cholangiocyte organoids.[88,89] Gkven the oncogenic potential of Notch pathway overexpression, any therapy designed to increase Notch signaling would need to be used with caution and preferably for a short window of time.

Work from the authors' group and others has shown in mouse models that *JAG1* and Notch signaling are crucial for normal skeletal development and fracture healing.[32,90,91] In a recent publication by Youngstrom and colleagues,[92] the investigators successfully delivered recombinant Jagged1 ligand to bone fracture sites in mice and demonstrated improved healing compared with controls. This approach has potential as a viable therapeutic intervention, not only for ALGS but also for complicated fractures in a broader patient population.

SUMMARY

ALGS is a complex multisystem autosomal dominant disorder with a wide variability in penetrance of clinical features. A majority of patients have pathogenic mutations in either the *JAG1* gene, encoding a Notch pathway ligand, or the receptor *NOTCH2*. No genotype-phenotype correlations have been found in any organ system. Liver disease is a major cause of morbidity in this population, whereas cardiac and vascular involvement account for most of the mortality. Current therapies are supportive, but the future is promising for the development of targeted interventions to augment Notch pathway signaling in involved tissues.

REFERENCES

1. Kamath BM, Bason L, Piccoli DA, et al. Consequences of JAG1 mutations. J Med Genet 2003;40(12):891–5.
2. Li L, Krantz ID, Deng Y, et al. Alagille syndrome is caused by mutations in human Jagged1, which encodes a ligand for Notch1. Nat Genet 1997;16(3):243–51.
3. Oda T, Elkahloun AG, Pike BL, et al. Mutations in the human Jagged1 gene are responsible for Alagille syndrome. Nat Genet 1997;16(3):235–42.

4. Kamath BM, Bauer RC, Loomes KM, et al. NOTCH2 mutations in Alagille syndrome. J Med Genet 2012;49(2):138–44.

5. McDaniell R, Warthen DM, Sanchez-Lara PA, et al. NOTCH2 mutations cause Alagille syndrome, a heterogeneous disorder of the notch signaling pathway. Am J Hum Genet 2006;79(1):169–73.

6. Subramaniam P, Knisely A, Portmann B, et al. Diagnosis of Alagille syndrome-25 years of experience at King's college hospital. J Pediatr Gastroenterol Nutr 2011; 52(1):84–9.

7. Emerick KM, Rand EB, Goldmuntz E, et al. Features of Alagille syndrome in 92 patients: frequency and relation to prognosis. Hepatology 1999;29(3):822–9.

8. Lykavieris P, Hadchouel M, Chardot C, et al. Outcome of liver disease in children with Alagille syndrome: a study of 163 patients. Gut 2001;49(3):431–5.

9. Kamath BM, Munoz PS, Bab N, et al. A longitudinal study to identify laboratory predictors of liver disease outcome in Alagille syndrome. J Pediatr Gastroenterol Nutr 2010;50(5):526–30.

10. Hoffenberg EJ, Narkewicz MR, Sondheimer JM, et al. Outcome of syndromic paucity of interlobular bile ducts (Alagille syndrome) with onset of cholestasis in infancy. J Pediatr 1995;127(2):220–4.

11. Kamath BM, Wen Y, Goodrich N, et al. Characteristics and outcomes of pediatric cholestasis in alagille syndrome in the modern era: results of a multi-centre prospective observational study [abstract]. Hepatology 2017;66(1):60A.

12. Kahn E. Paucity of interlobular bile ducts. Arteriohepatic dysplasia and nonsyndromic duct paucity. Perspect Pediatr Pathol 1991;14:168–215.

13. McElhinney DB, Krantz ID, Bason L, et al. Analysis of cardiovascular phenotype and genotype-phenotype correlation in individuals with a JAG1 mutation and/or Alagille syndrome. Circulation 2002;106(20):2567–74.

14. Loomes KM, Underkoffler LA, Morabito J, et al. The expression of Jagged1 in the developing mammalian heart correlates with cardiovascular disease in Alagille syndrome. Hum Mol Genet 1999;8(13):2443–9.

15. Kamath BM, Spinner NB, Emerick KM, et al. Vascular anomalies in Alagille syndrome: a significant cause of morbidity and mortality. Circulation 2004;109(11):1354–8.

16. Lykavieris P, Crosnier C, Trichet C, et al. Bleeding tendency in children with Alagille syndrome. Pediatrics 2003;111(1):167–70.

17. Connor SE, Hewes D, Ball C, et al. Alagille syndrome associated with angiographic moyamoya. Childs Nerv Syst 2002;18(3–4):186–90.

18. Emerick KM, Krantz ID, Kamath BM, et al. Intracranial vascular abnormalities in patients with Alagille syndrome. J Pediatr Gastroenterol Nutr 2005;41(1):99–107.

19. Carpenter CD, Linscott LL, Leach JL, et al. Spectrum of cerebral arterial and venous abnormalities in Alagille syndrome. Pediatr Radiol 2018. https://doi.org/10.1007/s00247-017-4043-2.

20. Jones EA, Clement-Jones M, Wilson DI. JAGGED1 expression in human embryos: correlation with the Alagille syndrome phenotype. J Med Genet 2000; 37(9):658–62.

21. Alagille D, Estrada A, Hadchouel M, et al. Syndromic paucity of interlobular bile ducts (Alagille syndrome or arteriohepatic dysplasia): review of 80 cases. J Pediatr 1987;110(2):195–200.

22. Kamath BM, Podkameni G, Hutchinson AL, et al. Renal anomalies in Alagille syndrome: a disease-defining feature. Am J Med Genet A 2012;158A(1):85–9.

23. Sanderson E, Newman V, Haigh SF, et al. Vertebral anomalies in children with Alagille syndrome: an analysis of 50 consecutive patients. Pediatr Radiol 2002;32(2):114–9.

24. Deprettere A, Portmann B, Mowat AP. Syndromic paucity of the intrahepatic bile ducts: diagnostic difficulty; severe morbidity throughout early childhood. J Pediatr Gastroenterol Nutr 1987;6(6):865–71.

25. Quiros-Tejeira RE, Ament ME, Heyman MB, et al. Variable morbidity in alagille syndrome: a review of 43 cases. J Pediatr Gastroenterol Nutr 1999;29(4):431–7.

26. Kamath BM, Loomes KM, Oakey RJ, et al. Facial features in Alagille syndrome: specific or cholestasis facies? Am J Med Genet 2002;112(2):163–70.

27. Berrocal T, Gamo E, Navalon J, et al. Syndrome of Alagille: radiological and sonographic findings. A review of 37 cases. Eur Radiol 1997;7(1):115–8.

28. Okuno T, Takahashi H, Shibahara Y, et al. Temporal bone histopathologic findings in Alagille's syndrome. Arch Otolaryngol Head Neck Surg 1990;116(2):217–20.

29. Olsen IE, Ittenbach RF, Rovner AJ, et al. Deficits in size-adjusted bone mass in children with Alagille syndrome. J Pediatr Gastroenterol Nutr 2005;40(1):76–82.

30. Bales CB, Kamath BM, Munoz PS, et al. Pathologic lower extremity fractures in children with Alagille syndrome. J Pediatr Gastroenterol Nutr 2010;51(1):66–70.

31. Kung AW, Xiao SM, Cherny S, et al. Association of JAG1 with bone mineral density and osteoporotic fractures: a genome-wide association study and follow-up replication studies. Am J Hum Genet 2010;86(2):229–39.

32. Youngstrom DW, Dishowitz MI, Bales CB, et al. Jagged1 expression by osteoblast-lineage cells regulates trabecular bone mass and periosteal expansion in mice. Bone 2016;91:64–74.

33. Humphreys R, Zheng W, Prince LS, et al. Cranial neural crest ablation of Jagged1 recapitulates the craniofacial phenotype of Alagille syndrome patients. Hum Mol Genet 2012;21(6):1374–83.

34. Rennie CA, Chowdhury S, Khan J, et al. The prevalence and associated features of posterior embryotoxon in the general ophthalmic clinic. Eye (Lond) 2005;19(4):396–9.

35. Nischal KK, Hingorani M, Bentley CR, et al. Ocular ultrasound in Alagille syndrome: a new sign. Ophthalmology 1997;104(1):79–85.

36. Hingorani M, Nischal KK, Davies A, et al. Ocular abnormalities in Alagille syndrome. Ophthalmology 1999;106(2):330–7.

37. Kim BJ, Fulton AB. The genetics and ocular findings of Alagille syndrome. Semin Ophthalmol 2007;22(4):205–10.

38. Rovner AJ, Schall JI, Jawad AF, et al. Rethinking growth failure in Alagille syndrome: the role of dietary intake and steatorrhea. J Pediatr Gastroenterol Nutr 2002;35(4):495–502.

39. Sokol RJ, Stall C. Anthropometric evaluation of children with chronic liver disease. Am J Clin Nutr 1990;52(2):203–8.

40. Hoffenberg EJ, Smith DJ, Sauaia A, et al. Growth is not related to the presence of vertebral anomalies in alagille syndrome [abstract]. J Pediatr Gastroenterol Nutr 1998;27(4):469.

41. Chong SK, Lindridge J, Moniz C, et al. Exocrine pancreatic insufficiency in syndromic paucity of interlobular bile ducts. J Pediatr Gastroenterol Nutr 1989;9(4):445–9.

42. Kamath BM, Piccoli DA, Magee JC, et al, Childhood Liver Disease Research and Education Network. Pancreatic insufficiency is not a prevalent problem in Alagille syndrome. J Pediatr Gastroenterol Nutr 2012;55(5):612–4.

43. Gliwicz D, Jankowska I, Wierzbicka A, et al. Exocrine pancreatic function in children with Alagille syndrome. Sci Rep 2016;6:35229.

44. Alagille D, Odievre M, Gautier M, et al. Hepatic ductular hypoplasia associated with characteristic facies, vertebral malformations, retarded physical, mental, and sexual development, and cardiac murmur. J Pediatr 1975;86(1):63–71.

45. Elisofon SA, Emerick KM, Sinacore JM, et al. Health status of patients with Alagille syndrome. J Pediatr Gastroenterol Nutr 2010;51(6):759–65.

46. Kamath BM, Yin W, Miller H, et al. Outcomes of liver transplantation for patients with Alagille syndrome: the studies of pediatric liver transplantation experience. Liver Transpl 2012;18(8):940–8.

47. Leung DH, Sorensen LG, Ye W, et al. Neurocognitive status in alagille syndrome: results of a mult-center prospective observational study [abstract]. Hepatology 2017;66(1):647A.

48. Costa RM, Honjo T, Silva AJ. Learning and memory deficits in Notch mutant mice. Curr Biol 2003;13(15):1348–54.

49. Crosnier C, Driancourt C, Raynaud N, et al. Mutations in JAGGED1 gene are predominantly sporadic in Alagille syndrome. Gastroenterology 1999;116(5):1141–8.

50. Krantz ID, Piccoli DA, Spinner NB. Alagille syndrome. J Med Genet 1997;34(2):152–7.

51. Spinner NB, Leonard LD, Krantz ID. Alagille syndrome. In: Adam MP, Ardinger HH, Pagon RA, et al, editors. GeneReviews((R)). Seattle (WA): University of Washington, Seattle; 2013.

52. Bray SJ. Notch signalling in context. Nat Rev Mol Cell Biol 2016;17(11):722–35.

53. Grochowski CM, Loomes KM, Spinner NB. Jagged1 (JAG1): structure, expression, and disease associations. Gene 2016;576(1 Pt 3):381–4.

54. Penton AL, Leonard LD, Spinner NB. Notch signaling in human development and disease. Semin Cell Dev Biol 2012;23(4):450–7.

55. Stenson PD, Mort M, Ball EV, et al. The human gene mutation database: towards a comprehensive repository of inherited mutation data for medical research, genetic diagnosis and next-generation sequencing studies. Hum Genet 2017; 136(6):665–77.

56. Lindsell CE, Shawber CJ, Boulter J, et al. Jagged: a mammalian ligand that activates Notch1. Cell 1995;80(6):909–17.

57. Warthen DM, Moore EC, Kamath BM, et al. Jagged1 (JAG1) mutations in Alagille syndrome: increasing the mutation detection rate. Hum Mutat 2006;27(5):436–43.

58. McCright B, Lozier J, Gridley T. A mouse model of Alagille syndrome: notch2 as a genetic modifier of Jag1 haploinsufficiency. Development 2002;129(4):1075–82.

59. Vilarinho S, Choi M, Jain D, et al. Individual exome analysis in diagnosis and management of paediatric liver failure of indeterminate aetiology. J Hepatol 2014;61(5): 1056–63.

60. Tamura K, Taniguchi Y, Minoguchi S, et al. Physical interaction between a novel domain of the receptor Notch and the transcription factor RBP-J kappa/Su(H). Curr Biol 1995;5(12):1416–23.

61. Dhorne-Pollet S, Deleuze JF, Hadchouel M, et al. Segregation analysis of Alagille syndrome. J Med Genet 1994;31(6):453–7.

62. Elmslie FV, Vivian AJ, Gardiner H, et al. Alagille syndrome: family studies. J Med Genet 1995;32(4):264–8.

63. Izumi K, Hayashi D, Grochowski CM, et al. Discordant clinical phenotype in monozygotic twins with Alagille syndrome: possible influence of non-genetic factors. Am J Med Genet A 2016;170A(2):471–5.

64. Shulman SA, Hyams JS, Gunta R, et al. Arteriohepatic dysplasia (Alagille syndrome): extreme variability among affected family members. Am J Med Genet 1984;19(2):325–32.

65. Krantz ID, Colliton RP, Genin A, et al. Spectrum and frequency of jagged1 (JAG1) mutations in Alagille syndrome patients and their families. Am J Hum Genet 1998; 62(6):1361–9.

66. Spinner NB, Colliton RP, Crosnier C, et al. Jagged1 mutations in alagille syndrome. Hum Mutat 2001;17(1):18–33.

67. Mouzaki M, Bass LM, Sokol RJ, et al. Early life predictive markers of liver disease outcome in an International, Multicentre cohort of children with Alagille syndrome. Liver Int 2016;36(5):755–60.

68. Bauer RC, Laney AO, Smith R, et al. Jagged1 (JAG1) mutations in patients with tetralogy of Fallot or pulmonic stenosis. Hum Mutat 2010;31(5):594–601.

69. Lu F, Morrissette JJ, Spinner NB. Conditional JAG1 mutation shows the developing heart is more sensitive than developing liver to JAG1 dosage. Am J Hum Genet 2003;72(4):1065–70.

70. Morrissette JD, Colliton RP, Spinner NB. Defective intracellular transport and processing of JAG1 missense mutations in Alagille syndrome. Hum Mol Genet 2001; 10(4):405–13.

71. Fernandez-Valdivia R, Takeuchi H, Samarghandi A, et al. Regulation of mammalian Notch signaling and embryonic development by the protein O-glucosyltransferase Rumi. Development 2011;138(10):1925–34.

72. Jafar-Nejad H, Leonardi J, Fernandez-Valdivia R. Role of glycans and glycosyltransferases in the regulation of Notch signaling. Glycobiology 2010;20(8): 931–49.

73. Ryan MJ, Bales C, Nelson A, et al. Bile duct proliferation in Jag1/fringe heterozygous mice identifies candidate modifiers of the Alagille syndrome hepatic phenotype. Hepatology 2008;48(6):1989–97.

74. Takeuchi H, Yu H, Hao H, et al. O-Glycosylation modulates the stability of epidermal growth factor-like repeats and thereby regulates Notch trafficking. J Biol Chem 2017;292(38):15964–73.

75. Thakurdas SM, Lopez MF, Kakuda S, et al. Jagged1 heterozygosity in mice results in a congenital cholangiopathy which is reversed by concomitant deletion of one copy of Poglut1 (Rumi). Hepatology 2016;63(2):550–65.

76. Tsai EA, Gilbert MA, Grochowski CM, et al. THBS2 is a candidate modifier of liver disease severity in alagille syndrome. Cell Mol Gastroenterol Hepatol 2016;2(5): 663–675 e2.

77. Narkewicz MR, Smith D, Gregory C, et al. Effect of ursodeoxycholic acid therapy on hepatic function in children with intrahepatic cholestatic liver disease. J Pediatr Gastroenterol Nutr 1998;26(1):49–55.

78. Zellos A, Roy A, Schwarz KB. Use of oral naltrexone for severe pruritus due to cholestatic liver disease in children. J Pediatr Gastroenterol Nutr 2010;51(6): 787–9.

79. Emerick KM, Whitington PF. Partial external biliary diversion for intractable pruritus and xanthomas in Alagille syndrome. Hepatology 2002;35(6):1501–6.

80. Mattei P, von Allmen D, Piccoli D, et al. Relief of intractable pruritus in Alagille syndrome by partial external biliary diversion. J Pediatr Surg 2006;41(1):104–7 [discussion: 104–7].

81. Modi BP, Suh MY, Jonas MM, et al. Ileal exclusion for refractory symptomatic cholestasis in Alagille syndrome. J Pediatr Surg 2007;42(5):800–5.

82. Shneider BL, Spino C, Kamath BM, et al. Results of ITCH, A multicenter randomized double-blind placebo-controlled trial of maralixibat, an ileal apical sodium-dependent bile acid transporter inhibitor (ASBTi), for pruritus in alagille syndrome (ALGS) [abstract]. Hepatology 2017;66(1):84A.

83. Kamath BM, Schwarz KB, Hadzic N. Alagille syndrome and liver transplantation. J Pediatr Gastroenterol Nutr 2010;50(1):11–5.

84. Kasahara M, Kiuchi T, Inomata Y, et al. Living-related liver transplantation for Alagille syndrome. Transplantation 2003;75(12):2147–50.
85. Andersson ER, Lendahl U. Therapeutic modulation of Notch signalling–are we there yet? Nat Rev Drug Discov 2014;13(5):357–78.
86. Keeling KM, Xue X, Gunn G, et al. Therapeutics based on stop codon readthrough. Annu Rev Genomics Hum Genet 2014;15:371–94.
87. Najimi M, Defresne F, Sokal EM. Concise review: updated advances and current challenges in cell therapy for inborn liver metabolic defects. Stem Cells Transl Med 2016;5(8):1117–25.
88. Sampaziotis F, Justin AW, Tysoe OC, et al. Reconstruction of the mouse extrahepatic biliary tree using primary human extrahepatic cholangiocyte organoids. Nat Med 2017;23(8):954–63.
89. Ghanekar A, Kamath BM. Cholangiocytes derived from induced pluripotent stem cells for disease modeling. Curr Opin Gastroenterol 2016;32(3):210–5.
90. Lawal RA, Zhou X, Batey K, et al. The notch ligand jagged1 regulates the osteoblastic lineage by maintaining the osteoprogenitor pool. J Bone Miner Res 2017; 32(6):1320–31.
91. Dishowitz MI, Mutyaba PL, Takacs JD, et al. Systemic inhibition of canonical Notch signaling results in sustained callus inflammation and alters multiple phases of fracture healing. PLoS One 2013;8(7):e68726.
92. Youngstrom DW, Senos R, Zondervan RL, et al. Intraoperative delivery of the Notch ligand Jagged-1 regenerates appendicular and craniofacial bone defects. NPJ Regen Med 2017;2:32.

Alpha-1-Antitrypsin Deficiency Liver Disease

Dhiren Patel, MD[a], Jeffrey H. Teckman, MD[a,b],*

KEYWORDS

- Alpha 1 antitrypsin • Autophagy • Proteolysis • ERAD • Protein polymer • siRNA

KEY POINTS

- Homozygous ZZ alpha-1-antitrypsin (AAT) deficiency is a common genetic metabolic liver disease primarily affecting adults but also, rarely, children. The clinical manifestations are highly variable, with many patients remaining healthy or exhibiting only mild biochemical abnormalities.
- Accumulation of the AAT mutant Z protein within hepatocytes activates an intracellular injury cascade of apoptotic liver cell death and compensatory hepatocellular proliferation, leading to end-organ injury.
- There is no specific treatment of AAT-associated liver disease; however, there are treatment options involving supportive measures and liver transplant.
- New technologies aimed at stimulating proteolysis via autophagy, small molecule chaperones, gene therapy, RNA technologies, gene repair, or cell transplantation may hold promise for the treatment of this disease.

INTRODUCTION

The liver is the primary site of synthesis of alpha-1-antitrypsin (AAT) protein, although it is also made in enterocytes and some mononuclear white blood cells.[1] Large quantities of AAT are secreted from the liver on a daily basis, second only to albumin as a mass of a single serum protein. Almost all liver disease is associated with homozygosity for the Z mutant of the AAT gene, although in some circumstances compound

Disclosure Statement: D. Patel has no disclosures. Dr J.H. Teckman is a consultant in the Alpha-1 patient community, and grant reviewer and advocate for the nonprofit Alpha-1 Foundation and the Alpha-1 Project. Dr J.H. Teckman is a consultant, site investigator, and/or grant recipient involved with the following companies: Alnylam Inc, Arrowhead Pharmaceuticals Inc, Dicerna Inc, Editas Pharmaceuticals, Gilead Pharmaceuticals, Intellia Corp, Proteostasis Inc, RestorBio, Third Rock Consulting, Triangle Insights, and Snyder Legal.
^a Department of Pediatrics, Division of Gastroenterology, Hepatology and Nutrition, Saint Louis University School of Medicine, 1465 South Grand Boulevard, St Louis, MO 63104, USA; ^b Department of Biochemistry and Molecular Biology, Saint Louis University School of Medicine, 1465 South Grand Boulevard, St Louis, MO 63104, USA
* Corresponding author. 1465 South Grand Boulevard, St Louis, MO 63104.
E-mail address: Jeff.teckman@health.slu.edu

Clin Liver Dis 22 (2018) 643–655
https://doi.org/10.1016/j.cld.2018.06.010
1089-3261/18/© 2018 Elsevier Inc. All rights reserved.

heterozygotes involving one Z gene are implicated in liver disease. During biosynthesis, the AAT mutant Z protein is appropriately transcribed and translated, and the nascent polypeptide chain is translocated into the endoplasmic reticulum (ER) lumen of the hepatocyte.[1,2] In the ER, the nascent polypeptide binds with a complex system of chaperone proteins, which not only assist in folding but also perform quality-control functions to identify abnormal proteins. Unlike the wild-type (WT) M, AAT protein, which rapidly folds into its final conformation and is secreted in minutes, the mutant Z form folds inefficiently: 85% of the molecules never reach a secretion-competent conformation and are retained in the hepatocyte. Individual, monomeric mutant Z molecules are held in the ER, which can last more than an hour before being directed to proteolysis pathways in experimental systems.[2] Some new data suggest that the molecules may be routed to the Golgi and then returned to the ER as part of the quality-control process. Some of the mutant Z molecules aggregate, or polymerize, into large masses surrounded by rough ER, although how the destiny of these molecules is determined and how the location in the ER is chosen remains unknown. Often, these inclusions, termed globules, are large enough to be seen by light microscopy as the classically described periodic acid-Schiff (PAS)–positive, digestion-resistant, hepatocellular inclusions characteristic of this disease (**Fig. 1**). It is this accumulation of AAT mutant Z protein in hepatocytes that is the inciting event in liver injury associated with AAT deficiency. Although this accumulation is the primary cause of liver damage, it is not sufficient because not all ZZ individuals develop liver disease despite the presence of mutant Z protein retained in the liver.[1,3] Therefore, there is likely a significant role for genetic and environmental disease modifiers, or second hits, which determine whether a given individual will develop liver injury and at what age this might occur.

CLINICAL PRESENTATION

Liver disease associated with AAT deficiency is highly variable and may have a variety of clinical presentations, including chronic hepatitis, cirrhosis, hepatocellular carcinoma (HCC), or the rare occurrence of fulminant hepatic failure[4–6] The pathogenesis of liver and lung disease seems to be independent and, therefore, it is likely that they are neither protective of each other nor a risk factor for each other. The peak

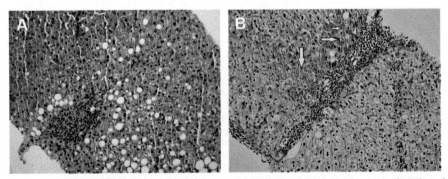

Fig. 1. Photomicrographs of human ZZ liver stained with (*A*) hematoxylin-eosin (H&E) and (*B*) PAS followed by diastase digestion (PASd). PASd stains accumulations of glycoproteins red, which can be easily identified on a neutral background. Normal liver is typically free of large, stainable glycoprotein masses. The globules (some highlighted by *arrows*), are variable in size and are not seen in all hepatocytes for unknown reasons.

incidence of diagnosis of liver and lung disease occurs at different ages in ZZ patients, which gives the impression to caretakers that one does not occur in the presence of the other. The risk of life-threatening liver disease in children is about 3% to 5%, although many children may have self-limited neonatal cholestasis or mild serum aminotransferase elevations.[1,7] In the neonatal period, the typical presentation is the neonatal hepatitis syndrome, which includes cholestatic jaundice, pruritus, poor feeding, poor weight gain, hepatomegaly, and splenomegaly.[7,8] Laboratory evaluation in infants may reveal elevated total or conjugated bilirubin, elevated serum aspartate transaminase (AST) and alanine transaminase (ALT), hypoalbuminemia, or coagulopathy due to vitamin K deficiency or liver synthetic dysfunction. There are rare reports of severe vitamin K–deficient coagulopathic hemorrhage as the presenting feature of AAT deficiency in infants, which may result from impaired vitamin K absorption during subclinical neonatal cholestasis. Liver biopsy findings may be highly variable in infants, including giant cell transformation, lobular hepatitis, significant steatosis, fibrosis, hepatocellular necrosis, bile duct paucity, or bile duct proliferation.[4,5,9] Differentiation from other cholestatic liver diseases of infancy by liver biopsy alone is not reliable. Globular, eosinophilic inclusions in some but not all hepatocytes are usually seen under conventional hematoxylin-eosin (H&E) stain, which represent dilated ER membranes engorged with polymerized AAT mutant Z protein (see **Fig. 1**).[10] Staining with PAS followed by digestion with diastase, a technique which stains glycoproteins red, is used to highlight the globules (PAS-positive) within hepatocytes on a neutral background. Significant accumulations of PAS-positive material are not usually seen in normal hepatocytes. Examination of liver biopsies for PAS-positive globules should be done with caution, however, because similar structures have sometimes been described in other liver diseases (viral hepatitis, alcohol). Furthermore, the globules are not present in all hepatocytes or can be small and dust-like in small infants. Globules may be absent in the neonatal liver.

The best, prospective, unbiased data on the natural history of AAT deficiency are in the study by Sveger and colleagues, which screened 200,000 newborns in Sweden in the 1970s and identified 127 protease inhibitor (PI)-ZZ.[7] These data show that life-threatening liver disease occurs in about 3% to 5% of ZZ children in the first few months or years of life but that the 80% presenting with neonatal cholestasis are healthy and free of chronic disease by age 18 years.[11] However, there is concern that the outcomes reported might not be fully representative of a less homogenous genetic population, such as North America, which may carry a different array of modifier genes.[12]

In toddlers and older children, ZZ AAT deficiency may present as asymptomatic chronic hepatitis (isolated ALT and AST elevation); failure to thrive, possibly with poor feeding; or as isolated portal hypertension, hepatomegaly, or splenomegaly. The occurrence of various liver-related abnormalities ranged from 15% to 50% in the Swedish cohort, although many were mild enough to likely escape medical attention without newborn screening.[7] Many children are completely healthy, without evidence of liver injury, except for mild and usually clinically insignificant elevations of serum AST or ALT. The liver biopsy findings in later childhood often become more classic with easy-to-identify, large globules in many but not all hepatocytes, steatosis, possible lobular inflammation, and possible fibrosis. Occasionally, children with previously unrecognized chronic liver disease and cirrhosis present with ascites, gastrointestinal bleeding, or hepatic failure. There has also been a common observation that some children with severe liver disease in the first few months or years of life may enter a honeymoon period with few signs or symptoms and normal growth before entering a period of renewed progressive injury and decompensation as teenagers. However, even ZZ children with established cirrhosis and portal hypertension may remain stable and grow normally for years or decades with minimal intervention.[5,13–15]

Progressive liver disease in young and middle-aged ZZ adults seems to be uncommon. Although this is mostly anecdotal, the risk of cirrhosis seems to increase with advancing age. There are very little published data on adult AAT liver disease.[6,11,16,17] Adults may develop chronic hepatitis, with or without cirrhosis; however, the risk of clinically significant disease likely increases with advancing age.[16] The biochemical and histopathologic findings in ZZ adult may be similar to those of alcoholic liver disease, which may lead to diagnostic confusion if specific serum testing for AAT deficiency is not performed in patients undergoing evaluation for unexplained liver disease. Liver biopsy findings in adults may include lobular inflammation; variable hepatocellular necrosis; fibrosis; cirrhosis; steatosis; and PAS-positive, diastase-resistant globules in some but not all, hepatocytes; however, rare patients may lack globules.[5] These findings can be similar to those of alcoholic liver disease if the globular inclusions are misinterpreted. There also may be an increased risk of HCC in ZZ adults, although the magnitude of the risk is unclear.[9,16,18] Autopsy studies show that histologically significant but possibly clinically undetected liver injury and cirrhosis may be present in 40% of elderly ZZ adults.[16] As middle aged emphysema is more effectively treated, or prevented as a result of decreased smoking, it is possible that additional older adults with ZZ liver disease will come to medical attention.[16]

DIAGNOSIS AND MANAGEMENT

The diagnosis of AAT deficiency does not require liver biopsy. The gold standard for the diagnosis of AAT deficiency is the analysis of the phenotype of AAT protein in a patient's serum or the genotype analysis of genomic DNA.[1] The phenotype gel analysis is technically demanding and, therefore, is best performed in an experienced reference laboratory. It is common in some liver clinics to use a serum AAT level as a screening test and then perform the gold standard test if the result is outside the normal range. Isolated, single AAT level results should be interpreted with caution, however, because AAT is an acute-phase reactant and even a ZZ patient will have modest increases in serum levels during times of systemic inflammation. Serum AAT levels also seem to be higher in the neonatal period and then rapidly decrease to the more typical expected ranges later in the first year of life, which may not be reflected in the reference ranges of some laboratories. Care should also be taken not to obtain serum for a level or phenotype if the patient has recently had a plasma transfusion, which is sometimes used to treat patients with severe liver disease, because the result will reflect the status of the plasma donor and not the host patient. The same is true if a serum phenotype test is performed on a patient already receiving protein replacement for AAT-associated adult emphysema. Liver biopsy during a liver disease evaluation can be an important tool to assess the degree of liver injury and is still regarded as the gold standard to determine the extent of hepatic fibrosis and to diagnose cirrhosis.

Given the unpredictability of disease progression, many authorities suggest regular monitoring of all ZZ individuals for liver disease, on at least an annual basis, by a physician familiar with liver disease and its complications.[4] Monitoring should include history and physical examination sensitive for liver disease, such as a focus on the detection of splenomegaly, and laboratory examination, including white blood cell count, platelet count, AST, ALT, alkaline phosphatase, albumin, bilirubin, and international normalized ratio. Some data suggest that gamma-glutamyl transpeptidase may be an especially sensitive indicator of liver disease. Granulocytopenia, thrombocytopenia, climbing enzymes and bilirubin, and coagulopathy often accompany progressive liver injury in children and adults. However, care should be taken not to be overly reassured by normal liver blood tests because it is well known that individuals with life-threatening cirrhosis and portal hypertension can sometimes have normal blood tests. As in many liver diseases, a baseline liver ultrasound is considered useful as an adjunct to the physical examination to confirm spleen size and other signs of hepatobiliary health. The American Association for the Study of Liver Diseases (AASLD) guidelines for the detection of HCC recommend a liver ultrasound every 6 months for individuals at greater than 2% per year risk of HCC.[19] Although data for the magnitude of HCC risk in AAT deficiency are lacking, this is often interpreted to apply to AAT individuals with evidence of cirrhosis, portal hypertension, or persistently large elevations of liver tests.

There is no specific treatment of AAT liver disease. Current treatment of progressive liver injury is primarily supportive with attention to the prevention of malnutrition, rickets, coagulopathy, or managing the complications of portal hypertension, such as ascites or variceal bleeding. It is not uncommon for children or adults with AAT-associated cirrhosis to remain stable and compensated, with minimal signs and symptoms for years to decades. Studies show that children with cirrhosis usually have normal growth, development, and anthropometric measures. However, the recognition of the presence of cirrhosis with portal hypertension is critical, even if the patient is minimally symptomatic, so that they can be cautioned against splenic injury from contact sports, advised to abstain from alcohol, supplemented as needed with fat-soluble vitamins, surveyed for variceal bleeding, and cautioned to avoid nonsteroidal antiinflammatory drugs (NSAIDs) because this can result in life-threatening bleeding even in well-compensated individuals. NSAID avoidance is typical advice for cirrhosis of any cause; however, studies in animal models of AAT deficiency suggest that NSAIDs may be uniquely toxic to the ZZ liver even if cirrhosis is not present. This is because AAT is an acute-phase reactant such that the baseline constitutive high level of synthesis is increased in the presence of inflammation. In the case of AAT, the inflammation-linked synthesis is released by prostaglandin inhibition.[1] Therefore, NSAIDs would be predicted to increase AAT synthesis and, in the case of ZZ, would increase hepatic accumulation and augment liver injury. Although never tested in humans, this process of increased ZZ liver injury associated with NSAIDs has been observed in model systems of AAT disease. Although high doses of acetaminophen might also be injurious, normal doses seem less likely to be toxic than normal doses of NSAIDs. Therefore, many authorities suggest overall NSAID avoidance in favor of moderate doses of acetaminophen for mild pain or fever in ZZ patients. There are no data regarding alcohol consumption in ZZ individuals who have no evidence of liver injury. AASLD guidelines for adults with hepatitis C without evidence of liver injury suggest that up to 3 alcoholic drinks per week may be safe.

If progressive liver failure or uncompensated cirrhosis is present and becomes life-threatening, then liver transplantation is considered. In the United States, cadaveric organs are allocated by empirically derived severity scores for both children and adults, which are correlated with increasing risk of mortality without transplant. Early evaluation at a transplant center is recommended for patients with signs or symptoms of deterioration, although early listing and time on the list do not influence the severity scores in the United States. Listing and transplantation in other countries is highly variable and is often influenced by referral, waiting, and center-specific factors. Many centers have reported excellent liver transplant outcomes for AAT deficiency, often better than the median benchmark outcomes for other liver diseases. Living related liver transplants in infants (left lateral segment) and adults (split liver) are also reported as successful, including anecdotes of success when 1 of the donors is heterozygous, MZ for AAT.

All patients with AAT deficiency, regardless of the presence of lung disease or liver disease, are urgently cautioned to avoid cigarette smoke and other inhalation exposures. Some studies suggest that exposure to even secondhand smoke and environmental air pollutants in childhood are important risk factors for the development AAT deficiency–associated adult emphysema.[6,20,21] Therefore, ZZ children and their household contacts are urgently cautioned against smoking, even if they come to medical attention primarily because of liver disease. Children with ZZ AAT deficiency generally do not develop clinically detectable emphysema, although they may be at increased risk for childhood asthma and may report various respiratory symptoms.[22,23] ZZ children are commonly referred to an adult pulmonologist at age 18 years for a baseline evaluation, unless asthma or other respiratory symptoms are present, in which case an earlier pulmonary evaluation is recommended.

HETEROZYGOTES AND OTHER GENOTYPES

It is commonly accepted that individuals who are compound heterozygotes for the S and the Z alleles of AAT (SZ) may develop liver disease identical to ZZ patients, including PAS-positive, diastase-resistant globules. However, the magnitude of the risk of disease in SZ patients is not well-established. The S allele is common in North American and Western European populations, especially in Spain and Portugal. Studies have shown that the AAT mutant S protein can heteropolymerize intracellularly only when it is coexpressed with the mutant Z protein, which may explain the occurrence of liver injury in SZ patients when liver disease is absent in SS individuals.[6,24,25] More than 100 other rare mutations in the AAT gene have been described, some of which yield a gene product with a normal M migration on the phenotype test gel and lack point mutations that define Z or S; however, when present in the heterozygous state with a Z allele, can accumulate within the liver and have been associated with liver disease.[6,26,27] Two examples are the M Duarte and M Malton alleles.[6,26] Serum deficiency states caused by null genes, or other unusual alleles that do not direct the synthesis of a protein product that accumulates within the liver, are not associated with liver disease.[6]

Individuals who are heterozygous for AAT, carrying 1 normal M allele and 1 mutant Z allele (PIMZ or MZ), representing 2% of white populations, are generally considered asymptomatic and healthy with regard to liver and lung disease.[6] However, data from retrospective, referral center studies report a 3-fold to 5-fold overrepresentation of MZ patients in groups with chronic liver diseases, such as cryptogenic cirrhosis, sometimes in association with concurrent viral hepatitis.[6,13] The most widely accepted explanation is that the MZ heterozygous state likely represents a genetic modifier of other liver diseases. There are anecdotal case reports of rare MZ adults developing liver disease, including the development of PAS-positive globules in hepatocytes, without other apparent risk factors for liver disease, although the possible genetic or environmental influences on the development of this injury remains controversial.[6,28–30] MZ children seem to be completely healthy and, even in adults, an MZ phenotype result is not readily accepted as the cause of otherwise unexplained liver disease without extensive further evaluation.

MOLECULAR AND CELLULAR PATHOPHYSIOLOGY OF ALPHA-1-ANTITRYPSIN ZZ LIVER DISEASE

The understanding of liver injury in this disease has been a lengthy process, and identification of critical modifiers is still underway. However, there are a few seminal observations that have driven the field and now provide insights into potential therapies. The first was the original recognition by Sharp and colleagues that pediatric ZZ patients can develop liver disease.[31] Then, studies of patient tissues by Perlmutter and colleagues showed reduced intracellular clearance of mutant Z protein correlated to life-threatening liver disease, which gave strong support to the hypothesis that accumulation of the mutant Z protein in the liver was the key trigger of liver injury.[32] The accumulation hypothesis was also dramatically illustrated in various studies of mice transgenic for the human mutant Z gene. These mice retain their endogenous antiprotease genes but develop liver injury very similar to ZZ humans, which seems to be caused by hepatic accumulation of mutant Z protein. At the same time, the polymerized conformation was discovered by Lomas and Carrell, which focused the field on the key concepts of protein conformation and trafficking.[33] More recently, the discovery by Teckman and Perlmutter that autophagy was an important route of intracellular degradation for the mutant Z protein, when combined with these other concepts, has led to multiple new therapeutic approaches.[2] Many investigators have studied the role of intracellular degradation in liver injury, with the findings of Sifers and colleagues being especially informative regarding mutant protein trafficking, degradation involving ER-associated degradation (ERAD), the MAN1B1, and identification of factors associated with susceptibility to liver disease. Finally, documentation by Teckman and Perlmutter of the hepatocellular apoptosis and compensatory proliferation in the liver revealed how mutant Z protein accumulation was likely linked to cirrhosis and HCC.[34,35] Following is a review of how these discoveries led to the current concept of the mechanism of AAT liver injury.

Accumulation of the mutant Z protein in hepatocytes is the inciting event of liver injury, although most of the retained mutant Z protein molecules are eventually directed to intracellular proteolysis pathways and degraded into their constituent amino acids (**Fig. 2**).[2] The cell uses a variety of proteolytic processes in an attempt to reduce the intracellular mutant Z protein burden and reduce injury. These include ubiquitin-dependent and ubiquitin-independent proteasomal pathways, as well as other mechanisms sometimes referred to as ERAD.[36] It is thought that the proteasomal pathways as a part of ERAD are the primary route for degradation for AAT mutant Z monomeric molecules in the nonpolymerized conformation. Although many of the mechanistic steps in the degradation process, and their specific sequence, are still being investigated, previous work has shown that 2 molecules present in the ER, calnexin and ER ManlBl, are likely to be critical points of control.[36,37] Calnexin is a transmembrane ER chaperone that binds AAT mutant Z, becomes targeted for degradation by linkage to ubiquitin, and then is degraded as this trimolecular complex (AAT mutant Z-calnexin-ubiquitin) by the proteasome.[38] Studies in human fibroblast cell lines established from ZZ homozygous patients show that patients susceptible to liver disease have less efficient ERAD of AAT mutant Z protein than ZZ patients without liver disease.[25,39] The reduced efficiency of degradation in liver disease patients presumably leads to a greater steady-state burden of mutant Z protein within liver cells and increased liver injury. Studies of the enzyme ManlBl also suggest that it may have a critical role in directing AAT mutant Z molecules to the proteasome for degradation. These data raise the possibility that allelic variations in these genes, or in other genes involved in the quality-control or proteolytic systems, might alter susceptibility to liver injury by changing the efficiency of degradation. There has been a report that susceptibility to liver disease might also be related to allelic variations in the AAT gene itself, which would not otherwise be considered disease-associated mutations.[40] Another important proteolytic pathway seems to be autophagy. Autophagy is a highly conserved degradation system in which specialized vacuoles degrade abnormal proteins and larger

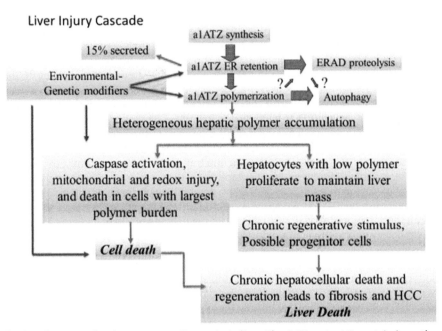

Fig. 2. Injury cascade of AAT mutant Z protein in liver. The AAT mutant Z protein is synthesized but then 85% of the molecules are retained in the ER of hepatocytes rather than secreted. Quality-control processes direct most of the mutant Z protein molecules to intracellular proteolysis (ERAD). However, some of the mutant Z protein molecules escape proteolysis and may attain a polymerized conformation, forming inclusions in the ER. Autophagy is activated to degrade mutant Z polymer; however, for reasons that are still unclear, some cells remain engorged with large amounts of mutant Z polymerized protein. In the population of cells with the largest polymer accumulations, hepatocellular death results from an uninhibited apoptotic cascade, redox injury, and possibly other mechanisms. Compensatory hepatocellular regeneration is stimulated to preserve functional liver mass. The chronic cycle of liver cell death and regenerations leads to fibrosis, HCC and end-organ injury. Given the variable nature of clinical liver injury between individuals with this same genotype, there are likely to be important genetic modifiers affecting the rate and magnitude of these processes.

structures such as senescent organelles. Studies show that the accumulation of the polymerized AAT mutant Z protein within cells induces an autophagic response and that autophagy is an important route for the degradation of AAT mutant Z polymers.[2] In experimental systems, liver injury can be reduced by increased autophagic degradation of mutant Z polymer protein.[41–43]

Several other lines of evidence support this model of injury from mutant Z protein accumulation. Studies in cell culture models and mouse models, show that there is a dose–response relationship between AAT mutant Z intracellular protein accumulation and cell and liver injury.[44] Several experimental systems have been used to increase mutant Z protein intracellular accumulation, such as inhibitors of degradation or enhanced inflammation, which result in increased cell injury markers. Likewise, interventions to reduce mutant Z intracellular accumulation, including silencing RNA (siRNA) to reduce synthesis and drugs to enhance degradation, have a profoundly positive effect on protecting cells from injury and can even eliminate the liver injury in a mouse model.

Clinically, liver injury in ZZ humans is usually a slow process that takes place over years to decades, and analysis of human livers have shown that accumulation of AAT mutant Z protein is very heterogeneous among individual hepatocytes.[3,45] In the past, it was difficult to reconcile these clinical data with in vitro, cell biological mechanistic studies. New insights from recent studies show that a cellular injury cascade is triggered within the small population of hepatocytes, with the largest AAT mutant Z polymerized protein accumulation. Hepatocytes with the largest AAT mutant Z protein accumulation, perhaps only a few percent of the total hepatocytes, have increased caspase activation and increased susceptibility to apoptosis.[1,35] There is also a newly recognized component of oxidative injury.[44] These processes cause a low but higher than normal baseline rate of hepatocyte death in ZZ liver tissue compared with normal liver. The cells with low polymer accumulation then proliferate to maintain the functional liver mass. Over time, the continued stress, death, and repair leads to liver fibrosis, cirrhosis, HCC, and chronic organ injury. Environmental and genetic modifiers of protein secretion, degradation, apoptosis, or regeneration would then by hypothesized to influence the progression of liver disease in an individual patient.[35]

NEW THERAPEUTIC TECHNOLOGIES

Many new approaches are currently being examined for potential value in the treatment of AAT deficiency. Extensive studies have been published using in vitro analyses of molecular structure, and more than 10 different compounds have been shown to block liver injury in the PiZ mouse model of AAT liver disease, although none are yet approved for human use.[35,42,43,46] First, at the point of synthesis, several applications of RNA inhibition technology are being examined to prevent mutant Z protein synthesis and thereby prevent accumulation and liver injury. In the PiZ mouse model, these methods have been shown to eliminate liver injury and to return the liver to WT health.[47] Two different phase I human trials of siRNA inhibition of mutant Z protein synthesis as liver disease therapy have been performed and will soon be expanded to phase II. Several gene repair technologies are also being investigated, including the recently developed clustered regularly interspersed short palindromic repeats (CRISPR) method but no human trials have yet begun and in vitro reports are still limited. However, the promise of this approach, which might be a long-term answer to both lung and liver disease, is exciting.

There has been longstanding interest in chemical chaperone approaches to improve proper folding and to augment secretion of AAT mutant Z, instead of intrahepatic protein retention. Such an approach might treat the lung and the liver, as well. The primary barrier to this approach is the sheer mass of AAT protein synthesized, which is up to 2 g/d in an adult. If a 1-to-1 binding stoichiometry is needed as part of the mechanism, then a huge mass of drug would need to be delivered to the ER of the hepatocytes. Nevertheless, studies in cell cultures have shown that several compounds promote the secretion of AAT and, of these, 4-phenyl butyrate was effective in the mouse model.[48] A pilot human trial was conducted but no effect on secretion was detected, likely due to peak drug levels not able to reach the therapeutic range documented in the mouse.[49] Strategies designed in silico or cell-free systems for therapeutic disruption of mutant Z protein polymerization, likely an event distal to the protein-retention signal, have also been examined in several studies.[46,50] However, many of the compounds examined have not had the predicted effect when examined in cell culture and there have been chemical hurdles to creating medicinal molecules for trials in animal models.

Extensive studies have also examined methods to accelerate the intracellular degradation of mutant Z protein as a treatment of the liver. Several successful cell culture and mouse experiments have shown that enhanced autophagic degradation reduces the burden of mutant Z protein in the liver and reduces liver injury.[1–3] Autophagy is an intracellular degradation pathway known to play an important role in trying to compensate for the accumulation of misfolded mutant Z protein in the liver. Sirolimus, carbamazepine, and the bile acid or ursodeoxycholic acid, plus a genetic approach to augment expression of key autophagy regulators, have all been shown to reduce mutant Z protein accumulation within cells via enhanced autophagy and to reduce liver cell injury in model system. Basic science studies have also suggested similar effects from fluphenazine, pimozide, suberoylanilide, hydroxamic acid (SAHA), tat-beclin-1 peptide, ezetimibe, spermidine, and stattic, among others. However, excessively high doses of all of these agents were required to show an effect. A human trial of low-dose carbamazepine in ZZ patients with cirrhosis was begun but has been closed with no results released. Finally, several studies, including human trials, have examined strategies to synthesize WT AAT in tissues outside the liver, which might increase serum levels to protect the lung but which would not change the risk of liver injury.[51,52] To date, these studies have only been able to generate less than 5% of the WT serum AAT level thought to be needed for therapeutic benefit.

SUMMARY

Homozygous ZZ AAT deficiency is a common genetic metabolic liver disease primarily affecting adults but also, rarely, children. The clinical manifestations are highly variable, with many patients remaining healthy or exhibiting only mild biochemical abnormalities. Accumulation of the AAT mutant Z protein within hepatocytes activates an intracellular injury cascade of apoptotic liver cell death and compensatory hepatocellular proliferation, leading to end-organ injury. Genetic and environmental disease modifiers are thought to be important but remain generally unidentified. There is no specific treatment of AAT-associated liver disease; however, there are treatment options involving supportive measures and liver transplant. New technologies aimed at stimulating proteolysis via autophagy, small molecule chaperones, gene therapy, RNA technologies, gene repair, or cell transplantation may hold promise for the treatment of this disease. Future research is likely to lead to studies of these new approaches, although the high degree of clinical variability will pose a challenge to the design of clinical trials.

REFERENCES

1. Teckman JH, Mangalat N. Alpha-1 antitrypsin and liver disease: mechanisms of injury and novel interventions. Expert Rev Gastroenterol Hepatol 2015;9(2): 261–8.
2. Teckman JH, Perlmutter DH. Retention of mutant alpha(1)-antitrypsin Z in endoplasmic reticulum is associated with an autophagic response. Am J Physiol Gastrointest Liver Physiol 2000;279(5):G961–74.
3. Teckman JH, Rosenthal P, Abel R, et al. Baseline analysis of a young alpha-1-antitrypsin deficiency liver disease cohort reveals frequent portal hypertension. J Pediatr Gastroenterol Nutr 2015;61(1):94–101.
4. Nelson DR, Teckman J, Di Bisceglie AM, et al. Diagnosis and management of patients with a(1)-antitrypsin (A1AT) deficiency. Clin Gastroenterol Hepatol 2011. https://doi.org/10.1016/j.cgh.2011.12.028.

5. Perlmutter DH. Alpha-1-antitrypsin deficiency: diagnosis and treatment. Clin Liver Dis 2004;8(4):839–59, viii–ix.

6. American Thoracic Society, European Respiratory Society. American Thoracic Society/European Respiratory Society statement: standards for the diagnosis and management of individuals with alpha-1 antitrypsin deficiency. Am J Respir Crit Care Med 2003;168(7):818–900.

7. Sveger T. Liver disease in alpha1-antitrypsin deficiency detected by screening of 200,000 infants. N Engl J Med 1976;294(24):1316–21.

8. Sveger T. Alpha 1-antitrypsin deficiency in early childhood. Pediatrics 1978;62(1): 22–5.

9. Eriksson S. Alpha 1-antitrypsin deficiency. J Hepatol 1999;30(Suppl 1):34–9.

10. Alboni P, Gianfranchi L, Pacchioni F, et al. Antiarrhythmic drugs in patients with recurrent atrial fibrillation: where are we? Ital Heart J 2005;6(3):169–74.

11. Sveger T, Eriksson S. The liver in adolescents with alpha 1-antitrypsin deficiency. Hepatology 1995;22(2):514–7.

12. Cruz PE, Mueller C, Cossette TL, et al. In vivo post-transcriptional gene silencing of alpha-1 antitrypsin by adeno-associated virus vectors expressing siRNA. Lab Invest 2007;87(9):893–902.

13. Sveger T. The natural history of liver disease in alpha 1-antitrypsin deficient children. Acta Paediatr Scand 1988;77(6):847–51.

14. Mowat AP. Alpha 1-antitrypsin deficiency (PiZZ): features of liver involvement in childhood. Acta Paediatr Suppl 1994;393:13–7.

15. Pittschieler K, Massi G. Alpha 1 antitrypsin deficiency in two population groups in north Italy. Padiatr Padol 1988;23(4):307–11.

16. Eriksson S. Alpha-1-antitrypsin deficiency: natural course and therapeutic strategies. In: Boyer JL, Blum HE, Maier KP, et al, editors. Falk symposium 115: liver cirrhosis and its development. Dordrecht (Netherlands): Kluwer Academic Publishers; 2001. p. 307–15.

17. Eriksson S. A 30-year perspective on alpha 1-antitrypsin deficiency. Chest 1996; 110(6 Suppl):237S–42S.

18. Eriksson S, Lindmark B, Olsson S. Lack of association between hemochromatosis and alpha-antitrypsin deficiency. Acta Med Scand 1986;219(3):291–4.

19. He XX, Li Y, Ren HP, et al. 2010 guideline for the management of hepatocellular carcinoma recommended by the American Association for the Study of Liver Diseases. Zhonghua Gan Zang Bing Za Zhi 2011;19(4):249–50 [in Chinese].

20. Piitulainen E, Sveger T. Respiratory symptoms and lung function in young adults with severe alpha(1)-antitrypsin deficiency (PiZZ). Thorax 2002;57(8):705–8.

21. Sveger T, Thelin T, McNeil TF. Young adults with alpha 1-antitrypsin deficiency identified neonatally: their health, knowledge about and adaptation to the high-risk condition. Acta Paediatr 1997;86(1):37–40.

22. Sveger T, Piitulainen E, Arborelius M Jr. Lung function in adolescents with alpha 1-antitrypsin deficiency. Acta Paediatr 1994;83(11):1170–3.

23. Eden E, Hammel J, Rouhani FN, et al. Asthma features in severe alpha1-antitrypsin deficiency: experience of the National Heart, lung, and blood Institute Registry. Chest 2003;123(3):765–71.

24. Mahadeva R, Chang WS, Dafforn TR, et al. Heteropolymerization of S, I, and Z alpha1-antitrypsin and liver cirrhosis. J Clin Invest 1999;103(7):999–1006.

25. Teckman JH, Perlmutter DH. The endoplasmic reticulum degradation pathway for mutant secretory proteins alpha1-antitrypsin Z and S is distinct from that for an unassembled membrane protein. J Biol Chem 1996;271(22):13215–20.

26. Lomas DA, Elliott PR, Sidhar SK, et al. Alpha 1-Antitrypsin Mmalton (Phe52-deleted) forms loop-sheet polymers in vivo. Evidence for the C sheet mechanism of polymerization. J Biol Chem 1995;270(28):16864–70.

27. Lomas DA, Finch JT, Seyama K, et al. Alpha 1-antitrypsin Siiyama (Ser53–>Phe). Further evidence for intracellular loop-sheet polymerization. J Biol Chem 1993; 268(21):15333–5.

28. Pittschieler K. Liver disease and heterozygous alpha-1-antitrypsin deficiency. Acta Paediatr Scand 1991;80(3):323–7.

29. Kaserbacher R, Propst T, Propst A, et al. Association between heterozygous alpha 1-antitrypsin deficiency and genetic hemochromatosis. Hepatology 1993; 18(3):707–8.

30. Propst T, Propst A, Dietze O, et al. High prevalence of viral infection in adults with homozygous and heterozygous alpha 1-antitrypsin deficiency and chronic liver disease. Ann Intern Med 1992;117(8):641–5.

31. Sharp HL, Bridges RA, Krivit W, et al. Cirrhosis associated with alpha-1-antitrypsin deficiency: a previously unrecognized inherited disorder. J Lab Clin Med 1969; 73(6):934–9.

32. Wu Y, Whitman I, Molmenti E, et al. A lag in intracellular degradation of mutant alpha 1-antitrypsin correlates with the liver disease phenotype in homozygous PiZZ alpha 1-antitrypsin deficiency. Proc Natl Acad Sci U S A 1994;91(19):9014–8.

33. Lomas DA, Evans DL, Finch JT, et al. The mechanism of Z alpha 1-antitrypsin accumulation in the liver. Nature 1992;357(6379):605–7.

34. Rudnick DA, Liao Y, An JK, et al. Analyses of hepatocellular proliferation in a mouse model of alpha-1-antitrypsin deficiency. Hepatology 2004;39(4):1048–55.

35. Lindblad D, Blomenkamp K, Teckman J. Alpha-1-antitrypsin mutant Z protein content in individual hepatocytes correlates with cell death in a mouse model. Hepatology 2007;46(4):1228–35.

36. Sifers RN. Medicine. Clearing conformational disease. Science 2010;329(5988): 154–5.

37. Sifers RN. Resurrecting the protein fold for disease intervention. Chem Biol 2013; 20(3):298–300.

38. Qu D, Teckman JH, Omura S, et al. Degradation of a mutant secretory protein, alpha1-antitrypsin Z, in the endoplasmic reticulum requires proteasome activity. J Biol Chem 1996;271(37):22791–5.

39. Perlmutter DH. Alpha-1-antitrypsin deficiency: importance of proteasomal and autophagic degradative pathways in disposal of liver disease-associated protein aggregates. Annu Rev Med 2011;62:333–45.

40. Sifers RN. Intracellular processing of alpha1-antitrypsin. Proc Am Thorac Soc 2010;7(6):376–80.

41. Pastore N, Blomenkamp K, Annunziata F, et al. Gene transfer of master autophagy regulator TFEB results in clearance of toxic protein and correction of hepatic disease in alpha-1-anti-trypsin deficiency. EMBO Mol Med 2013;5(3):397–412.

42. Kaushal S, Annamali M, Blomenkamp K, et al. Rapamycin reduces intrahepatic alpha-1-antitrypsin mutant Z protein polymers and liver injury in a mouse model. Exp Biol Med (Maywood) 2010;235(6):700–9.

43. Hidvegi T, Ewing M, Hale P, et al. An autophagy-enhancing drug promotes degradation of mutant alpha1-antitrypsin Z and reduces hepatic fibrosis. Science 2010; 329(5988):229–32.

44. Marcus NY, Blomenkamp K, Ahmad M, et al. Oxidative stress contributes to liver damage in a murine model of alpha-1-antitrypsin deficiency. Exp Biol Med (Maywood) 2012;237(10):1163–72.

45. Teckman JH. Liver disease in alpha-1 antitrypsin deficiency: current understanding and future therapy. COPD 2013;10(Suppl 1):35–43.

46. Mahadeva R, Dafforn TR, Carrell RW, et al. 6-mer peptide selectively anneals to a pathogenic serpin conformation and blocks polymerization. Implications for the prevention of Z alpha(1)-antitrypsin-related cirrhosis. J Biol Chem 2002;277(9): 6771–4.

47. Guo S, Booten SL, Aghajan M, et al. Antisense oligonucleotide treatment ameliorates alpha-1 antitrypsin-related liver disease in mice. J Clin Invest 2014;124(1): 251–61.

48. Burrows JA, Willis LK, Perlmutter DH. Chemical chaperones mediate increased secretion of mutant alpha 1-antitrypsin (alpha 1-AT) Z: a potential pharmacological strategy for prevention of liver injury and emphysema in alpha 1-AT deficiency. Proc Natl Acad Sci U S A 2000;97(4):1796–801.

49. Teckman JH. Lack of effect of oral 4-phenylbutyrate on serum alpha-1-antitrypsin in patients with alpha-1-antitrypsin deficiency: a preliminary study. J Pediatr Gastroenterol Nutr 2004;39(1):34–7.

50. Parfrey H, Dafforn TR, Belorgey D, et al. Inhibiting polymerization: new therapeutic strategies for Z alpha1-antitrypsin-related emphysema. Am J Respir Cell Mol Biol 2004;31(2):133–9.

51. Loring HS, Flotte TR. Current status of gene therapy for alpha-1 antitrypsin deficiency. Expert Opin Biol Ther 2015;15(3):329–36.

52. Flotte TR, Trapnell BC, Humphries M, et al. Phase 2 clinical trial of a recombinant adeno-associated viral vector expressing alpha1-antitrypsin: interim results. Hum Gene Ther 2011;22(10):1239–47.

Progressive Familial Intrahepatic Cholestasis

Laura N. Bull, PhD[a],*, Richard J. Thompson, MD, PhD[b]

KEYWORDS

- Cholestasis • Genetics • Bile acids • Pediatrics • PFIC

KEY POINTS

- Progressive familial intrahepatic cholestasis (PFIC) is an umbrella term and describes the severest form of a number of genetically discrete diseases.
- Mechanisms of cholestasis include defects of canalicular transport, tight junction integrity, nuclear signaling, vesicular trafficking, and membrane maintenance.
- Human bile acids are highly detergent and most cellular and organ damage in PFIC is mediated through a failure of bile acid and lipid homeostasis.
- Genetic technology has helped reveal disease mechanisms, and can now be incorporated in new diagnostic algorithms.

INTRODUCTION

Bile was recognized by the ancient Greeks as 1 of the 4 humors; its importance is still recognized in twenty-first century medicine, although maybe only by hepatologists. Bile formation is essential for normal liver and gastrointestinal functions. Jaundice is the most frequent manifestation of liver disease, and exemplifies the importance of bile in the disposal of a major waste product, bilirubin. Bile is in truth a complex liquid. It is an alkali solution, rich in a variety of lipids, containing numerous organic anions. Many of the latter are metabolites of drugs and other xenobiotics that have been conjugated and excreted by the liver. The lipids are largely composed of bile acids, which are themselves amphipaths with powerful detergent properties. Human bile acids are particularly powerful detergents. The biliary tree, like every other epithelium, is composed of cells, themselves defined by the lipid plasma membrane. The normal lipid composition of the canalicular and cholangiocyte apical membrane renders the cells more resistant to detergent damage than most epithelia. Furthermore, the

Disclosure Statement: R.J. Thompson has undertaken consultancy work for Shire, Albireo, Arcturus, Alexion, Retrophin, GSK, and Qing Bile Therapeutics. L.N. Bull has nothing to disclose.
[a] Department of Medicine and Institute for Human Genetics, University of California San Francisco, UCSF Liver Center Laboratory, Zuckerberg San Francisco General, 1001 Potrero Avenue, Building 40, Room 4102, San Francisco, CA 94110, USA; [b] Institute of Liver Studies, King's College London, King's College Hospital, Denmark Hill, London SE5 9RS, UK
* Corresponding author.
E-mail address: Laura.Bull@ucsf.edu

Clin Liver Dis 22 (2018) 657–669
https://doi.org/10.1016/j.cld.2018.06.003

detergent effect of bile acids is significantly moderated through packaging into mixed micelles, the other major component of which is phosphatidylcholine (PC).

The diseases described in this article are collectively known as progressive familial intrahepatic cholestasis, or PFIC. This term predates our understanding of the different disease mechanisms. It also fails to acknowledge that nearly all the genetic deficiencies that we describe occur in spectra, ranging from infrequent symptoms, often precipitated by exogenous factors, through to severe early-onset disease. For most diseases described, those with the most severe disease manifest autosomal recessive inheritance and could be labeled as having PFIC. The diseases described represent defects in major processes involved in bile acid handling (bile acid synthesis defects are described elsewhere). Bile salt transport out of the liver is mediated by the bile salt export pump (BSEP) located in the canalicular membrane; BSEP expression is regulated by farnesoid X receptor (FXR). Correct localization of apical membrane transporters, such as BSEP, is dependent on intracellular trafficking processes, mediated in part by myosin 5B (MYO5B). Inclusion of PC into bile is dependent on MDR3. Familial intrahepatic cholestasis 1 (FIC1) is important for distribution of lipids between the 2 leaflets of the apical membrane. The canaliculi themselves are sealed by tight junctions, themselves dependent on intracellular anchors, including TJP2. The major genes underlying the different types of PFIC, and typical phenotypes, are summarized in **Table 1**.

Table 1
Summary of the typical features of progressive familial intrahepatic cholestasis associated with different genetic etiologies

Deficiency	Mutated Gene	Typical Clinical Characteristics	Characteristic Histology at Diagnosis	Typical Clinical Outcomes
FIC1	ATP8B1	Multisystem disease Normal γGT Only modest elevation of transaminases	Bland canalicular cholestasis Coarsely granular canalicular bile	Moderate rate of progression Posttransplant hepatic steatosis and diarrhea
BSEP	ABCB11	Normal γGT High risk of HCC High incidence of gallstones	Giant cell transformation	Moderate to rapid progression Allo-antibody formation after transplantation in some
MDR3	ABCB4	Progressive cholangiopathy Elevated γGT	Cholangiolytic changes	Highly variable rate of progression
TJP2	TJP2	Some extrahepatic features Near-normal γGT	Bland cholestasis	Rapid progression
FXR	NR1H4	Early-onset coagulopathy Normal γGT Markedly elevated AFP	Intralobular cholestasis Ductular reaction Giant cell transformation	Very rapid progression Posttransplant hepatic steatosis
MYO5B	MYO5B	Normal γGT Variable degree of intestinal involvement	Giant cell change Hepatocellular and canalicular cholestasis	Slow progression

Abbreviations: γGT, γ-glutamyltranspeptidase; AFP, α-fetoprotein; HCC, hepatocellular carcinoma.

FAMILIAL INTRAHEPATIC CHOLESTASIS 1 DEFICIENCY

FIC1, encoded by *ATP8B1*, is a member of the P4 family of P-type ATPases, ATP-dependent membrane transporters known as phospholipid "flippases."[1] Flippases translocate phospholipids in from the external, to the cytoplasmic, membrane leaflet. Floppases move phospholipids out, in the opposite direction. Although the identification of *ATP8B1* as a cholestasis gene occurred early in the focused application of genetics to hereditary cholestasis,[2] it has been challenging to determine the precise mechanism(s) whereby FIC1 deficiency results in cholestasis.

FIC1 is expressed in a variety of tissues, including the liver and intestine.[2,3] Some early data suggested FIC1 transports phosphatidylserine, but accumulating data more strongly support PC as a preferred substrate.[4–6] When FIC1 is not available to help maintain normal distribution of lipids between the 2 membranes of the lipid bilayer, the canalicular membrane may become vulnerable to damage by bile acids in the canaliculus.[7] Proteins in this membrane, including BSEP, also may have impaired function[7]; such impaired BSEP function would be expected to contribute to cholestasis. Through its phospholipid flippase function, FIC1 also may play a role in membrane trafficking and vesicular transport, functions that if impaired, could contribute to cholestasis.[1] Some studies suggest that loss of FIC1 impairs FXR signaling, although other studies do not support that mechanism.[8–13] FIC1 may also play a role in the innate immune response, attenuating the inflammatory response, perhaps through a role in endocytosis.[14]

Autosomal recessive mutations in *ATP8B1* can result in cholestatic disease along a continuum of severity, with PFIC typically diagnosed in patients with likely complete loss of FIC1 function.[2] Patients with milder phenotypes, including episodic cholestasis, also have been found to harbor mutations in *ATP8B1*. Such patients have been labeled as BRIC, or benign recurrent intrahepatic cholestasis. It is important to realize that lateness of onset does not preclude disease progression.[15]

In PFIC due to FIC1 deficiency, patients typically present with jaundice within the first few months of life. At or near presentation, patients also may have clinically significant diarrhea. Biochemically, patients have hyperbilirubinemia, normal serum γ-glutamyltranspeptidase (γGT) activities, high serum bile acids, and mildly elevated transaminase activities. Consistent with the broad tissue distribution of FIC1, patients often have extrahepatic manifestations during the course of disease, such as diarrhea, pneumonia, hearing loss, pancreatic disease, resistance to parathyroid hormone, and growth impairment beyond that attributable to cholestasis.[2,16–19]

Early in disease course, histologic findings are of bland intracanalicular cholestasis, without signs of significant hepatocyte injury. As disease progresses, inflammation, fibrosis, bile duct proliferation, and cirrhosis may become apparent. Ultrastructural evaluation using transmission electron microscopy may demonstrate coarsely granular bile in the canaliculus.[20] Immunostaining for FIC1 has not been established for routine clinical use. However, surrogate markers of FIC1 deficiency are fairly widely used. In particular, reduced canalicular staining for ectoenzymes, such as γGT, CD10, and carcinoembryonic antigen, is typical. Staining for membrane transporter proteins including BSEP and MDR3 is maintained.[21]

Disease is often managed with medication or nontransplant surgical interventions, such as partial external biliary diversion.[17,22] When end-stage liver disease occurs, liver transplantation is required for survival. After liver transplantation, patients with FIC1 deficiency usually develop marked graft steatosis, and inflammation.[17,22,23] The liver graft abnormalities can be greatly improved by creating a total external biliary diversion, which many would now perform at the time of transplantation.[24–26] Many patients also suffer diarrhea, which can be worse than before the transplant.[17,22,24] Given the roles of FIC1 in many tissues, and these posttransplant manifestations, liver transplantation is not curative of FIC1 deficiency.

BILE SALT EXPORT PUMP DEFICIENCY

BSEP is encoded by *ABCB11*.[27] Severe BSEP deficiency is the most frequently seen form of PFIC. At any moment in time there is either enough bile acid–transporting capacity, in which case there is no accumulation of bile acids within the hepatocyte, or there is not enough, and bile acids do accumulate and disease ensues. Patients who have a very significant reduction in BSEP function, and hence PFIC, generally present in the first few months of life, and manifest jaundice, high serum bile acids and transaminases, normal serum γGT levels, fat-soluble vitamin deficiency, and, in due course, pruritus.[16,17] Histology of the liver, at this stage, shows marked intracellular cholestasis and, usually, obvious giant cell transformation. BSEP antibody staining is widely available, and is abnormal or absent in more than 90% of severe cases.[28]

Individuals with later-onset disease caused by biallelic mutations in *ABCB11* have been identified, presenting as late as the third decade.[15,29,30] Some have gone on to need liver transplantation, despite presenting after infancy.

Patients with cholestasis can have various milder phenotypes caused by mutations in one or both copies of this gene.[29] Patients with reduced transport capacity may have adequate BSEP function most of the time. A true pathogenic mutation may be present on only 1 allele, although polymorphisms (such as p.V444A) influencing levels of protein expression or function on the other allele probably mean that such individuals have reduced function on both alleles.[31] Somewhere nearer 25% of ideal BSEP function is probably the threshold for patients at risk of cholestasis, be that induced by drugs, pregnancy, viruses, malignancy, or less obvious precipitants.

Two mutations, relatively common among European patients with BSEP deficiency, appear to result in some residual function.[32] Patients with at least 1 copy of either of these mutations (p.E297G or p.D482G) can present with either PFIC or a less severe phenotype.[15,29,30] They also have been shown to have better outcomes, and improved responses to some treatments, compared with other patients with early-onset BSEP deficiency.[17,22,33]

Most drugs treatments, to date, have not shown significant impact on the disease in patients with severe BSEP deficiency. Ursodeoxycholic acid (UDCA) is widely prescribed, and in a few cases, a significant improvement has been described.[17] Partial external biliary diversion (PEBD) helps a proportion of patients.[17,22,33] PEBD relies on the presence of bile acids in bile and has shown a better response in those shown to have some residual BSEP function. In particular, good response has been seen in 60% of individuals with at least one copy of either of the variants p.E297G or p.D482G.[22]

Missense mutations are typically annotated using the predicted change of amino acid. This could be taken to infer that it is the change in amino acid that causes the loss of function. We know, however, that many such mutations actually have their effect at an RNA level.[34] Many others do not so much interfere with transport function, for instance, but actually reduce the amount of protein getting to the correct cellular location. Incorrectly localized apical proteins, such as BSEP and indeed cystic fibrosis transmembrane conductance regulator (CFTR), are potential targets for drug treatment.[35,36] A number of small molecules have been tested in both conditions as chaperones,[37,38] and in the case of CFTR, are now licensed. This is certainly an area for further laboratory and clinical research.

BSEP deficiency, manifesting as PFIC, typically progresses to end-stage liver disease within a few years. Many patients have actually been transplanted due to severe pruritus before they reach end-stage disease. Despite the early use of transplantation, as many as 15% have developed hepatocellular carcinoma, either clinically or at explant.[39] Most of the cancers have occurred by 5 years of age. Transplantation is therefore widely and successfully used to treat severe BSEP deficiency. As the protein is expressed only in the liver, transplantation should be an excellent treatment. However, an unusual complication has become apparent. Some patients have been noted to have recurrence of exactly the same symptoms that they had before transplantation.[40,41] It transpires that this is secondary to allo-reactive antibodies, specific to one extracellular loop of the protein, which block the function of the normal protein in the transplanted liver.[42] Most patients with this condition have responded to modest increases in immunosuppression. Some patients have proved to have resistant disease and have required B-cell depletion for a number of years until they have regained control with conventional immunosuppression.[43,44]

MDR3 DEFICIENCY

MDR3 is encoded by *ABCB4*. Perhaps the disease caused by mutations in this gene should not be called PFIC at all, as it is really a cholangiopathy.[45] MDR3 transports PC from the inner to the outer leaflet of the canalicular membrane, where it is then available for incorporation into bile micelles.[46] Deficiency of PC in bile means that there are free bile acids, resulting in a detergent bile, injurious to cholangiocyte membranes. Unlike BSEP deficiency, the primary defect in MDR3 deficiency does not cause retention of bile acids in the hepatocyte, and therefore does not directly cause cholestasis. Symptoms occur only as a consequence of the damage resulting from the ensuing cholangiopathy.[47] Even complete deficiency of MDR3 can take several years before presenting clinically.[48] At presentation, the serum γGT level is usually markedly elevated, and histology shows cholangiolytic changes, and occasionally, clefts where cholesterol crystals have been. Immunohistochemical staining for MDR3 is not quantitative and is negative only in the complete absence of protein.[49]

A partial loss of MDR3 function will lead to a more slowly progressive disease; there is a very wide range of diseases, manifestations, and ages of presentation.[48,49] Unfortunately, 50% function, as seen in heterozygotes for complete loss of function alleles, is sufficient impairment for damage to occur in some individuals.[48] If investigated, such individuals may have evidence of disease in the first few decades; however, clinical presentation may only be with end-stage disease, or hepatobiliary malignancy. Heterozygous relatives of patients with MDR3 deficiency are therefore at increased risk of slowly progressive disease. Many patients have also been described without intrinsic cholangiopathy, but with a reduction in biliary PC such that they are highly predisposed to cholesterol precipitation and stone formation.[50] Such individuals can develop extensive intrahepatic cholelithiasis and be extremely difficult to manage.

The cholangiopathy in MDR3 deficiency is caused by biliary bile acids. Reduction of the bile acid pool size, via PEBD, has been rarely attempted and has probably never been undertaken early enough in the disease process to prevent progression. Instead, a reduction in the detergent nature of the bile has been achieved through supplementation with UDCA.[49] Enrichment of the bile salt pool by UDCA is probably limited by its inability to suppress the synthesis of endogenous bile salts, via FXR.[51] In milder forms of MDR3 deficiency, UDCA frequently achieves very significant biochemical improvement. It is not yet clear if this results in an improvement in long-term clinical outcomes. Treatment of severe MDR3 deficiency by all current modalities, short of transplantation, probably has been frustrated by the relatively late diagnosis. It is, however, a disease that may well respond to the use of highly hydrophilic bile acids, FXR agonists, and endogenous bile salt depletion, possibly in combination. Transplantation is a very effective treatment of end-stage MDR3 deficiency, with one proviso. The clinical manifestations described in heterozygotes, do mean that many first-degree relatives do not make good living-related donors. When there are no other options, UDCA should certainly be maintained, and close surveillance observed.

TJP2 DEFICIENCY

Most of the conditions described here have been identified in their severest forms first. TJP2 deficiency is an exception. Homozygosity for a particular missense change manifests as hypercholanemia among the Amish, with reduced penetrance.[52] These patients did not manifest chronic liver disease. On the other hand, severe progressive liver disease was later attributed to biallelic mutations predicted to cause complete loss of TJP2 function.[53] Patients with intermediate loss of function have subsequently been identified (unpublished data, R. Thompson and L. Bull, 2017).

The tight junction proteins (1, 2, and 3) are not part of the tight junction itself, but are cytoplasmic. They are closely associated with the proteins that do form tight junctions, such as the claudins. Deficiency of Claudin-1 has been described, associated with a cholangiopathy, as might be expected.[54–56] By contrast, deficiency of TJP2 is associated with cholestasis, but not a cholangiopathy, suggesting that the tight junction barrier function is not badly disrupted. The disease mechanism is not known, but tight junctions have a number of other functions. They form a selective barrier, allowing passage of some molecules and not others. They also form a fence between the basolateral and apical membranes; these 2 membranes differ markedly in both protein and lipid composition. Last, TJP2 has been shown to have a quite separate function, traveling to the nucleus, where it is transcriptionally active and inhibits cell cycle progression.

The patients so far described with complete loss of function of TJP2 have all had early-onset progressive liver disease, most requiring liver transplantation within the first few years of life. At presentation, these patients have had near-normal levels of γGT. Several cases have developed extrahepatic disease; respiratory and neurologic most frequently (Sambrotta and colleagues[53] and the author's unpublished data). This is consistent with the widespread expression of TJP2, and the general importance of tight junctions. Histology has shown rather nonspecific features, with intracellular cholestasis and scant giant cells early in disease course, although immunohistochemical staining for TJP2 itself has been useful in identifying cases. Patients with TJP2 deficiency and hepatocellular carcinoma have been described.[57,58]

FARNESOID X RECEPTOR DEFICIENCY

The FXR, encoded by *NR1H4*, is a nuclear receptor and transcription factor, for which bile acids are the natural ligand. Along with a wider role in metabolic regulation, it plays an important role in bile acid homeostasis.[59–61] If hepatic bile acid levels are high, FXR represses bile acid synthesis and uptake, and increases export of bile acids out of the hepatocyte. In intestinal cells, in response to bile acids, FXR induces expression of FGF19, which then travels to the liver, where it represses bile acid synthesis. FXR is involved in regulation of other known cholestasis genes, including *ABCB11* and to a lesser degree, *ABCB4*.[62,63] Based on the understood roles of FXR, it has been anticipated that complete loss of function of FXR would result in severe cholestasis and liver damage; the first, and only, cases of PFIC attributable to autosomal recessive FXR mutation reported to date are those of 2 pairs of affected siblings.[64] FXR deficiency thus appears to be a relatively rare cause of PFIC.

One pair of affected siblings was homozygous for a mutation that prematurely truncates the protein in the FXR's DNA binding domain (p.R176*). The other pair of affected siblings was compound heterozygous for an in-frame insertion into the DNA binding domain, and a large deletion, which eliminated the first 2 coding exons of FXR. Evidence in all patients indicated loss of FXR protein expression and function.

Three of the patients presented with cholestasis by 7 weeks of age, whereas the fourth presented at birth with ascites, pleural effusions, and intraventricular hemorrhage; the latter patient died of an aortic thrombus at age 5 weeks. At initial biochemical evaluation, patients demonstrated conjugated hyperbilirubinemia, substantially elevated serum transaminases, and γGT activities normal for age. Serum bile acids were measured in only one patient, and were elevated. Coagulation was also impaired. Characterization of the coagulopathy determined that these patients had severe vitamin K–independent coagulopathy with early onset, occurring well before endstage liver failure. This finding is consistent with evidence for a role of FXR in regulation of coagulation.[64,65] Alpha-fetoprotein (AFP) was assayed in 3 patients and found very elevated in 2. Early-onset vitamin K–independent coagulopathy and markedly elevated AFP levels may help to distinguish FXR deficiency from other genetic forms of PFIC. In liver of patients with FXR deficiency, intralobular cholestasis was seen, along with ductular reaction, giant cell transformation, and hepatocyte ballooning. Fibrosis, infiltration by inflammatory cells, and cirrhosis appeared as disease progressed. Immunohistochemical studies found expression of BSEP and FXR undetectable in all 4 patients, consistent with the important role of FXR in inducing expression of BSEP, while MDR3 was detected.

The 3 patients presenting with cholestasis had particularly rapid progression to endstage liver disease, in comparison with other genetically understood forms of PFIC. Two underwent liver transplantation (at ages 22 months and 4 months), whereas the third died at 8 months of age while awaiting transplantation. After liver transplantation, serum γGT remained normal, but alanine aminotransferase was sometimes elevated, and one patient developed mild conjugated hyperbilirubinemia. These findings were accompanied by histologically diagnosed hepatic steatosis, reminiscent of that seen in many patients with FIC1 deficiency after liver transplantation. The steatosis and mild biochemical abnormalities seen in FXR deficiency after liver transplantation may be a consequence of lack of induction of FGF19 by intestinal FXR.

MYOSIN 5B DEFICIENCY

Myosin 5B (MYO5B) plays a role in plasma membrane recycling, transcytosis, and epithelial cell polarization in multiple tissues, including enterocytes and respiratory epithelial cells, as well as hepatocytes.[66–70] In hepatocytes, MYO5B interacts with RAB11A to facilitate normal trafficking of ABC transporter proteins, including BSEP, to the canalicular membrane.[71,72] Autosomal recessive mutations in MYO5B were initially identified in a proportion of patients with microvillus inclusion disease (MVID).[68,73] A subset of patients with MVID with MYO5B mutations developed cholestasis as well.[71] Most recently, mutations in MYO5B have been reported in some patients diagnosed with cholestasis, in the absence of obvious features of MVID.[74,75]

Fifteen patients bearing autosomal recessive MYO5B mutations, with cholestasis but without an MVID diagnosis, have been reported.[74,75] Some of these patients have manifested chronic cholestasis, although typically without rapid progression, whereas others have had recurrent bouts of cholestasis, or a single transient bout of cholestasis to date. Comparison of mutation profiles in patients with MYO5B deficiency with MVID diagnosis, versus those with isolated cholestasis diagnosis, suggests that patients with MVID are more likely to have biallelic severe mutations, and biallelic mutations affecting the MYO5B-RAB11A interaction domain.[75] Thus, milder MYO5B deficiency may tend more often to manifest as cholestasis in the absence of notable intestinal disease.

In cholestasis due to MYO5B deficiency, patients typically present within the first 2 years of life with jaundice, pruritus, and hepatomegaly. Conjugated hyperbilirubinemia is accompanied by high serum bile salts, low-to-normal serum γGT activity, and mild-to-moderately elevated transaminases.

Histologic evaluation revealed giant cell change, and hepatocellular and canalicular cholestasis; fibrosis was sometimes present. Immunohistochemical studies revealed that MYO5B and RAB11A in these patients typically demonstrate abnormal staining, with reduced canalicular staining and increased cytoplasmic staining, the latter showing a granular appearance. BSEP and MDR3 staining also was abnormal, with the suggestion of patchy subcanalicular staining; in other patients, BSEP was not detected or staining was weak.

In most patients with MYO5B deficiency with isolated cholestasis, their condition was managed with medications, including ursodeoxycholic acid, and/or rifampicin, cholestyramine, or traditional Chinese medicine. However, one patient underwent PEBD, and another died aged 2.6 years, while awaiting liver transplantation.

It is likely that MYO5B deficiency results in cholestasis at least partially through decreased targeting of BSEP to the canalicular membrane; the cell membrane is likely also dysfunctional in other ways.

GENETICS

Genetics has allowed the discovery and definition of the diseases described here. For many years, diagnosis has relied on assembly of clinical features, often supported by liver histology and immunohistochemistry data. It was often then possible to match patients with the original published descriptions and confirm the diagnosis by Sanger sequencing of the appropriate gene.

In recent years, genetic technology has developed such that a quite different diagnostic algorithm is possible. Next generation sequencing technology makes it possible to sequence multiple genes, in multiple individuals, simultaneously. Its most comprehensive form is whole genome sequencing (WGS). Whole exome sequencing (WES) restricts sequencing to the exons of most genes. WES is a widely used research technique, responsible for the identification of some of the genes in this article. Over the next few years, WES will become a routine diagnostic tool, followed by WGS.[76] In 2018, the most widely used strategy is targeted panels of genes. For cholestatic liver disease, such panels typically include all the PFIC-related genes, genes underlying Alagille syndrome, Arthrogryposis, Renal Dysfunction and Cholestasis Syndrome and Dubin-Johnson syndrome, those causative of Niemann-Pick disease, and the genes underlying the inborn errors bile acid synthesis. Such a panel can now be used much earlier in a diagnostic pathway, perhaps as soon as biliary atresia and structural defects have been excluded. Biochemical and other phenotype-based testing for some of these disorders can now be avoided, or perhaps used only selectively to confirm the genetic diagnosis.

One consequence of using genetics in this way is that we are learning that not everyone with a given genetic etiology has the same phenotype as was originally described. This is most notably the case for patients with partial Alagille syndrome, but it has also become clear that FIC1 and MDR3 deficiencies both have very broad ranges of presentation, and there are clearly patients with mutations in ABCC2 that do not have a Dubin-Johnson phenotype. A minority of PFIC cases elude genetic diagnosis using current methods. Some probably have mutations in the known PFIC genes that are not detectable by routine clinical testing, and others will have mutations in genes not currently implicated in PFIC.

SUMMARY

PFIC is an ever-growing family of diseases. Genetics has helped unravel the disease mechanisms, and we can better understand the spectra of phenotypes associated with mutations in each gene. Different responses to medical and surgical management, based on genetic etiology and molecular mechanisms, are becoming apparent. A precision medicine approach to treatment is now realistic. Current genetic technology is greatly speeding diagnoses and improving our understanding of the full impact of mutations in these genes in children and adults.

REFERENCES

1. Andersen JP, Vestergaard AL, Mikkelsen SA, et al. P4-ATPases as phospholipid flippases—structure, function, and enigmas. Front Physiol 2016;7:275.
2. Bull LN, van Eijk MJ, Pawlikowska L, et al. A gene encoding a P-type ATPase mutated in two forms of hereditary cholestasis. Nat Genet 1998;18(3):219–24.
3. Ujhazy P, Ortiz D, Misra S, et al. Familial intrahepatic cholestasis 1: studies of localization and function. Hepatology 2001;34(4 Pt 1):768–75.
4. Paulusma CC, Folmer DE, Ho-Mok KS, et al. ATP8B1 requires an accessory protein for endoplasmic reticulum exit and plasma membrane lipid flippase activity. Hepatology 2008;47(1):268–78.
5. Paulusma CC, Groen A, Kunne C, et al. Atp8b1 deficiency in mice reduces resistance of the canalicular membrane to hydrophobic bile salts and impairs bile salt transport. Hepatology 2006;44(1):195–204.
6. Takatsu H, Tanaka G, Segawa K, et al. Phospholipid flippase activities and substrate specificities of human type IV P-type ATPases localized to the plasma membrane. J Biol Chem 2014;289(48):33543–56.
7. Paulusma CC, de Waart DR, Kunne C, et al. Activity of the bile salt export pump (ABCB11) is critically dependent on canalicular membrane cholesterol content. J Biol Chem 2009;284(15):9947–54.
8. Frankenberg T, Miloh T, Chen FY, et al. The membrane protein ATPase class I type 8B member 1 signals through protein kinase C zeta to activate the farnesoid X receptor. Hepatology 2008;48(6):1896–905.
9. Martinez-Fernandez P, Hierro L, Jara P, et al. Knockdown of ATP8B1 expression leads to specific downregulation of the bile acid sensor FXR in HepG2 cells: effect of the FXR agonist GW4064. Am J Physiol Gastrointest Liver Physiol 2009; 296(5):G1119–29.
10. Pawlikowska L, Groen A, Eppens EF, et al. A mouse genetic model for familial cholestasis caused by ATP8B1 mutations reveals perturbed bile salt homeostasis but no impairment in bile secretion. Hum Mol Genet 2004;13(8): 881–92.
11. Cai SY, Gautam S, Nguyen T, et al. ATP8B1 deficiency disrupts the bile canalicular membrane bilayer structure in hepatocytes, but FXR expression and activity are maintained. Gastroenterology 2009;136(3):1060–9.

12. Chen F, Ellis E, Strom SC, et al. ATPase Class I Type 8B Member 1 and protein kinase C zeta induce the expression of the canalicular bile salt export pump in human hepatocytes. Pediatr Res 2010;67(2):183–7.
13. van der Mark VA, de Waart DR, Ho-Mok KS, et al. The lipid flippase heterodimer ATP8B1-CDC50A is essential for surface expression of the apical sodium-dependent bile acid transporter (SLC10A2/ASBT) in intestinal Caco-2 cells. Biochim Biophys Acta 2014;1842(12 Pt A):2378–86.
14. van der Mark VA, Ghiboub M, Marsman C, et al. Phospholipid flippases attenuate LPS-induced TLR4 signaling by mediating endocytic retrieval of Toll-like receptor 4. Cell Mol Life Sci 2017;74(4):715–30.
15. van Ooteghem NA, Klomp LW, van Berge-Henegouwen GP, et al. Benign recurrent intrahepatic cholestasis progressing to progressive familial intrahepatic cholestasis: low GGT cholestasis is a clinical continuum. J Hepatol 2002;36(3): 439–43.
16. Pawlikowska L, Strautnieks S, Jankowska I, et al. Differences in presentation and progression between severe FIC1 and BSEP deficiencies. J Hepatol 2010;53(1): 170–8.
17. Davit-Spraul A, Fabre M, Branchereau S, et al. ATP8B1 and ABCB11 analysis in 62 children with normal gamma-glutamyl transferase progressive familial intrahepatic cholestasis (PFIC): phenotypic differences between PFIC1 and PFIC2 and natural history. Hepatology 2010;51(5):1645–55.
18. Nagasaka H, Yorifuji T, Kosugiyama K, et al. Resistance to parathyroid hormone in two patients with familial intrahepatic cholestasis: possible involvement of the ATP8B1 gene in calcium regulation via parathyroid hormone. J Pediatr Gastroenterol Nutr 2004;39(4):404–9.
19. Stapelbroek JM, Peters TA, van Beurden DH, et al. ATP8B1 is essential for maintaining normal hearing. Proc Natl Acad Sci U S A 2009;106(24):9709–14.
20. Bull LN, Carlton VE, Stricker NL, et al. Genetic and morphological findings in progressive familial intrahepatic cholestasis (Byler disease [PFIC-1] and Byler syndrome): evidence for heterogeneity. Hepatology 1997;26(1):155–64.
21. Knisely AS, Bull LN, Shneider BL. ATP8B1 deficiency. In: Adam MP, Ardinger HH, Pagon RA, et al, editors. GeneReviews®. Seattle (WA): University of Washington, Seattle; 2014.
22. Bull LN, Pawlikowska L, Strautnieks S, et al. Outcomes of surgical management of familial intrahepatic cholestasis 1 and bile salt export protein deficiencies. Hepatol Commun 2018;2(5):515–28.
23. Miyagawa-Hayashino A, Egawa H, Yorifuji T, et al. Allograft steatohepatitis in progressive familial intrahepatic cholestasis type 1 after living donor liver transplantation. Liver Transpl 2009;15(6):610–8.
24. Usui M, Isaji S, Das BC, et al. Liver retransplantation with external biliary diversion for progressive familial intrahepatic cholestasis type 1: a case report. Pediatr Transplant 2009;13(5):611–4.
25. Nicastro E, Stephenne X, Smets F, et al. Recovery of graft steatosis and protein-losing enteropathy after biliary diversion in a PFIC 1 liver transplanted child. Pediatr Transplant 2012;16(5):E177–82.
26. Mali VP, Fukuda A, Shigeta T, et al. Total internal biliary diversion during liver transplantation for type 1 progressive familial intrahepatic cholestasis: a novel approach. Pediatr Transplant 2016;20(7):981–6.
27. Strautnieks SS, Bull LN, Knisely AS, et al. A gene encoding a liver-specific ABC transporter is mutated in progressive familial intrahepatic cholestasis. Nat Genet 1998;20(3):233–8.

28. Strautnieks SS, Byrne JA, Pawlikowska L, et al. Severe bile salt export pump deficiency: 82 different ABCB11 mutations in 109 families. Gastroenterology 2008; 134(4):1203–14.

29. Droge C, Bonus M, Baumann U, et al. Sequencing of FIC1, BSEP and MDR3 in a large cohort of patients with cholestasis revealed a high number of different genetic variants. J Hepatol 2017;67(6):1253–64.

30. van Mil SW, van der Woerd WL, van der Brugge G, et al. Benign recurrent intrahepatic cholestasis type 2 is caused by mutations in ABCB11. Gastroenterology 2004;127(2):379–84.

31. Dixon PH, van Mil SW, Chambers J, et al. Contribution of variant alleles of ABCB11 to susceptibility to intrahepatic cholestasis of pregnancy. Gut 2009; 58(4):537–44.

32. Hayashi H, Takada T, Suzuki H, et al. Two common PFIC2 mutations are associated with the impaired membrane trafficking of BSEP/ABCB11. Hepatology 2005; 41(4):916–24.

33. Wang KS, Tiao G, Bass LM, et al. Analysis of surgical interruption of the enterohepatic circulation as a treatment for pediatric cholestasis. Hepatology 2017; 65(5):1645–54.

34. Byrne JA, Strautnieks SS, Ihrke G, et al. Missense mutations and single nucleotide polymorphisms in ABCB11 impair bile salt export pump processing and function or disrupt pre-messenger RNA splicing. Hepatology 2009;49(2):553–67.

35. Brown CR, Hong-Brown LQ, Biwersi J, et al. Chemical chaperones correct the mutant phenotype of the delta F508 cystic fibrosis transmembrane conductance regulator protein. Cell Stress Chaperones 1996;1(2):117–25.

36. Vauthier V, Housset C, Falguieres T. Targeted pharmacotherapies for defective ABC transporters. Biochem Pharmacol 2017;136:1–11.

37. Gonzales E, Grosse B, Schuller B, et al. Targeted pharmacotherapy in progressive familial intrahepatic cholestasis type 2: evidence for improvement of cholestasis with 4-phenylbutyrate. Hepatology 2015;62(2):558–66.

38. Hayashi H, Naoi S, Hirose Y, et al. Successful treatment with 4-phenylbutyrate in a patient with benign recurrent intrahepatic cholestasis type 2 refractory to biliary drainage and bilirubin absorption. Hepatol Res 2016;46(2):192–200.

39. Knisely AS, Strautnieks SS, Meier Y, et al. Hepatocellular carcinoma in ten children under five years of age with bile salt export pump deficiency. Hepatology 2006;44(2):478–86.

40. Jara P, Hierro L, Martinez-Fernandez P, et al. Recurrence of bile salt export pump deficiency after liver transplantation. N Engl J Med 2009;361(14):1359–67.

41. Keitel V, Burdelski M, Vojnisek Z, et al. De novo bile salt transporter antibodies as a possible cause of recurrent graft failure after liver transplantation: a novel mechanism of cholestasis. Hepatology 2009;50(2):510–7.

42. Kubitz R, Droge C, Kluge S, et al. Autoimmune BSEP disease: disease recurrence after liver transplantation for progressive familial intrahepatic cholestasis. Clin Rev Allergy Immunol 2015;48(2–3):273–84.

43. Siebold L, Dick AA, Thompson R, et al. Recurrent low gamma-glutamyl transpeptidase cholestasis following liver transplantation for bile salt export pump (BSEP) disease (posttransplant recurrent BSEP disease). Liver Transpl 2010;16(7): 856–63.

44. Grammatikopoulos T, Knisely AS, Dhawan A, et al. Anti-CD20 monoclonal antibody therapy in functional bile salt export pump deficiency after liver transplantation. J Pediatr Gastroenterol Nutr 2015;60(6):e50–3.

45. Mauad TH, van Nieuwkerk CM, Dingemans KP, et al. Mice with homozygous disruption of the mdr2 P-glycoprotein gene. A novel animal model for studies of nonsuppurative inflammatory cholangitis and hepatocarcinogenesis. Am J Pathol 1994;145(5):1237–45.

46. Oude Elferink RP, Ottenhoff R, van Wijland M, et al. Regulation of biliary lipid secretion by mdr2 P-glycoprotein in the mouse. J Clin Invest 1995;95(1):31–8.

47. de Vree JM, Jacquemin E, Sturm E, et al. Mutations in the MDR3 gene cause progressive familial intrahepatic cholestasis. Proc Natl Acad Sci U S A 1998;95(1): 282–7.

48. Ziol M, Barbu V, Rosmorduc O, et al. ABCB4 heterozygous gene mutations associated with fibrosing cholestatic liver disease in adults. Gastroenterology 2008; 135(1):131–41.

49. Jacquemin E, De Vree JM, Cresteil D, et al. The wide spectrum of multidrug resistance 3 deficiency: from neonatal cholestasis to cirrhosis of adulthood. Gastroenterology 2001;120(6):1448–58.

50. Rosmorduc O, Hermelin B, Poupon R. MDR3 gene defect in adults with symptomatic intrahepatic and gallbladder cholesterol cholelithiasis. Gastroenterology 2001;120(6):1459–67.

51. Campena G, Pasini P, Roba A, et al. Regulation of ileal bile acid-binding protein expression in Caco-2 cells by ursodeoxycholic acid: role of the farnesoid X receptor. Biochem Pharmacol 2005;69(12):1755–63.

52. Carlton VE, Harris BZ, Puffenberger EG, et al. Complex inheritance of familial hypercholanemia with associated mutations in TJP2 and BAAT. Nat Genet 2003; 34(1):91–6.

53. Sambrotta M, Strautnieks S, Papouli E, et al. Mutations in TJP2 cause progressive cholestatic liver disease. Nat Genet 2014;46(4):326–8.

54. Grosse B, Cassio D, Yousef N, et al. Claudin-1 involved in neonatal ichthyosis sclerosing cholangitis syndrome regulates hepatic paracellular permeability. Hepatology 2012;55(4):1249–59.

55. Hadj-Rabia S, Baala L, Vabres P, et al. Claudin-1 gene mutations in neonatal sclerosing cholangitis associated with ichthyosis: a tight junction disease. Gastroenterology 2004;127(5):1386–90.

56. Paganelli M, Stephenne X, Gilis A, et al. Neonatal ichthyosis and sclerosing cholangitis syndrome: extremely variable liver disease severity from claudin-1 deficiency. J Pediatr Gastroenterol Nutr 2011;53(3):350–4.

57. Vij M, Shanmugam NP, Reddy MS, et al. Paediatric hepatocellular carcinoma in tight junction protein 2 (TJP2) deficiency. Virchows Arch 2017;471(5):679–83.

58. Zhou S, Hertel PM, Finegold MJ, et al. Hepatocellular carcinoma associated with tight-junction protein 2 deficiency. Hepatology 2015;62(6):1914–6.

59. Cariello M, Piccinin E, Garcia-Irigoyen O, et al. Nuclear receptor FXR, bile acids and liver damage: introducing the progressive familial intrahepatic cholestasis with FXR mutations. Biochim Biophys Acta 2018;1864(4 Pt B):1308–18.

60. Massafra V, van Mil SWC. Farnesoid X receptor: a "homeostat" for hepatic nutrient metabolism. Biochim Biophys Acta 2018;1864(1):45–59.

61. Schonewille M, de Boer JF, Groen AK. Bile salts in control of lipid metabolism. Curr Opin Lipidol 2016;27(3):295–301.

62. Ananthanarayanan M, Balasubramanian N, Makishima M, et al. Human bile salt export pump promoter is transactivated by the farnesoid X receptor/bile acid receptor. J Biol Chem 2001;276(31):28857–65.

63. Huang L, Zhao A, Lew JL, et al. Farnesoid X receptor activates transcription of the phospholipid pump MDR3. J Biol Chem 2003;278(51):51085–90.

64. Gomez-Ospina N, Potter CJ, Xiao R, et al. Mutations in the nuclear bile acid receptor FXR cause progressive familial intrahepatic cholestasis. Nat Commun 2016;7:10713.
65. Zhan L, Liu HX, Fang Y, et al. Genome-wide binding and transcriptome analysis of human farnesoid X receptor in primary human hepatocytes. PLoS One 2014; 9(9):e105930.
66. Knowles BC, Roland JT, Krishnan M, et al. Myosin Vb uncoupling from RAB8A and RAB11A elicits microvillus inclusion disease. J Clin Invest 2014;124(7): 2947–62.
67. Lapierre LA, Kumar R, Hales CM, et al. Myosin vb is associated with plasma membrane recycling systems. Mol Biol Cell 2001;12(6):1843–57.
68. Muller T, Hess MW, Schiefermeier N, et al. MYO5B mutations cause microvillus inclusion disease and disrupt epithelial cell polarity. Nat Genet 2008;40(10): 1163–5.
69. Thoeni CE, Vogel GF, Tancevski I, et al. Microvillus inclusion disease: loss of Myosin vb disrupts intracellular traffic and cell polarity. Traffic 2014;15(1):22–42.
70. Wakabayashi Y, Dutt P, Lippincott-Schwartz J, et al. Rab11a and myosin Vb are required for bile canalicular formation in WIF-B9 cells. Proc Natl Acad Sci U S A 2005;102(42):15087–92.
71. Girard M, Lacaille F, Verkarre V, et al. MYO5B and bile salt export pump contribute to cholestatic liver disorder in microvillous inclusion disease. Hepatology 2014;60(1):301–10.
72. Wakabayashi Y, Lippincott-Schwartz J, Arias IM. Intracellular trafficking of bile salt export pump (ABCB11) in polarized hepatic cells: constitutive cycling between the canalicular membrane and rab11-positive endosomes. Mol Biol Cell 2004;15(7):3485–96.
73. Ruemmele FM, Muller T, Schiefermeier N, et al. Loss-of-function of MYO5B is the main cause of microvillus inclusion disease: 15 novel mutations and a CaCo-2 RNAi cell model. Hum Mutat 2010;31(5):544–51.
74. Gonzales E, Taylor SA, Davit-Spraul A, et al. MYO5B mutations cause cholestasis with normal serum gamma-glutamyl transferase activity in children without microvillous inclusion disease. Hepatology 2017;65(1):164–73.
75. Qiu YL, Gong JY, Feng JY, et al. Defects in myosin VB are associated with a spectrum of previously undiagnosed low gamma-glutamyltransferase cholestasis. Hepatology 2017;65(5):1655–69.
76. Nicastro E, D'Antiga L. Next generation sequencing in pediatric hepatology and liver transplantation. Liver Transplant 2018;24(2):282–93.

Inborn Errors of Bile Acid Metabolism

James E. Heubi, MD[a,b],*, Kenneth D.R. Setchell, PhD[a,b], Kevin E. Bove, MD[a,b]

KEYWORDS

- Neonatal cholestasis • Cirrhosis • Liver • Zellweger spectrum disorder

KEY POINTS

- Inborn errors of bile acid metabolism are rare causes of neonatal cholestasis and liver disease in older children and adults.
- Diagnosis of inborn errors of bile acid metabolism requires a high index of suspicion with low serum bile acids in the presence of hyperbilirubinemia or advanced liver disease.
- Diagnosis is based on either genetic testing using available panels of genes associated with neonatal cholestasis and/or urine liquid secondary ionization mass spectrometry (LCIMS).
- Therapy for single enzyme defects with cholic acid is very effective for most inborn errors of bile acid metabolism except conjugation defects or oxysterol-7α-hydroxylase deficiency.

INTRODUCTION

Bile acids are synthesized by the liver from cholesterol through a complex series of reactions involving at least 15 enzymatic steps. Failure to perform any of these reactions will block bile acid production with failure to produce normal bile acids and, instead, the accumulation of unusual bile acids and intermediary metabolites. Failure to synthesize bile acids leads to reduced bile flow and decreased intraluminal solubilization of fat and fat-soluble vitamins. The intermediates created because of blockade in the bile acid biosynthetic pathway may be toxic to hepatocytes. Multiple recognized inborn errors of bile acid metabolism have been identified and caused by enzyme deficiencies and impaired bile acid synthesis in infants, children, and adults. Patients may present with neonatal cholestasis, neurologic disease, advanced liver disease,

Disclosures: Drs J.E. Heubi and K.D.R. Setchell have equity interests in Asklepion Pharmaceuticals, LLC and have consulting agreements with Retrophin, Inc, which markets cholic acid.
[a] Division of Pediatric Gastroenterology, Hepatology and Nutrition, Cincinnati Children's Hospital Medical Center, University of Cincinnati College of Medicine, 240 Sabin Way, Cincinnati, OH 45229, USA; [b] Division of Pathology, Cincinnati Children's Hospital Medical Center, University of Cincinnati College of Medicine, 240 Sabin Way, Cincinnati, OH 45229, USA
* Corresponding author. Center for Clinical and Translational Science and Training, Cincinnati Children's Hospital Medical Center, 240 Sabin Way, S 2. 518, Cincinnati, OH 45229-3039.
E-mail address: james.heubi@cchmc.org

or fat and fat-soluble vitamin malabsorption. If untreated, progressive liver disease may develop or reduced intestinal bile acid concentrations may lead to serious morbidity or mortality. This review focuses on a description of the disorders of bile acid synthesis that are directly related to defects in the metabolic pathway and their proposed pathogenesis, treatment, and prognosis.

CHEMISTRY AND PHYSIOLOGY

The bile acids belong to the steroid class classified as acidic sterols. In humans, the principal bile acids synthesized by the liver have hydroxyl groups substituted in the nucleus at the carbon positions C-3, C-7, and C-12.[1,2] During early development, alternative pathways for bile acid synthesis and metabolism become quantitatively important, as is evident from the findings of relatively high proportions of bile acids hydroxylated at the C-1, C-2, C-4, and C-6 positions of the nucleus.[3,4] The two principal bile acids synthesized by the liver and referred to as the primary bile acids are cholic acid (3α,7α,12α-trihydroxy-5β-cholanoic acid [CA]) and chenodeoxycholic acid (3α,7α-dihydroxy-5β-cholanoic acid [CDCA]). These bile acids are almost extensively conjugated to the amino acids glycine and taurine.[5] The biosynthetic pathway for bile acids is depicted in **Fig. 1**.

Bile acids perform several important functions. Bile acids are the major catabolic pathways for the elimination of cholesterol from the body.[1,6] Bile acids provide the primary driving force for the secretion of bile and are essential to the development of the

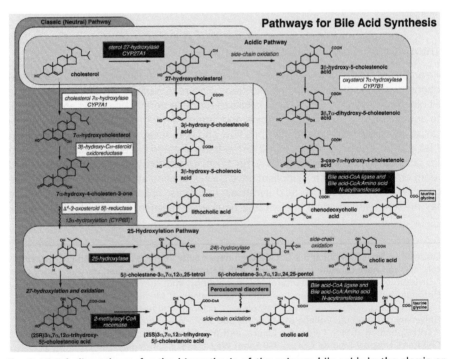

Fig. 1. Metabolic pathway for the biosynthesis of the primary bile acids in the classic or neutral pathway and the alternative or acidic pathway. Recognized inborn errors are shown in boxes in the pathways. (*From* Bove KE, Daugherty CC, Tyson W, et al. Bile acid synthetic defects and liver disease. Pediatr Dev Pathol 2000;3(1):1–16; with permission.)

biliary excretory route for the elimination of endogenous and exogenous toxic substances, including bilirubin, xenobiotics, and drug metabolites.[7] Within the intestinal lumen, the detergent action of bile acids facilitates the absorption of fats and fat-soluble vitamins.

Physiologically, the normal bile acid pool size in the adult is 2 to 4 g, but the effectiveness of this pool is increased by an efficient enterohepatic recycling (10–12 times per day) stimulated by postprandial gallbladder contraction.[8] Conservation of the bile acid pool occurs by an efficient reabsorption, principally from the small intestine, and an effective hepatic extraction from the portal venous circulation so that each day less than 20% of the pool is lost in the stool. This bile acid loss is compensated for by hepatic synthesis of newly formed bile acids. A fraction of the pool is deconjugated and then converted to secondary bile acids (deoxycholic and lithocholic acid) by intestinal bacteria with most recycled within the enterohepatic circulation and reconjugated in the liver. Although term and preterm neonates are born with a relatively reduced-size corrected bile acid pool, rapid expansion of the pool in the first months of life ensures adequate intraluminal concentrations for fat and fat-soluble vitamin absorption and promotion of bile flow.[9–12]

INBORN ERRORS IN BILE ACID SYNTHESIS

Disorders in bile acid synthesis and metabolism can be broadly classified as primary or secondary. Primary enzyme defects involve congenital deficiencies in enzymes responsible for catalyzing key reactions in the synthesis of cholic and chenodeoxycholic acids. The primary defects reported thus far include cholesterol 7-hydroxylase deficiency, 3β-hydroxy-C_{27}-steroid oxidoreductase deficiency (3β-HSD), Δ^4-3-oxosteroid 5β-reductase deficiency (5β-reductase deficiency), oxysterol 7α-hydroxylase deficiency, 27-hydroxylase deficiency or cerebrotendinous xanthomatosis (CTX), 2-methylacyl-coenzyme A (CoA) racemase deficiency, trihydroxycholestanoic acid CoA oxidase deficiency, amidation defects involving a deficiency in the bile acid–CoA ligase or bile acid CoA, amino acid N-acyl transferase, acyl CoA oxidase deficiency, ATP binding cassette subfamily D member 3 (ABCD3) deficiency, and a side-chain oxidation defect in the 25-hydroxylation pathway. Secondary metabolic defects that impact primary bile acid synthesis include peroxisomal disorders, such as Zellweger spectrum disorder (ZSD), and Smith-Lemli-Opitz syndrome caused by a deficiency of Δ^{7-} desaturase.

The biochemical presentation of these bile acid synthetic defects includes a markedly reduced or complete lack of cholic and chenodeoxycholic acids in the serum, bile, and urine with elevated concentrations of atypical bile acids and sterols that retain the characteristic structure of the substrates for the deficient enzyme. These signature metabolites are generally not detected by the routine or classic methods for bile acid measurement, and mass spectrometric techniques presently provide the most appropriate means of characterizing defects in bile acid synthesis. Screening procedures using liquid secondary ionization mass spectrometry (LSIMS) done in Cincinnati have found that inborn errors in bile acid synthesis accounted for 2.1% of the screened cases of cholestatic liver disease in infants, children, and adolescents.[13] Screening patients in Saudi Arabia using LSIMS in patients with cholestasis, cirrhosis, or liver failure presenting with low routine serum bile acids concentrations Al-Hussaini and colleagues[14] have found an incidence of 2.7%. Other estimates have been as high as 6.3%, but these differences likely represent the characteristics of the pool of samples from which the estimates were derived.[15] Although recent studies from Europe have suggested that the overall incidence may be 1.13 cases per 10 million based on surveys from 39 centers, this is likely an underestimate because it is unclear how many cases may have gone unrecognized.[16] The investigators think that the overall incidence of the primary defects is unknown even with the European data; however, it is likely that they have an incidence of 1 per 50,000 to 100,000 with an increased incidence in more inbred populations. All defects are inherited as autosomal recessive mutations of genes coding for the enzymatic defect. Typical LSIMS scans for healthy and cholestatic infants are shown in **Fig. 2**. The distribution of the inborn errors diagnosed using LSIMS techniques over the last 30 years in Cincinnati are shown in **Fig. 3**. Clinical experience with patients with inborn errors of bile acid metabolism has borne out the observation that defects affecting the steroid nucleus of the bile acid molecule tend to present with liver disease and potential early mortality, whereas defects that affect the side chain of the bile acid molecule tend to present with multiorgan disease with coagulopathies and neurologic disease, with or without cholestasis. This review focuses on these defects that are of primary interest to the hepatologist.

3β-HYDROXY-C_{27}-STEROID OXIDOREDUCTASE DEFICIENCY

This defect is the most common of the bile acid synthetic defects presenting in cholestasis in infancy and childhood involving the conversion of 7α-hydroxycholesterol to 7α-hydroxy-4-cholesten-3-one, a reaction catalyzed by a 3β-hydroxy-C_{27}-steroid oxidoreductase (HSD3B7). Although the clinical presentation of this disorder is somewhat heterogeneous, most patients present as neonates with elevated serum

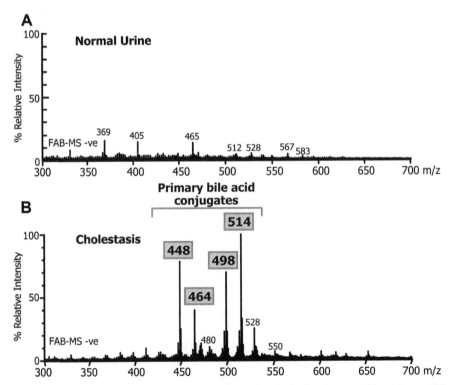

Fig. 2. Negative-ion LSIMS mass spectrum analysis of typical urine from a (A) healthy and (B) cholestatic infant. FAB-MS, fast atom bombardment ionization mass spectrometry.

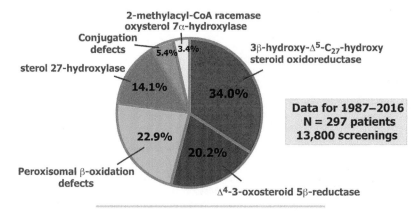

□ **Age at diagnosis and clinical presentation is highly variable ranging from early infancy to adulthood - Can be a cause of late-onset chronic cholestasis**

Fig. 3. Distribution of defects identified by LSIMS from 1987 to 2016 in Cincinnati.

aminotransferases, conjugated hyperbilirubinemia, and normal serum gamma glutamyl transpeptidase (GGT).[17–21] Clinical features include hepatomegaly, with or without splenomegaly, fat-soluble vitamin malabsorption, and mild steatorrhea. Pruritus is usually absent. The liver histology findings include cholangiolcentric hepatitis with giant cells and evidence of cholestasis[17–21] (**Fig. 4**A, B). The heterogeneity in the clinical course of those with early onset disease is illustrated by some patients who initially resolve their jaundice and are identified later in life with persistent small duct injury to those with progressive liver disease, eventuating in cirrhosis, death, or transplantation (**Fig. 5**A, B). The median age of presentation in the registration trial for CA was 3 years; increasingly, idiopathic late-onset chronic cholestasis has been explained by this disorder with cirrhotic adults identified with this defect.[21–23] In such patients, liver disease is not always evident initially and patients may have

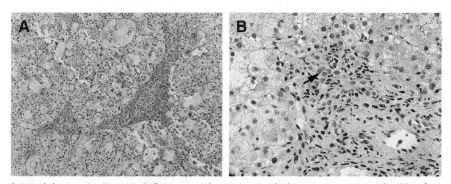

Fig. 4. (A) Liver in 3β-HSD deficiency with persistent cholestasis in a 6-month-old infant. Prominent ballooned multinucleate hepatocytes surround expanded inflamed portal areas (hematoxylin-eosin stain, original magnification ×150). (B) Liver in 3β-HSD deficiency with persistent cholestasis in a 6-month-old infant. Portal inflammatory infiltrate includes neutrophils oriented to swollen cholangiocytes (*arrow*) of small bile ducts and ductules along limiting plate (hematoxylin-eosin stain, original magnification ×250).

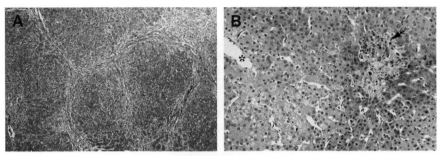

Fig. 5. (A) Liver in 3β-HSD deficiency with mild hyperbilirubinemia presenting at 2 years of age. Three portal areas in this field show variable inflammatory infiltrate. Pattern of incomplete septal cirrhosis is well established (Masson trichrome stain, original stain ×100). (B) Liver in 3β-HSD deficiency with mild hyperbilirubinemia presenting at 11 years of age. Portal area (*arrow*) contains heavily pigmented macrophages clustered near barely perceptible duct remnant. Lobular hepatocytes are uniformly normal. Central vein (*asterisk*) (hematoxylin-eosin stain, original magnification ×150).

fat-soluble vitamin malabsorption and rickets, which are corrected with vitamin supplementation. Serum liver enzymes in this subset of patients are often normal or minimally abnormal in the early stages of the disease that later have progressive increases in liver chemistries with evidence of progressive hepatic fibrosis. Definitive diagnosis of 3β-HSD deficiency requires either mass spectrometric analysis of urine with a characteristic ion pattern seen (**Fig. 6**) using LSIMS, formerly referred to as fast atom

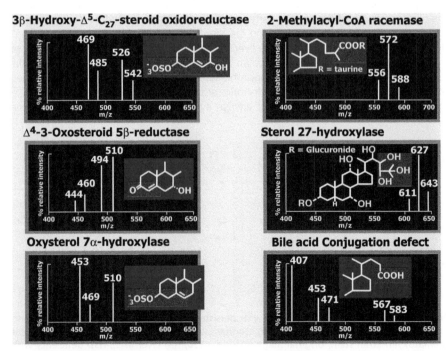

Fig. 6. Typical LCIMS findings in 3β-HSD deficiency, 2-methylacyl-CoA racemase deficiency and ZSD, 5β-reductase deficiency, sterol 27-hydroxylase deficiency (CTX), oxysterol 7α-hydroxylase deficiency, and bile acid conjugation defects.

bombardment ionization mass spectrometry (FAB-MS),[2] by electrospray ionization tandem mass spectrometry[24–26] or specific gene testing for HSD3B7 or testing of panels of genes that cause cholestasis at multiple Clinical Laboratory Improvement Amendments–certified commercial laboratories. The mechanism of cholestasis and liver injury is thought to result from failure to synthesize adequate amounts of primary bile acids that are essential to the promotion and secretion of bile and the increased production of unusual bile acids with hepatotoxic potential.[27,28] Treatment with CA leads to gradual resolution of biochemical and histologic abnormalities with an excellent long-term prognosis. In selected older children/adolescents presenting with extensive fibrosis or cirrhosis, CA therapy has prevented progression of disease.[21,29,30]

Δ⁴-3-OXOSTEROID 5β-REDUCTASE DEFICIENCY

Deficiency of Δ^4-3-oxosteroid 5β-reductase, which catalyzes the conversion of the intermediates 7α-hydroxy-4-cholesten-3-one and 7α,12α -dihydroxy-4-cholesten-3-one to the corresponding 3-oxo-5β(H) intermediates[31] is responsible for 5β-reductase deficiency. The clinical presentation is similar to 3β-HSD deficiency; however, the average age at diagnosis is 3 months in patients with 5β-reductase deficiency.[21] In contrast to 3β-HSD, infants with 5β-reductase deficiency tend to have more severe liver disease with rapid progression to cirrhosis and death without intervention. 5β-Reductase deficiency has since been found in several patients presenting with what was formerly presumed to be neonatal hemochromatosis that may now be considered to have gestational alloimmune liver disease. These cases most likely had reduced 5β-reductase activity due to end-stage liver disease rather than a primary enzyme deficiency.[32] Infants with 5β-reductase deficiency present with elevations in serum aminotransferases, markedly elevated serum conjugated bilirubin, and coagulopathy. Liver histologic[20,33] findings include marked lobular disarray as a result of giant cell and pseudoacinar transformation of hepatocytes, hepatocellular and canalicular bile stasis, and extramedullary hematopoiesis (**Fig. 7**A). On electron microscopy, bile canaliculi were small and sometimes slitlike in appearance and showed few or absent microvilli containing electron-dense material.[33] Diagnosis of this defect is possible by LSIMS and gas chromatography–mass spectrometry (GC-MS) analysis

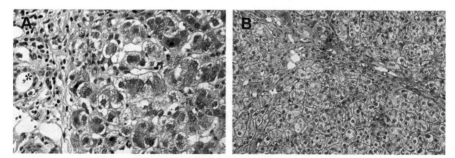

Fig. 7. (*A*) Liver in 5β-reductase deficiency, neonatal jaundice with liver biopsy at 3 weeks of age. Periportal hepatocytes are swollen and cholestatic with acinar change and scattered necrotic cells. Portal area contains a light inflammatory infiltrate and a duct (*asterisk*) lined by reactive cholangiocytes (hematoxylin-eosin stain, original magnification ×250). (*B*) Liver in 5β-reductase deficiency after 16 months of therapy with CA demonstrates resolution of previous cholestatic changes in hepatocytes and portal inflammation with residual mild fibrosis (Masson trichrome stain, original magnification ×150).

of the urine or by genetic testing for mutations in *AKR1D1*. LSIMS spectra reveal a characteristic ion profile consistent with increased production of Δ^4-3-oxo bile acids (see **Fig. 6**) in patients with severe liver disease[34] but because these bile acids are also excreted in elevated levels by infants during the first few weeks of life[35] it is, therefore, important to perform a repeat analysis of urine when there is a suspected 5β-reductase deficiency because, on rare occasions, a resolution of the liver disease occurs and these atypical bile acids disappear. Similarly, complementing mass spectrometry analysis with genetic analysis permits confirmation of the presence or absence of primary enzyme deficiency.

The liver injury in this defect is likely due to diminished primary bile acid synthesis and the hepatotoxicity of the accumulated Δ^4-3-oxo bile acids. The lack of canalicular secretion can be explained by the relative insolubility of oxo-bile acids, and the cholestatic effects of the taurine conjugate of 7α-dihydroxy-3-oxo-4-cholenoic acid have been demonstrated in rat canalicular plasma membrane vesicles.[28] The unique morphologic findings in these patients[33] may indicate that maturation of the canalicular membrane and the transport system for bile acid secretion may require a threshold concentration of primary bile acids in early development. Treatment with CA leads to resolution of histologic and biochemical abnormalities with an excellent long-term prognosis (**Fig. 7**B).[21,29]

CHOLESTEROL 27-HYDROXYLASE DEFICIENCY: CEREBROTENDINOUS XANTHOMATOSIS

CTX is a rare inherited lipid-storage disease, with an estimated prevalence of 1 in 70,000, first described in adults in 1937.[36] Characteristic features of the disease in adults include progressive neurologic dysfunction, dementia, ataxia, cataracts, and xanthomata in the brain and tendons. Affected patients may present with neonatal cholestasis, diarrhea during infancy, and juvenile cataracts. In the second and third decades of life they may develop neurologic symptoms and xanthomata. Patients with CTX have significantly reduced primary bile acid synthesis; elevations in biliary, urinary, and fecal excretion of bile alcohol glucuronides; low plasma cholesterol concentration, with deposition of cholesterol and cholestanol in the tissues; and marked elevations in cholestanol. Point mutations in *CYP27A1* have been identified that lead to reduced sterol 27-hydroxylase and clinical findings characteristic of CTX.[37] Impaired oxidation of the cholesterol side chain results in accelerated cholesterol synthesis and metabolism that leads to greatly increased production and excretion of bile alcohol glucuronides detectable by LSIMS[38] (see **Fig. 6**). The elevation in 5α-cholestan-3β-ol (cholestanol) in the nervous system of patients with CTX and the high plasma concentrations of this sterol are unique features of the disease. CDCA is effective in arresting progression of neurologic disease in adults with CTX.[39] Early diagnosis of this disorder, which is readily achieved by mass spectrometry analysis of the urine or by sequencing of the *CYP27A1* gene, is crucial to prevent the progressive accumulation of cholestanol and cholesterol in tissues in the long-term. Several infants and children have been identified with sterol 27-hydroxylase deficiency because they presented with elevated serum aminotransferases and total and conjugated bilirubin with normal serum GGT.[21,40] In the identified patients, liver dysfunction normalized over time, which was likely independent of CA therapy; however, early introduction of CA likely prevents the long-term extrahepatic complications of CTX. The histopathology findings on liver biopsy in these young patients are similar to those observed in idiopathic neonatal hepatitis. A recent report suggests that sterol 27-hydroxylase may not be a benign condition in infancy. Gong and colleagues[41] reported biochemical and genetic findings in a group of 8 Chinese infants with neonatal chole-stasis with a very rapidly progressive liver resulting in the death or transplantation in 5 with clearance of jaundice in the remaining 3.

DEFECTIVE AMIDATION: BILE ACID-COENZYME A LIGASE DEFICIENCY AND BILE ACID-COENZYME A: AMINO ACID N-ACYL TRANSFERASE DEFICIENCY

The final step in bile acid synthesis involves conjugation with the amino acids glycine and taurine. Two enzymes catalyze the reactions leading to amidation of bile acids. In the first, a CoA thioester is formed by the rate-limiting bile acid-CoA ligase (BACL), af-ter which glycine or taurine is coupled in a reaction catalyzed by a cytosolic bile acid-CoA:amino acid N-acyltransferase (BAAT). A defect in BACL, caused by homozygous disease causing mutations in *SLC27A5* with biochemical findings consistent with fail-ure to conjugate bile acids found in urine and plasma, was described in 2 Pakistani siblings. The index case presented with conjugated hyperbilirubinemia and elevated serum aminotransferases with normal serum GGT activity and fat-soluble vitamin defi-ciency. Biochemical resolution occurred by 49 weeks without therapy. The sibling, with the same mutation in *SLC27A5*, did not have cholestasis; both are well without therapy.[42] Patients with the second amidation enzyme deficiency BAAT typically pre-sent with neonatal cholestasis, fat-soluble vitamin deficiency, and growth failure. In 10 patients identified by the authors, the diagnosis was based on the LSIMS analysis of the urine and serum and bile revealing a typical pattern devoid of conjugated bile acids but including bile acids conjugated with glucuronide and sulfates (see **Fig. 6**).[43] Hadzic and colleagues[44] have described a single case and Carlton and colleagues[45] have described a kindred of Amish descent with mutations in the BAAT. Patients with ho-mozygous mutations of BAAT have increased serum bile acids and variable growth failure and coagulopathy without jaundice and normal serum GGT concentrations. Ho-mozygotes have only unconjugated bile acids in serum, whereas heterozygotes had increased amounts unconjugated serum bile acids. Treatment of 5 patients with BAAT with the conjugated primary bile acid glycocholic acid improved their growth and corrected their fat-soluble vitamin malabsorption.[46] The recognition that genetic defects in bile acid synthesis are associated with fat-soluble vitamin malabsorption warrants a more concerted effort to explore this type of patient population, particularly because conjugated bile acids in the form of glycocholic acid are available under a treatment Investigational New Drug (IND) from the US Food and Drug Administration.

OXYSTEROL 7α-HYDROXYLASE DEFICIENCY

The genetic defect (*CYP8B1*) in oxysterol 7α-hydroxylase[47] established the acidic pathway as a quantitatively important pathway for bile acid synthesis in early life. This defect has been found in a limited number of infants. Patients present with severe progressive cholestasis, hepatosplenomegaly, cirrhosis, and liver synthetic failure in early infancy. Serum aminotransferases are markedly elevated, and serum GGT is normal. Liver biopsy findings included cholestasis, bridging fibrosis, extensive giant cell transformation, and proliferating bile ductules.[48–50] In these patients, analysis of the urine by LSIMS reveals a pattern consisting of glycol-sulfate conjugates of 3β-hy-droxy-5-cholenoic and 3β-hydroxy-5-cholestenoic acids (see **Fig. 6**) shown to be extremely cholestatic that likely explains the severe liver disease in affected patients.[51] Alternatively, the condition may be diagnosed by genetic testing for mutations in *CYP8B1*. Unlike the other two nuclear defects in bile acid synthesis, the oxysterol 7α-hydroxylase deficiency is particularly severe and is unresponsive to cholic acid; however, in one report, CDCA was reported to be effective.[52]

2-METHYLACYL-COENZYME A RACEMASE DEFICIENCY

2-Methylacyl-CoA racemase is a crucial enzyme that is uniquely responsible for the racemization of (25R) 3α,7β,12α-trihydroxy-5β-cholestanoic acid (THCA)-CoA to its (25S) enantiomer, while also performing the same reaction on the branched-chain fatty acid (2R) pristanoyl-CoA. Defects in this enzyme, therefore, have profound effects on both the bile acid and the fatty acid pathways. Mutations in the gene encoding 2-methylacyl-CoA racemase (AMARC) were first reported in 3 adults who presented with a sensory motor neuropathy[53] and later in a 10-week-old infant who had severe fat-soluble vitamin deficiencies, hematochezia, and mild cholestatic liver disease.[54] With the infantile presentation, liver histologic findings include cholestasis and giant cell transformation with modest inflammation. The infant had the same missense mutation (S52P) described in 2 adult patients, yet was seemingly phenotypically quite different. Two of the adult patients had neurologic symptoms but were asymptomatic until the fourth decade of life, whereas the other adult was described as having the typical features of Niemann-Pick type C disease at 18 months of age and presumably had liver dysfunction. With the expansion of whole-exome sequencing, additional neurologic phenotypes in children have been observed (J.E.H., K.D.R.S, personal observations, 2016.). It is possible that patients presenting later in life could have had subclinical mild liver disease and fat-soluble vitamin absorption early in life that, if undiagnosed in infancy, would likely lead to a neuropathy owing to the tissue accumulation of phytanic and pristanic acids. Diagnosis is based on urinary, serum, and biliary bile acid analysis by LSIMS (electrospray ionization–tandem mass spectrometry) and GC-MS, which reveal subnormal levels of primary bile acids and markedly increased concentrations of cholestanoic acids, which are characteristically found as major bile acids of the alligator, other reptiles, and amphibians.[55] The mass spectrum and gas chromatography profiles in this defect closely resemble those observed in peroxisomal disorders impacting bile acid synthesis, such as ZSD (see **Fig. 6**). Alternatively, genetic analysis for mutations in the AMARC gene may be used for diagnostic purposes. Primary bile acid therapy with CA is effective in normalizing liver enzymes and preventing the onset of neurologic symptoms in the infant coupled with dietary restriction of phytanic acid and pristanic acids, which are necessary to prevent neurotoxicity from their accumulation in the brain.

ACYL-COENZYME A OXIDASE AND 3α,7β,12α-TRIHYDROXY-5β-CHOLESTANOIC ACID–COENZYME A OXIDASE DEFICIENCY

A limited number of patients have been reported to have side-chain oxidation defects involving the THCA-CoA oxidase.[56,57] The clinical presentation differs; although all impact on primary bile acid synthesis, neurologic disease is the main clinical feature.[12] Whether these are primary bile acid defects or secondary to single-enzyme defects in peroxisomal β-oxidation is unclear. Two distinct acyl-CoA oxidases have been identified in humans.[57] The human acyl-CoA oxidase (ACOX2) active on bile acid C_{27} cholestanoic acid intermediates has been found to be the same enzyme that catalyzes the oxidation of 2-methyl branched-chain fatty acids. Of the case reports of proposed THCA-CoA oxidase deficiency, phytanic and pristanic acids were elevated.[56–58] All had ataxia as a primary feature of the disease, with its onset occurring at about 3.0 to 3.5 years of age. None had evidence of liver disease. It is possible, with the exception of the patient described by Clayton and colleagues,[56] that these patients had a 2-methylacyl-CoA racemase deficiency; but the analysis of the cholestanoic acids was not sufficiently detailed to permit the diastereoisomers of THCA and 3α,7α-dihydroxy-5β-cholestanoic acid (DHCA) or pristanic acid to be measured. In the case of the patient reported by Clayton and colleagues,[56] 2-methylacyl-CoA racemase deficiency was excluded as an explanation for the clinical presentation. ACOX2 deficiency as a cause of liver dysfunction, ataxia, and cognitive impairment has been recently described.[59] A case report described an 8 year old who presented at 8 months with elevated serum aminotransferases with normal GGT levels without jaundice and reduced vitamin A and E levels. At 6 years of age, liver biopsy findings included fibrous septa, swollen hepatocytes, and focal acinar transformation. He grew normally but developed cognitive impairment and ataxia, slurred speech, and dysmetria by 6.5 years of age. His exome sequencing revealed homozygous T207A mutations in ACOX2. Urine and serum analysis revealed increased DHCA and THCA, commonly found in peroxisomal disorders. Unlike more generalized peroxisomal disorders, elevated serum pristanic, phytanic acids, and very long chain fatty acids (VLCFAs) were not observed.

ADENOSINE TRIPHOSPHATE BINDING CASSETTE SUBFAMILY D MEMBER 3 DEFICIENCY

ATP binding cassette transporters catalyze metabolic pathways of fatty acids and bile acids in the peroxisome. A case report has described a patient with ABCD3 deficiency, which caused mild neonatal jaundice with recurrence of jaundice at 6 months of age with the development of hepatosplenomegaly at 18 months of age with anemia, thrombocytopenia, elevated aminotransferases, mild conjugated hyperbilirubinemia with normal serum GGT, and coagulopathy unresponsive to parenteral vitamin K. Liver histology findings included fibrosis with minimal inflammation. Plasma DHCA and THCA and VLCFA were elevated, and phytanic and pristanic acid levels were normal; plasmalogens were reduced but not deficient. Her liver synthetic dysfunction deteriorated, and she underwent liver transplantation but died postoperatively.[60]

SIDE-CHAIN OXIDATION DEFECT IN THE ALTERNATE 25-HYDROXYLATION PATHWAY

A defect in side-chain oxidation in the 25-hydroxylation pathway has been proposed by Clayton and colleagues[61] for a 9-week-old infant presenting with familial giant cell hepatitis and severe intrahepatic cholestasis. Reduced serum CA and CDCA, concomitant with high concentrations of serum and urine bile alcohol glucuronides, were observed. Although the profile resembled that seen in patients with CTX, it was concluded based on the liver disease (not previously reported for CTX at that time) that this represented a different side-chain defect and that it was possibly an oxidation defect downstream of the 25-hydroxylation step in this minor pathway for bile acid synthesis. The implications of the findings are that it could indicate that the 25-hydroxylation pathway, considered of negligible importance in adults,[62] may be an important pathway for infants. The patient was treated with CDCA and CA with normalization in serum aminotransferases and suppression in production of bile alcohols.

SECONDARY DEFECTS OF BILE ACID SYNTHESIS RELATED TO IMPAIRED PEROXISOMAL FUNCTION

Peroxisomal biogenesis disorders, a genetically heterogeneous group of autosomal recessive traits, have a generalized or specific defect in peroxisome function that interferes with fatty acid β-oxidation, bile acid synthesis, ether phospholipid biosynthesis, fatty acid α-oxidation, glyoxylate detoxification, and/or L-pipecolic acid degradation.[63,64] Clinical features that may occur across the spectrum of ZSD severity include developmental delay and neurologic abnormalities, seizures, liver dysfunction and hepatomegaly, vision and hearing impairment, adrenocortical dysfunction, and dentition enamel hypoplasia.[65] In these conditions, there is evidence of peroxisomal dysfunction of bile acid metabolism, including the presence of increased urinary and serum elevation of DHCA and THCA (as found in 2-methylacyl-CoA racemase deficiency, see **Fig. 4**) and fatty acid metabolism with elevated serum pristanic and phytanic acids, VLCFAs, and reduced plasmalogens. Liver disease in ZSDs has been associated with the accumulation of C_{27}-bile acid synthesis intermediates (DHCA, THCA), which have peroxisomal toxicity ameliorated by bile acid treatment in a mouse model.[64,66–68] In ZSDs, bile acid synthesis is dysregulated because of the lack of peroxisomal β-oxidation of C_{27}-bile acid intermediates that cannot undergo side-chain oxidation to form normal C_{24}-primary bile acids. Patients with ZSD commonly present with liver dysfunction characterized by variable increases in serum aminotransferases with or without conjugated hyperbilirubinemia with variable synthetic defects as evidenced by coagulopathy or hypalbuminemia. In the registration trial, 20 patients with ZSD were treated with CA with the total duration of treatment of all patients of 145 weeks with a range of 0 to 545 weeks.[21,69] The median age at the time of treatment of patients with Zellweger syndrome was 6 years and for neonatal adrenoleukodystrophy was 2 years. Treatment seems to prevent progression of liver disease.[21] There have been concerns raised that patients with advanced liver disease may have adverse outcomes with treatment with CA; however, it is likely the liver disease was so advanced that CA therapy was not as effective as has been observed in patients with single enzyme defect.[21,70]

DIAGNOSIS AND TREATMENT OF INBORN ERRORS IN BILE ACID SYNTHESIS

Diagnosis of inborn errors of metabolism should be considered in infants with conjugated hyperbilirubinemia with low serum GGT in a neonate and low or normal serum bile acids measured by conventional testing methods; however, patients with chronic liver disease may also present later in life. Accurate identification of inborn errors currently can be done by 2 different but complementary methods. The use of LSIMS, in conjunction with genetic testing, confirms the biochemical diagnosis as well as serves as an effective means to assess biochemical response and compliance to therapy.[2,71,72] Urine LSIMS screening may be the quickest means to identify inborn errors of bile acid metabolism with turnaround times typically faster than gene analysis. As a screening test, in assessing infants with conjugated hyperbilirubinemia, it may be practical to measure serum bile acids by a standard laboratory technique that will identify primary and secondary bile acids but not the metabolites typically seen in the inborn errors of bile acid metabolism. If the serum bile acids by this technique are elevated, one can safely assume you have ruled out the more life-threatening defects, such as *HSD3B7*, *AKR1D1*, and *CYP8B1* deficiencies. This simple screen would not necessarily rule out defects of amidation, which typically present with fat and fat-soluble vitamin malabsorption, or sterol 27-hydroxylase deficiency; mass spectrometry or genetic analysis would be essential for screening. When assessing for bile acid metabolites in the urine, it is also essential to note that if ursodeoxycholic acid (UCDA) is being administered during the screening with either the urine FAB-MS or conventional serum bile acid methods, the results may be difficult to interpret, so all specimens should be collected after a period of at least 4 to 5 days off UDCA.

The earliest experience with using primary bile acid therapy was for CTX, even though chronic liver disease is not typically seen. Long-term treatment with

CDCA (750 mg/d) normalizes plasma cholestanol concentrations, markedly reduces the urinary excretion of bile alcohols, and improves the clinical condition.[39] More recently, because it is recognized that patients with CTX may present with neonatal cholestasis, CA has been shown to be effective in reducing toxic metabolites produced in this condition.[21] Oral bile acid therapy is a safe and effective treatment of patients with the 3β-hydroxy-Δ^5-C_{27}-steroid oxidoreductase deficiency, 5β-reductase deficiency, and 2-methylacyl-CoA racemase deficiency and may provide stabilization of liver disease in patients with ZSD.[21,29,30] Cholic acid, marketed as Cholbam, is the therapy of choice and has been shown to be effective in a dosage range of 10 to 15 mg per kilogram of body weight per day.[21] Although UDCA may lead to improvement in serum aminotransferase and potentially liver histology in some patients with the 3β-hydroxy-Δ^5-C_{27}-steroid oxidoreductase deficiency,[18] it does not suppress the synthesis of atypical 3β-hydroxy-Δ^5 bile acids, which over the long-term is important given that these bile acids are cholestatic and interfere with canalicular bile acid transport.[27,28] UDCA should not be used in combination with cholic acid, because UDCA competitively inhibits the ileal uptake of CA, reduces the pool of CA acid, and compromises its therapeutic effectiveness.

The success of CA for patients with multiple defects in the bile acid biosynthetic pathway is well documented; however, some treatment failures have occurred for patients with oxysterol 7α-hydroxylase deficiency and amidation defects as well as patients with very advanced liver disease as commonly found in 5β-reductase deficiency.[21,29] Patients with a bile acid conjugation (amidation) defect[42–45] who synthesize cholic acid almost exclusively may be treated under a treatment IND with glycocholic acid (available from the authors) or potentially do not require treatment with close attention to growth and fat-soluble vitamins with appropriate interventions as needed to address deficiencies.

After initiation of treatment with CA, patients should be monitored frequently with serum liver chemistries until they normalize and thereafter every 6 to 12 months with concomitant urine LSIMS analysis. Bile acid therapy is lifelong for the responsive conditions, and adherence should be periodically confirmed by using LSIMS or in circumstances when liver chemistries become abnormal. Because of concerns regarding the long-term risks of hepatocellular carcinoma even in the presence of apparent health, annual ultrasound and serum alpha fetoprotein should be considered after the first 5 years of treatment.

REFERENCES

1. Russell DW, Setchell KDR. Bile acid biosynthesis. Biochemistry 1992;31: 4737–49.
2. Setchell KDR, Heubi JE, Bove KE. Bile acid synthesis and metabolism. In: Kleinman RE, Sanderson IR, Goulet O, et al, editors. Walker's pediatric gastrointestinal disease. Pathophysiology, diagnosis, management. Hamilton (Ontario): BC Decker Inc; 2008. p. 1069–94.
3. Lester R, St. Pyrek J, Little JM, et al. Diversity of bile acids in the fetus and newborn infant. J Pediatr Gastroenterol Nutr 1983;2:355–64.
4. Setchell KDR, Dumaswala R, Colombo C, et al. Hepatic bile acid metabolism during early development revealed from the analysis of human fetal gallbladder bile. J Biol Chem 1988;263:16637–44.
5. Sjovall J. Dietary glycine and taurine conjugation in man. Proc Soc Exp Biol Med 1959;100:676–8.

6. Bjorkhem I. Mechanism of bile acid biosynthesis in mammalian liver. In: Danielsson H, Sjovall J, editors. Sterols and bile acids. Amsterdam (Netherlands): BV Elsevier Science Publishers; 1985. p. 231–77.

7. Boyer JL. New concepts of mechanisms of hepatocyte bile formation. Physiol Rev 1980;60:303–26.

8. LaRusso NF, Korman MG, Hoffman NE, et al. Dynamics of the enterohepatic circulation of bile acids. Postprandial serum concentrations of conjugates of cholic acid in health, cholecystectomized patients, and patients with bile acid malabsorption. N Engl J Med 1974;291:689–92.

9. Watkins JB, Ingall D, Szczepanik P, et al. Bile-salt metabolism in the newborn. Measurement of pool size and synthesis by stable isotope technique. N Engl J Med 1973;288:431–4.

10. Watkins JB, Szczepanik P, Gould JB, et al. Bile salt metabolism in the human premature infant. Preliminary observations of pool size and synthesis rate following prenatal administration of dexamethasone and phenobarbital. Gastroenterology 1975;69:706–13.

11. Heubi JE, Balistreri WF, Suchy FJ. Bile salt metabolism in the first year of life. J Lab Clin Med 1982;100:127–36.

12. Watkins JB, Jarvenpaa AL, Szczepanik-Van Leeuwen P, et al. Feeding the low-birth weight infant: V. Effects of taurine, cholesterol, and human milk on bile acid kinetics. Gastroenterology 1983;85:793–800.

13. Setchell KDR, Heubi JE. Defects in bile acid biosynthesis-diagnosis and treatment. J Pediatr Gastroenterol Nutr 2006;43(1):S17–22.

14. Al-Hussaini A, Setchell KDR, AlSaleem B, et al. Bile acid synthesis disorders in Arabs: a 10-year screening study. J Pediatr Gastroenterol Nutr 2017;65(6): 613–20.

15. Nittono H, Takei H, Unno A, et al. Diagnostic determination system for high-risk screening for inborn errors of bile acid metabolism based on an analysis of urinary bile acids using gas chromatography-mass spectrometry: results for 10 years in Japan. Pediatr Int 2009;51:535–43.

16. Jahnel J, Zohrer E, Fischler B, et al. Attempt to determine the prevalence of two inborn errors of primary bile acid synthesis: results of a European survey. J Pediatr Gastroenterol Nutr 2017;64:864–8.

17. Clayton PT, Leonard JV, Lawson AM, et al. Familial giant cell hepatitis associated with synthesis of 3 beta, 7 alphadihydroxy-and 3 beta,7 alpha, 12 alpha-trihydroxy-5-cholenoic acids. J Clin Invest 1987;79:1031–8.

18. Jacquemin E, Setchell KD, O'Connell NC, et al. A new cause of progressive intra-hepatic cholestasis: 3 beta-hydroxy-C27-steroid dehydrogenase/isomerase deficiency. J Pediatr 1994;125:379–84.

19. Setchell KDR, Flick R, Watkins JB, et al. Chronic hepatitis in a 10 yr old due to an inborn error in bile acid synthesis—diagnosis and treatment with oral bile acid. Gastroenterology 1990;98:A578.

20. Bove KE, Heubi JE, Balistreri WF, et al. Bile acid synthetic defects and liver disease: a comprehensive review. Pediatr Dev Pathol 2004;7:315–34.

21. Heubi JE, Bove KE, Setchell KDR. Oral cholic acid is efficacious and well tolerated in patients with bile acid synthetic and Zellweger Spectrum disorders. J Pediatr Gastroenterol Nutr 2017;65:321–6.

22. Fischler B, Bodin K, Stjernman H, et al. Cholestatic liver disease in adults may be due to an inherited defect in bile acid biosynthesis. J Intern Med 2007;262: 254–62.

23. Molho-Pessach V, Rios JJ, Xing C, et al. Homozygosity identifies a bile acid biosynthetic defect in an adult with cirrhosis of unknown etiology. Hepatology 2012;55:1139–45.

24. Lemonde HA, Johnson AW, Clayton PT. The identification of unusual bile acid metabolites by tandem mass spectrometry: use of low-energy collision-induced dissociation to produce informative spectra. Rapid Commun Mass Spectrom 1999;13:1159–64.

25. Libert R, Hermans D, Draye JP, et al. Bile acids and conjugates identified in metabolic disorders by fast atom bombardment and tandem mass spectrometry. Clin Chem 1991;37:2102–10.

26. Mushtaq I, Logan S, Morris M, et al. Screening of newborn infants for cholestatic hepatobiliary disease with tandem mass spectrometry. BMJ 1999;319: 471–7.

27. Javitt NB, Emerman S. Effect of sodium taurolithocholate on bile flow and bile acid excretion. J Clin Invest 1968;47:1002–14.

28. Stieger B, Zhang J, O'Neill B, et al. Transport of taurine conjugates of 7alpha-hydroxy-3-oxo-4-cholenoic acid and 3beta,7alpha-dihydroxy-5-cholenoic acid in rat liver plasma membrane vesicles. In: Van Berge-Henegouwen GP, Van Hock B, De Groote J, et al, editors. Cholestatic liver diseases. Dordrecht (Netherlands): Kluwer Academic Press; 1994. p. 82–7.

29. Gonzales E, Gerhardt MF, Fabre M, et al. Oral cholic acid for hereditary defects of primary bile acid synthesis: a safe and effective long-term therapy. Gastroenterology 2009;137(4):1310–20.

30. Riello L, D'Antiga L, Guido M, et al. Titration of bile acid supplements in 3β-Hydroxy-Δ5-C27-steroid dehydrogenase/isomerase deficiency. J Pediatr Gastroenterol Nutr 2010;50:655–60.

31. Setchell KDR, Suchy FJ, Welsh MB, et al. Delta 4-3-oxosteroid 5 beta-reductase deficiency described in identical twins with neonatal hepatitis. A new inborn error in bile acid synthesis. J Clin Invest 1988;82:2148–57.

32. Shneider BL, Setchell KDR, Whitington PF, et al. Delta 4-3-oxosteroid 5 beta-reductase deficiency causing neonatal liver failure and hemochromatosis. J Pediatr 1994;124:234–8.

33. Daugherty CC, Setchell KD, Heubi JE, et al. Resolution of liver biopsy alterations in three siblings with bile acid treatment of an inborn error of bile acid metabolism (delta 4-3-oxosteroid 5 beta-reductase deficiency). Hepatology 1993;18: 1096–101.

34. Clayton PT, Patel E, Lawson AM, et al. 3-oxo bile acids in liver disease. [letter]. Lancet 1988;1:1283–4.

35. Wahlen E, Egestad B, Strandvik B, et al. Ketonic bile acids in urine of infants during the neonatal period. J Lipid Res 1989;30:1847–57.

36. Van Bogaert L, Scherer HJ, Epstein E. Une forme cerebrale de la cholesterinose generalisee. Paris: Masson et Cie; 1937.

37. Cali JJ, Russell DW. Characterization of human sterol 27-hydroxylase. A mitochondrial cytochrome P-450 that catalyzes multiple oxidation reaction in bile acid biosynthesis. J Biol Chem 1991;266:7774–8.

38. Egestad B, Pettersson P, Skrede S, et al. Fast atom bombardment mass spectrometry in the diagnosis of cerebrotendinous xanthomatosis. Scand J Clin Lab Invest 1985;45:443–6.

39. Berginer VM, Salen G, Shefer S. Long-term treatment of cerebrotendinous xanthomatosis with chenodeoxycholic acid. N Engl J Med 1984;311:1649–52.

40. Clayton PT, Verrips A, Sistermans E, et al. Mutations in the sterol 27-hydroxylase gene (CYP27A) cause hepatitis of infancy as well as cerebrotendinous xanthomatosis. J Inherit Metab Dis 2002;25:501–13.
41. Gong J-Y, Setchell KDR, Zhao J, et al. Severe neonatal cholestasis in cerebrotendinous xanthomatotic: genetics, immunostaining, mass spectrometry. J Pediatr Gastroenterol Nutr 2017;65:561–8.
42. Chong CPK, Mills PB, McClean P, et al. Bile acid-CoA ligase deficiency- a new inborn error of bile acid metabolism. J Inherit Metab Dis 2012;35:521–30.
43. Setchell KDR, Heubi JE, Shah S, et al. Genetic defects in bile acid conjugation cause fat soluble vitamin deficiency. Gastroenterology 2013;144:945–55.
44. Hadzic N, Bull LN, Clayton PT, et al. Diagnosis in bile acid-CoA: amino acid N-acyltransferase deficiency. World J Gastroenterol 2012;18:3322–6.
45. Carlton VE, Harris BZ, Puffenberger EG, et al. Complex inheritance of familial hypercholanemia with associated mutations in TJP2 and BAAT. Nat Genet 2003; 34(1):91–6.
46. Heubi JE, Setchell KDR, Jha P, et al. Treatment of bile acid amidation defects with glycocholic acid. Hepatology 2015;61(1):268–74.
47. Setchell KDR, Schwarz M, O'Connell NC, et al. Identification of a new inborn error in bile acid synthesis: mutation of the oxysterol 7alpha-hydroxylase gene causes severe neonatal liver disease. J Clin Invest 1998;102:1690–703.
48. Dai D, Millls PB, Footitt E, et al. Liver disease in infancy caused by oxysterol 7α-hydroxylase deficiency: successful treatment with chenodeoxycholic acid. J Inherit Metab Dis 2014;37:851–61.
49. Mizuochi T, Kimura A, Suzuki M, et al. Successful heterozygous living donor liver transplant for an oxysterol 7α-hydroxylase deficiency in a Japanese Patient. Liver Transpl 2011;17:1059–65.
50. Ueki I, Kimura A, Nishiyori A, et al. Neonatal cholestatic liver disease in an Asian patient with homozygous mutation in the oxysterol 7α-hydroxylase gene. J Pediatr Gastroenterol Nutr 2008;46:465–9.
51. Mathis U, Karlaganis G, Preisig R. Monohydroxy bile salt sulfates: tauro-3 beta-hydroxy-5-cholenoate-3-sulfate induces intrahepatic cholestasis in rats. Gastroenterology 1983;85:674–81.
52. Clayton PT, Mills KA, Johnson AW, et al. Delta 4-3-oxosteroid 5 beta-reductase deficiency: failure of ursodeoxycholic acid treatment and response to chenodeoxycholic acid plus cholic acid. Gut 1996;38:623–8.
53. Ferdinandusse S, Denis S, Clayton PT, et al. Mutations in the gene encoding peroxisomal 2-methyl-acyl racemase cause adult-onset sensory motor neuropathy. Nat Genet 2000;24:188–91.
54. Setchell KDR, Heubi JE, Bove KE, et al. Liver disease caused by failure to racemize trihydroxycholestanoic acid: gene mutation and effect of bile acid therapy. Gastroenterology 2003;124:217–32.
55. Haslewood GA. Bile salt evolution. J Lipid Res 1967;8:535–50.
56. Clayton PT, Johnson AW, Mills KA, et al. Ataxia associated with increased plasma concentrations of pristanic acid, phytanic acid and C27 bile acids but normal fibroblast branched-chain fatty acid oxidation. J Inherit Metab Dis 1996;19: 761–8.
57. Vanhove GF, Van Veldhoven PP, Fransen M, et al. The CoA esters of 2-methyl-branched chain fatty acids and of the bile acid intermediates di- and trihydroxycoprostanic acids are oxidized by one single peroxisomal branched chain acyl-CoA oxidase in human liver and kidney. J Biol Chem 1993;268:10335–44.

58. Christensen E, Van Eldere J, Brandt NJ, et al. A new peroxisomal disorder: di- and trihydroxycholestanaemia due to a presumed trihydroxycholestanoyl-CoA oxidase deficiency. J Inherit Metab Dis 1990;13:363–6.
59. Vilarinho S, Sari S, Mazzacuva F, et al. ACOX2 deficiency: a disorder of bile acid synthesis with transaminase elevation, liver fibrosis, ataxia, and cognitive impairment. Proc Natl Acad Sci U S A 2016;113:11289–93.
60. Ferinandusse S, Jimenez-Sanchez G, Koster J, et al. A novel bile acid biosynthesis defect due to a deficiency of peroxisomal ABCD3. Hum Mol Genet 2015;24:361–70.
61. Clayton PT, Casteels M, Mieli-Vergani G, et al. Familial giant cell hepatitis with low bile acid concentrations and increased urinary excretion of specific bile alcohols: a new inborn error of bile acid synthesis? Pediatr Res 1995;37:424–31.
62. Duane WC, Pooler PA, Hamilton JN. Bile acid synthesis in man. In vivo activity of the 25-hydroxylation pathway. J Clin Invest 1988;82:82–5.
63. Waterham HR, Ferdinandusse S, Wanders RJ. Human disorders of peroxisome metabolism and biogenesis. Biochim Biophys Acta 2016;1863(5):922–33.
64. Wanders RJ, Ferdinandusse S. Peroxisomes, peroxisomal diseases, and the hepatotoxicity induced by peroxisomal metabolites. Curr Drug Metab 2012;13(10):1401–11.
65. Braverman NE, Raymond GV, Rizzo WB, et al. Peroxisome biogenesis disorders in the Zellweger spectrum: an overview of current diagnosis, clinical manifestations, and treatment guidelines. Mol Genet Metab 2016;117(3):313–21.
66. Baes M, Van Veldhoven PP. Hepatic dysfunction in peroxisomal disorders. Biochim Biophys Acta 2016;1863(5):956–70.
67. van Heijst AF, Verrips A, Wevers RA, et al. Treatment and follow-up of children with cerebrotendinous xanthomatosis. Eur J Pediatr 1998;157:313–6.
68. Keane MH, Overmars H, Wikander TM, et al. Bile acid treatment alters hepatic disease and bile acid transport in peroxisome-deficient *PEX2* Zellweger mice. Hepatology 2007;45:982–97.
69. Setchell KDR, Bragetti P, Zimmer-Nechemias L, et al. Oral bile acid treatment and the patient with Zellweger syndrome. Hepatology 1992;15(2):198–207.
70. Berendse K, Klouwer FC, Koot BG, et al. Cholic acid therapy in Zellweger spectrum disorders. J Inherit Metab Dis 2016;39(6):859–68.
71. Lawson AM, Setchell KDR. Mass spectrometry of bile acids. In: Setchell KDR, Kritchevsky D, Nair PP, editors. The bile acids: methods and applications, vol. 4. New York: Plenum Press; 1988. p. 167–268.
72. Lawson AM, Madigan MJ, Shortland D, et al. Rapid diagnosis of Zellweger syndrome and infantile Refsum's disease by fast atom bombardment–mass spectrometry of urine bile salts. Clin Chim Acta 1986;161:221–31.

Autoimmune Hepatitis, Sclerosing Cholangitis, and Autoimmune Sclerosing Cholangitis or Overlap Syndrome

Nanda Kerkar, MD[a],*, Albert Chan, MD[a,b]

KEYWORDS

- Autoimmune hepatitis • Immunosuppression • Sclerosing cholangitis
- Autoimmune sclerosing cholangitis • Children

KEY POINTS

- Autoimmune hepatitis is a diagnosis of exclusion and there is a scoring system in place for complicated cases.
- Sclerosing cholangitis is seen most commonly in association with inflammatory bowel disease.
- Autoimmune sclerosing cholangitis is the overlap of clinical, biochemical, and histologic features of autoimmune hepatitis and sclerosing cholangitis, seen most commonly in children.
- Immunosuppression is the current management for autoimmune liver disease in children and ursodeoxycholic acid is used in those diagnosed with sclerosing cholangitis.

INTRODUCTION

Autoimmune liver disease in pediatrics encompasses autoimmune hepatitis (AIH), autoimmune overlap with sclerosing cholangitis (SC), recurrence of AIH after liver transplantation, and the development of de novo AIH post-transplantation in patients transplanted for indications other than AIH.[1] Syndromes associated with AIH include autoimmune polyendocrinopathy candidiasis ectodermal dystrophy, immune dysregulation polyendocrinopathy enteropathy X-linked syndrome, common variable immunodeficiency, and hyperimmunoglobulin M syndrome.[2] An autoimmune phenotype has been described in association with drugs, and nitrofurantoin and

[a] Division of Gastroenterology, Hepatology and Nutrition, Golisano Children's Hospital, University of Rochester Medical Center, 601 Elmwood Avenue, Box 667, Rochester, NY 14642, USA;
[b] Division of Pediatric Gastroenterology, Hepatology and Nutrition, University of Florida, PO Box 100296, Gainesville, FL 32610, USA
* Corresponding author.
E-mail address: nanda_kerkar@urmc.rochester.edu

Clin Liver Dis 22 (2018) 689–702
https://doi.org/10.1016/j.cld.2018.06.005
1089-3261/18/© 2018 Elsevier Inc. All rights reserved.

minocycline are the most commonly implicated.[3] This article focuses on AIH, SC, and autoimmune overlap with SC.

DEFINITION AND TYPES OF AUTOIMMUNE HEPATITIS

Typically, AIH is described as a chronic inflammatory condition of the liver characterized by elevated serum aminotransferases and immunoglobulin G (IgG), presence of non-organ specific autoantibodies, and interface hepatitis with lymphoplasmacytic infiltration in the absence of known etiologic factors. Type 1 AIH is associated with antinuclear antibody (ANA) with or without smooth muscle antibody (SMA). Type 2 AIH is associated with liver kidney microsomal (LKM) antibody with or without anti-liver cytosol type 1. Both types 1 and 2 AIH may be associated with other types of autoimmune disease, including thyroiditis, celiac disease, and type 1 diabetes in up to 20% of patients. Family history of autoimmune disease is also reported to be present in up to 40% of patients with both types of AIH. The differences between types 1 and 2 AIH are illustrated in **Table 1**. Presence of soluble liver antigen signifies a worse prognosis in those with AIH.

Epidemiology and Pathogenesis

The prevalence of AIH has been reported as 1 per 200,000 in the US general population and 20 per 100,000 in female patients older than the age of 14 years in Spain.[4] The disease may be seen in all ethnic groups and ages but has a female preponderance. There is significant association with HLA DR3 and DR4. The pathogenesis of AIH is still not clear. The inflammation in the liver in AIH seems to be secondary to both cell-mediated (T-cell) and humoral (B-cell) activity. The stimulus that initiates the autoimmune inflammatory activity is unknown and may not be the same in all cases of AIH. Many viruses have been implicated and the identification of sequence homology between a virus and the target of antibodies has also been demonstrated in support of this mechanism of molecular mimicry.[5,6] The ability of T cells to proliferate is controlled by regulatory T (T-reg) cells, characterized by expression of CD4+, CD25 +, and nuclear expression of the forkhead transcription factor box P3 (FOXP3).[7] Reduced number and activity of these T-reg cells has been described in AIH.[8]

Table 1
Differences between type 1 and type 2 autoimmune hepatitis

	Type 1 AIH	Type 2 AIH
Age at presentation	Usually pubertal age	May present very early in life, much younger than type 1
Prevalence	Much more common than type 2	<1/3 of cases with AIH
Clinical features and course	Usually chronic	Acute liver failure presentation more common
Autoantibodies	ANA, SMA	LKM, Anti-liver cytosol type1
Autoimmune polyendocrinopathy candidiasis ectodermal dystrophy	No association	Association described
Histology	Cirrhosis more common	May have cell drop-out and necrosis in acute liver failure setting
Overlap with SC	Not uncommon	Very rare
Immunosuppression	May be weaned off	Need life-long immunosuppression

Scoring System

The first description of AIH appears in 1950 by Waldenstrom.[9] However, it was only after the discovery of the hepatitis C virus in 1989 that a scoring system was formulated to allow accurate diagnosis of AIH by the International Autoimmune Hepatitis group in Brighton, UK.[10] The scoring system has since been modified.[11] In the revised scoring system, points have been allocated to female gender, hepatitic liver chemistries, hypergammaglobulinemia, presence of autoantibodies (ANA, SMA, LKM), absence of viral markers, minimal alcohol intake, negative drug history, characteristic liver histology, possession of HLA DR3 or DR4 haplotype, presence of other defined antibodies, and complete or partial response to therapy. A score greater than 15 pretreatment and greater than 17 post-treatment was considered definite AIH, whereas a score of 10 to 15 pre-treatment and12 to 17 post-treatment was considered as probable AIH.[11] This revised scoring system has been further simplified to facilitate use in clinical practice.[12]

Diagnosis

Children with AIH, may present similar to an acute viral hepatitis with jaundice, abdominal pain, be picked up incidentally, have an acute liver failure presentation, or with a complication of portal hypertension, including ascites and gastrointestinal bleeding. Given that the presentation is variable and can be at any age, it is important to investigate for AIH in a timely manner in any child presenting with liver disease. The physical examination of these children varies from unremarkable to jaundiced with hepatosplenomegaly, depending on severity of disease. Laboratory testing may show evidence of hypersplenism with low white cell count and/or thrombocytopenia, impaired synthetic function with prolonged international normalized ratio and low serum albumin, elevated serum aminotransferases and serum bilirubin, elevated IgG, and positive autoantibodies. Imaging may show an enlarged liver and/or spleen, with ascites in advanced cases. Liver biopsy is an important tool and the histology typically shows a lymphoplasmacytic infiltration spilling over the limiting plate at the interface of the portal tract and the hepatocytes, which was previously known as piecemeal necrosis and now as interface hepatitis (**Fig. 1**). Emperipolesis and rosette formation are significantly associated with an autoimmune diagnosis.[1] In acute liver failure, the characteristic histology is not seen because there may be extensive necrosis and multilobular collapse. It is essential to rule out other etiologic factors, including viral hepatitis (A, B, C and E), Wilson disease, and alpha1-antitrypsin deficiency, before making a diagnosis of AIH. The scoring system is useful in complex cases and to compare subjects in research settings.

Management

Immunosuppression is the mainstay of therapy. It is conventional to start therapy with a steroid bolus, prednisone 2 mg/kg (maximum 40–60 mg), and preferable to give an antacid. Azathioprine (AZA) is usually added as a steroid-sparing agent but the start time can vary. Some clinicians like to start AZA at the beginning with the prednisone, others prefer to reserve it for instances when the serum aminotransferases flare during the steroid taper. It is not recommended to start AZA in the beginning when there is an acute liver failure presentation or severe liver disease with cirrhosis because hepatotoxicity may occur. The author's (Kerkar) preference is to check the thiopurine methyl transferase (TPMT) enzyme while commencing the steroid bolus and then starting the AZA when the results of the genetic study are available. The dose of AZA typically used in children is 1 to 2 mg/kg/d (maximum 50 mg at the start) and then titrated according

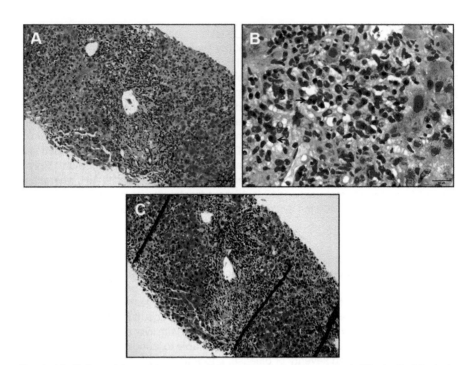

Fig. 1. (*A, B*) A portal tract is expanded by a chronic inflammatory infiltrate that includes plasma cells (seen at higher power in *B, arrows*) and extends beyond the limiting plate, consistent with interface hepatitis (hematoxylin-eosin, original magnification × 100). (*C*) Fibrosis that extends beyond the portal tract on trichrome stain (hematoxylin-eosin, original magnification × 400). (*Courtesy of* Philip J. Katzman, MD, University of Rochester Medical Center, Rochester, NY)

to the levels of the active metabolite, 6-thioguanine (6-TG). The dose of AZA may then be increased until 6-TG levels are between 240 to 400 pmol/8x10 (8) red blood cells, provided the levels of the hepatotoxic metabolite, 6-methylmercaptopurine (6-MMP) are below 5000 pmol/8 x10 (8) red blood cell.[13] In some situations when the dose of AZA is increased, instead of the 6-TG levels increasing, the levels of 6-MMP go up. Here, allopurinol may be used to divert the metabolism of AZA, so that 6-TG levels get to therapeutic levels without hepatotoxicity.[14] High 6-TG levels can cause bone-marrow toxicity. Pancreatitis is an idiosyncratic adverse event of AZA and checking the TPMT enzyme does not preclude its occurrence. When 6-TG is in the therapeutic range and the serum aminotransferases are in normal range, it is possible to wean the patient off the steroids completely. Some clinicians prefer to keep the patient on a combination of low-dose prednisone with AZA. Given the importance of achieving the full growth potential of the child, many prefer AZA monotherapy whenever feasible.

Remission and Relapse

Remission in AIH is said to occur when there is disappearance of symptoms, normal serum aminotransferases, bilirubin, and IgG with normal hepatic tissue or inactive cirrhosis histologically.[15] Once remission is achieved and maintained for several years, effort is often made to wean the patient off immunosuppression. The latter should not be attempted during puberty when autoimmune flares are common. Also, weaning immunosuppression off completely is not recommended in type 2 AIH because disease is more severe and relapse is almost inevitable. Relapse is defined as flare in serum aminotransferases after remission has been achieved. Usually, one has to repeat the liver biopsy and bolus the patient again with steroids. Checking adherence and reinforcing to the patient the importance of good adherence is essential for good outcomes.

Other Therapeutic Options

Mycophenolate mofetil (MMF) has been used successfully as rescue treatment in situations in which there have been adverse events with AZA or when AZA has not worked.[16] The adverse event profile of MMF includes gastrointestinal symptoms, bone marrow suppression, hair loss, and headaches. Budesonide may be a good option to consider when avoiding steroid side effects is the goal, because it has a high first-pass clearance in the liver. Budesonide, when used with AZA in a large multicenter study in adults, showed superior results to a combination of AZA with prednisone.[17] It is, however, recommended to not use budesonide alone as induction in AIH and to be aware that reactivation of AIH on budesonide monotherapy has been reported.[18] Calcineurin inhibitors (cyclosporine and tacrolimus) that are used as standard immunosuppression in transplant recipients to prevent rejection have been used successfully in controlling AIH.[11,19] Antitumor necrosis factor (TNF)-alpha has been used successfully as rescue treatment in difficult-to-treat AIH.[20] Recently, in a series of 11 children with juvenile autoimmune liver disease who received infliximab and/or adalimumab for their inflammatory bowel disease (IBD), all tolerated the treatment well without any impairment of liver function.[21] On the other hand, one must be aware that anti-TNF–related, drug-induced liver injury with autoimmune features have also been reported in children during management of IBD,[22] so careful monitoring of patients is necessary. Very recently, there have been reports in Japanese patients with AIH of using ursodeoxycholic acid (UDCA) monotherapy to successfully achieve and maintain remission[23]

Special Considerations

Autoimmune hepatitis with acute liver failure
In AIH presenting with acute liver failure and encephalopathy, medical management with immunosuppression is of little benefit and there is high risk of septic complications. The best option is to work the patient up for liver transplantation and list the patient. A trial of steroids may be tried cautiously in children, provided it is done by an experienced hepatologist in an institution with good intensive care facilities and liver transplantation capabilities. Success has been reported with immunosuppression in AIH with fulminant liver failure in some centers.[24,25]

Autoimmune hepatitis and liver transplantation
Liver transplantation is performed in 10% to 15% of children with AIH. Indications for transplantation include

1. Failure of medical treatment
2. Acute liver failure, particularly associated with encephalopathy
3. Development of hepatocellular carcinoma (rare).

AIH is the indication for transplantation in 2% to 3% of the liver transplants performed in the pediatric population in United States and Europe.[15] The patient and graft survival after liver transplantation are good and comparable to transplants for other indications. It is important to manage immunosuppression carefully after liver transplantation to minimize and possibly avoid recurrence of autoimmune disease in the allograft. Adding a third agent, AZA or MMF, to the calcineurin inhibitor and prednisone is helpful in achieving this. The risk of recurrent AIH has been reported to be between 15% and 40%.[26,27] The incidence increases as the interval from transplant increases and when there is nonadherence or another reason (eg, high Epstein-Barr virus polymerase chain reaction) for being on reduced immunosuppression. De novo AIH is the development of the classic features of AIH in patients not transplanted for AIH.[28] This was first described in children in 1989 and since then there have been numerous reports of its occurrence in the pediatric and adult population.[29] Although it is a rare cause of graft dysfunction, early diagnosis and appropriate management can help save grafts and lives. Ability to diagnose this accurately and early is contingent on a high degree of suspicion and on requesting an autoimmune panel with serum IgG and autoantibodies at the time of performing a liver biopsy after liver transplantation. The liver biopsy will show classic changes of AIH (as previously described). When AIH is diagnosed post transplant, either recurrent or de novo, management is with a bolus of steroids and the addition of another immunosuppressive agent such as AZA or MMF. The steroid taper, however, is much slower than that used to treat rejection, in line with that used in therapy of classic AIH.

Natural History and Prognosis

The natural history and prognosis of AIH depends on severity of the disease and is also influenced by adherence to medical management. Children diagnosed at an early age, with a strong family history, and advanced changes on histology are likely to require lifelong immunosuppression and even liver transplantation. Similarly, those presenting with acute liver failure and encephalopathy are more likely to have mortality without transplantation than those with mild disease. Almost all children should achieve remission within the first year of therapy. They can achieve excellent quality of life if their disease is under control on minimal immunosuppression. Too-rapid attempts to wean off immunosuppression or non-adherence can cause a high risk of relapse. It is important to monitor serum aminotransferases and the autoimmune panel intermittently, after stopping immunosuppression, so that a flare can be picked up early. Children with type 1 AIH are much more likely to have sustained remission off immunosuppression than type 2 AIH. An overall survival of 82% was noted in 34 children with AIH over a 6-year study period.[30] Risk factors for mortality include weight loss, jaundice, coagulopathy, and the presence of LKM; cirrhosis at presentation did not seem to influence outcome in this cohort. Hepatocellular carcinoma is a known complication of end-stage liver disease. Development of hepatocellular carcinoma with AIH in children is extremely rare compared with adults. Surveillance with alpha-fetoprotein and ultrasound scan may be done in patients with AIH and cirrhosis.

PEDIATRIC SCLEROSING CHOLANGITIS
Introduction

SC is a rare, chronic disease that afflicts the hepatobiliary system. It is characterized by an inflammatory process, leading to progressive fibrosis of the intrahepatic and/or extrahepatic bile ducts. Ultimately, it progresses toward end-stage liver disease, liver failure, biliary cirrhosis, cholangiocarcinoma, or a combination of these.[31] SC is widely known as primary SC, particularly in adults. In general, the term primary is used when the etiologic factors are unknown. In pediatrics, SC may be associated with several conditions, including ABCB4 (MDR3) gene mutation, cystic fibrosis, immunodeficiency, and Langerhans cell histiocytosis.[1] There is also autosomal recessive neonatal SC and overlap with AIH, the latter is known as autoimmune SC (ASC) (see later discussion).

Epidemiology

The incidence and prevalence of pediatric SC are estimated to be 0.2 and 1.5 cases per 100,000 children, respectively.[32] These numbers might be an underestimation because SC is often insidious and has subtle symptoms in the early stages.[33] Because it may have variable clinical presentation, SC may be difficult to detect early, and diagnosis is often made when obvious symptoms are present or complications arise. SC is seen more frequently in male patients by 2-fold. In addition, an increased prevalence in SC among first-degree relatives (0.7%), and more so in siblings (1.5%), has also been shown.[34] SC is often seen concurrently with AIH in children. It is associated with IBD in approximately 76% of children, with ranges reported typically from 33% to 90%.[35–38]

Primary Sclerosing Cholangitis–Inflammatory Bowel Disease

In pediatrics, the SC associated with IBD is widely referred to as primary SC (PSC). In patients with PSC and IBD, ulcerative colitis (UC) seems to be more common than Crohn disease. Whereas up to 90% of patients with SC have a diagnosis of IBD, most reports estimate that only about 4% of patients with IBD also have a diagnosis of PSC.[39] Interestingly, studies with longer term follow-up of IBD demonstrate higher rates of PSC. For example, the population of subjects with UC studied by Lindberg and colleagues[40] noted the prevalence of PSC in IBD to be 9.8%, and the mean time of onset from UC to PSC was about 12 years. Similarly, in centers where screening tests were performed more frequently, higher rates of PSC were found.[41] These studies suggest that the overall prevalence of PSC-IBD may actually be higher than what has typically been reported.

The intestinal inflammation of PSC-IBD may be different than the inflammation of non–PSC-IBD. When compared with non–PSC-UC, patients with PSC-UC are more likely to have pancolitis.[42] Similarly, those with PSC and Crohn disease tend to have Crohn colitis and those with PSC-UC had lower rates of IBD-related hospital admission and colectomies, suggesting a milder course of bowel disease. Studies suggest that the severity of disease in IBD does not predict the severity of disease in PSC, nor does treatment of IBD affect the overall course of PSC.[43]

Small-Duct Sclerosing Cholangitis

A diagnosis of small-duct SC is made in patients with typical symptoms of cholestasis, with biliary changes on liver histology consistent with SC, but without visible bile duct abnormalities on either endoscopic retrograde cholangiopancreatography (ERCP) or magnetic resonance cholangiopancreatography (MRCP).[44] The diagnosis of small-duct SC is more common in children (13%–36%) than adults (5%).[45,46] Small-duct SC seems to have better prognosis overall compared with classic or large-duct SC[47] and does not seem to lead to cholangiocarcinoma unless it converts to large-duct SC. A subset of patients with small-duct SC will require liver transplantation; however, there have been reports of post-transplant recurrence.

Diagnosis

In children, SC tends to have insidious onset, so early diagnosis can be difficult. Therefore, SC tends to be diagnosed only when obvious symptomatology or laboratory or imaging test abnormalities are present. The symptoms can include abdominal pain; decreased appetite and weight loss; growth delay; deficiencies in fat-soluble vitamins A, D, E, and K; fatigue; fever; jaundice; and pruritus.[35] Intractable pruritus is less common in children but remains an important indication for liver transplantation.[48]

On physical examination, hepatomegaly, splenomegaly, and/or jaundice may be present. Elevations of serum aminotransferases and γ-glutamyl transferase (GGT) can be seen and are typically significantly higher in children than in adults. Whereas ALP elevation is a useful marker in adults, GGT is more accurate in children because ALP can be affected by bone growth. In addition, GGT is already being used for prognostic purposes in other pediatric cholestatic diseases such as biliary atresia or parenteral nutrition–associated liver disease.

Imaging, such as MRCP or ERCP can show irregularity of the bile duct wall, multifocal dilatations, and intermittent strictures of the bile duct, showing a beaded appearance. MRCP is more commonly used in the pediatric population compared with ERCP owing to its lack of radiation, non-invasiveness, and its accuracy rate of 85%, making it a good screening test. Due to its invasive nature, ERCP has a higher risk of adverse events such as pancreatitis; yet, it has a definitive role in the management of SC. First, it may be needed for diagnosis if MRCP is non-diagnostic. Second, it can be therapeutic via dilation of dominant strictures within the bile ducts. Third, it is used to screen for cholangiocarcinoma because the risk for developing it is 9% at 10 years and 19% at 20 years after diagnosis.[49]

Liver biopsy can characteristically show periductal onion skin fibrosis (**Fig. 2**) but this finding is neither pathognomonic nor universally present (only seen in up to 40% of cases).[50] However, liver biopsy is warranted in the diagnosis of AIH–autoimmune overlap with SC and small-duct SC and thus may be more useful in children than in adults.[51] In the diagnosis of SC, it is important to think about secondary causes of SC. These may include but are not limited to choledocholithiasis, infectious causes (ascending cholangitis, sepsis), immunodeficiency, neoplasm, congenital causes (Caroli disease), or biliary injury.[52]

Management

The treatment of PSC is mostly supportive because there is no known medication that can stop the progression of this disease. Medications that have been used for the treatment of PSC-IBD include UDCA and vancomycin. UDCA is a hydrophilic bile acid that is already being used for many cholestatic liver diseases in children. It can protect liver cells from damage by inhibiting intestinal absorption of hepatotoxic bile acids, as well as by stimulating bile flow and secretion of bile acids, thus limiting cellular injury. UDCA may also have anti-inflammatory or immunomodulatory effects. UDCA has been shown to improve liver chemistries and cholestasis.[53] Unfortunately, there is no evidence that UDCA can improve liver outcomes in children or adults. Furthermore, high dosages of UDCA (30 mg/kg/d) have been shown to be associated with a 2-fold risk of death or transplant.[54] Based on these data, high dosages of UDCA should be avoided in children but smaller dosages could have some use (up to 20 mg/kg/d in divided doses). Discontinuation of UDCA could lead to deterioration in liver biochemistries.[55]

Vancomycin is a bactericidal antibiotic that mainly alters gram-positive bacteria by binding to precursor units of the cell wall. It is poorly absorbed in the gut, so its main area of effect is within the intestinal lumen. Data for vancomycin usage are conflicting and more studies need to be done. Davies and colleagues[56] reported a series of 14 subjects in whom use of vancomycin (50 mg/kg/d, treatment durations were variable) led to normalization of liver transaminases, GGT, and erythrocyte sedimentation rate in noncirrhotic children. Those with cirrhosis showed improvement of the same laboratory values but without complete normalization. It is important to recognize that 13 of the 14 subjects did have signs of colitis. Adult data are less promising. When weighing the use of vancomycin, it is important to consider long-term consequences of contributing to vancomycin-resistant enterococci, which could lead to rapid development of secondary SC.[57]

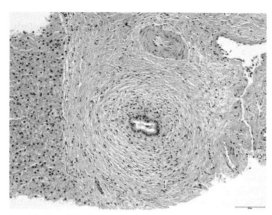

Fig. 2. Portal fibrosis with periductal concentric fibrosis and mild edema, also called "onion-skinning", is present in this liver needle core biopsy. These findings are consistent with primary sclerosing cholangitis (original magnification× 100). (*Courtesy of* Philip J. Katzman, MD, University of Rochester Medical Center, Rochester, NY)

ERCP can help to dilate dominant strictures. Balloon dilatation of dominant strictures could potentially slow down the development of end-stage liver disease and improve pre-transplant survival. Liver transplantation remains the definitive action for progressive SC and should be highly considered in patients with decompensated cirrhosis, hilar cholangiocarcinoma, intractable pruritus, or chronic cholangitis. Approximately 2% of all pediatric liver transplants are secondary to SC. However, SC can recur in about 20% of cases.[58] Survival of patients with liver transplantation are similar to survival rates of other organ transplants. There are differences in various medical societies regarding the screening of cholangiocarcinoma in patients with SC. Carbohydrate antigen 19-9 is the primary screening marker for cholangiocarcinoma, and carcinoembryonic antigen may also be abnormally elevated in 30% of patients with cholangiocarcinoma. However, although these tests may have high specificity, they have low sensitivity.[59]

Natural History and Outcomes

Descriptions of the natural history of pediatric SC are limited due to its relative rarity and a general lack of long-term follow-up studies. This led to the formation of a pediatric PSC consortium, which was a multicenter and international collaborative effort, enrolling 781 children as of 2017.[36] Data from the consortium showed that 38% of patients developed portal hypertension and 25% developed biliary complications after 10 years. Once these complications developed, the median survival rate with the native liver were 2.8 years and 3.5 years, respectively. In children, 1% developed cholangiocarcinoma. Event-free survival was 70% at 5 years and 53% at 10 years. The study also showed that high bilirubin, GGT, and high aspartate aminotransferase-to-platelet ratio typically led to worse outcomes. As in previous studies, subjects with PSC-IBD and small-duct SC had more favorable prognosis. In this study, long-term outcomes were not affected by age, gender, or AIH.

Pediatric Autoimmune Sclerosing Cholangitis or Overlap Syndrome

In hepatology, the term overlap syndrome is a clinical descriptor of various forms of autoimmune hepatobiliary diseases involving AIH, primary biliary cholangitis and PSC.[60] In pediatrics, the term ASC or overlap syndrome is being used to characterize patients with concomitant histologic and biochemical features of AIH, as well as those with SC.[1,61] In comparison with adults, ASC is described more commonly in children, perhaps due to the lack of burn-out of autoimmune-mediated inflammation in children. In ASC, patients tend to have improvement in serum transaminases with immunosuppressive medications.[46,61]

Male and female patients are equally affected by ASC, unlike AIH in which there is a female predilection. Association with IBD is more frequent with ASC than with AIH. In 2001, the King's group published a study in which cholangiographic studies were performed at diagnosis in children and adolescents with AIH, and ASC was noted to be as prevalent as AIH.[61] Due to the high prevalence of ASC in the pediatric population, patients who are diagnosed with SC may benefit from being screened for AIH. In ASC, perinuclear antineutrophil cytoplasmic antibody (p-ANCA), ANA, and SMA are frequently positive and serum IgG is elevated.[1,62] If laboratory testing is positive, obtaining a liver biopsy to assess for features of AIH, such as interface hepatitis, can be helpful.[51] Similarly, children diagnosed with AIH should be screened for SC with imaging such as MRCP or ERCP, particularly when the serum GGT is elevated, which may allow earlier diagnosis of autoimmune SC.

The current scoring systems are not useful in distinguishing between AIH and ASC. A new scoring system has recently been proposed in the European Society of Pediatric Gastroenterology, Hepatology and Nutrition (ESPGHAN) guidelines but requires validation.[1] In ASC, the immunosuppression therapy is similar to that used to treat AIH (see previous discussion). UDCA at a dosage of 10 mg/kg/d twice daily is added. It is not clear whether the biliary changes are reversible with this combination therapy. What is clear is that more multicenter studies are needed to better understand and manage ASC.

IgG subclasses should also be evaluated in patients with SC.[51] IgG4 is the least frequent IgG subclass, accounting for approximately 3% to 6% of total IgG in control subjects. Elevations of IgG4 may be found in a variety of conditions, notably autoimmune pancreatitis and IgG4-associated cholangitis (IAC).[63] Although it is important to rule out these entities as part of the workup for SC, up to 9% of SC patients have elevations of IgG4 but do not meet criteria for IAC. These patients seem to have a more aggressive phenotype and a shorter time to transplantation.[64]

SUMMARY

With the control of viral hepatitis, particularly hepatitis C, autoimmune liver disease is becoming an area of increased interest by both clinicians and researchers. It is important to have a high index of suspicion and screen appropriately for AIH because the spectrum of presentation is wide, from completely asymptomatic to acute liver failure. Ruling out other causes of liver disease and the presence of interface hepatitis on liver biopsy are key to making a diagnosis of AIH. Scoring systems are available for complicated cases or when diagnosis is in doubt. Management is with immunosuppression.

SC is rare in children. It has high morbidity and is progressive without a medical cure, leaving liver transplantation as the ultimate treatment despite potential recurrence of the disease posttransplantation. The diagnosis is made with imaging, laboratory tests, and sometimes liver biopsy, and by ruling out secondary causes. In children, compared with adults, there is a higher incidence of ASC and small-duct SC; hence liver biopsy may be of higher importance in children. There is a lower incidence of cholangiocarcinoma in pediatrics. The natural history of SC shows better prognosis in the IBD-PSC and small-duct subtypes. UDCA may improve liver biochemistries but does not seem to improve outcomes. Use of vancomycin lacks definitive data but, anecdotally, may be beneficial. There is overlap of AIH with SC, known as ASC or overlap syndrome, seen more commonly in children than adults.

REFERENCES

1. Mieli-Vergani G, Vergani D, Baumann U, et al. Diagnosis and management of pediatric autoimmune liver disease: ESPGHAN hepatology committee position statement. J Pediatr Gastroenterol Nutr 2018;66(2):345–60.
2. Kerkar N, Mack CL, Autoimmune Hepatitis. In: Suchy FJ, Sokol RJ, Balistreri WF, editors. Liver disease in children. 4th edition. Cambridge (UK): Cambridge University Press. p. 311–21.
3. de Boer YS, Kosinski AS, Urban TJ, et al. Features of autoimmune hepatitis in patients with drug-induced liver injury. Clin Gastroenterol Hepatol 2017;15(1):103–12.e2.
4. Mieli-Vergani G, Vergani D. Autoimmune hepatitis. Nat Rev Gastroenterol Hepatol 2011;8(6):320–9.
5. Kerkar N, Choudhuri K, Ma Y, et al. Cytochrome P4502D6(193-212): a new immunodominant epitope and target of virus/self cross-reactivity in liver kidney microsomal autoantibody type 1-positive liver disease. J Immunol 2003;170(3):1481–9.
6. Bogdanos DP, Choudhuri K, Vergani D. Molecular mimicry and autoimmune liver disease: virtuous intentions, malign consequences. Liver 2001;21(4):225–32.
7. Longhi MS, Ma Y, Mitry RR, et al. Effect of CD4+ CD25+ regulatory T-cells on CD8 T-cell function in patients with autoimmune hepatitis. J Autoimmun 2005;25(1):63–71.
8. Longhi MS, Ma Y, Mieli-Vergani G, et al. Aetiopathogenesis of autoimmune hepatitis. J Autoimmun 2010;34(1):7–14.
9. Waldenstrom J. Liver, blood proteins and nutritive protein. Dtsch Z Verdau Stoffwechselkr 1953;9:113–9.
10. Johnson PJ, McFarlane IG. Meeting report: international autoimmune hepatitis group. Hepatology 1993;18(4):998–1005.
11. Alvarez F, Berg PA, Bianchi FB, et al. International autoimmune hepatitis group report: review of criteria for diagnosis of autoimmune hepatitis. J Hepatol 1999;31(5):929–38.
12. Hennes EM, Zeniya M, Czaja AJ, et al. Simplified criteria for the diagnosis of autoimmune hepatitis. Hepatology 2008;48(1):169–76.
13. Rumbo C, Emerick KM, Emre S, et al. Azathioprine metabolite measurements in the treatment of autoimmune hepatitis in pediatric patients: a preliminary report. J Pediatr Gastroenterol Nutr 2002;35(3):391–8.
14. Dunkin D, Kerkar N, Arnon R, et al. Allopurinol salvage therapy in pediatric overlap autoimmune hepatitis-primary sclerosing cholangitis with 6-MMP toxicity. J Pediatr Gastroenterol Nutr 2010;51(4):524–6.
15. Manns MP, Czaja AJ, Gorham JD, et al. Diagnosis and management of autoimmune hepatitis. Hepatology 2010;51(6):2193–213.
16. Aw MM, Dhawan A, Samyn M, et al. Mycophenolate mofetil as rescue treatment for autoimmune liver disease in children: a 5-year follow-up. J Hepatol 2009;51(1):156–60.
17. Manns MP, Woynarowski M, Kreisel W, et al. Budesonide induces remission more effectively than prednisone in a controlled trial of patients with autoimmune hepatitis. Gastroenterology 2010;139(4):1198–206.
18. Lohse AW, Gil H. Reactivation of autoimmune hepatitis during budesonide monotherapy, and response to standard treatment. J Hepatol 2011;54(4):837–9.
19. Van Thiel DH, Wright H, Carroll P, et al. Tacrolimus: a potential new treatment for autoimmune chronic active hepatitis: results of an open-label preliminary trial. Am J Gastroenterol 1995;90(5):771–6.

20. Weiler-Normann C, Schramm C, Quaas A, et al. Infliximab as a rescue treatment in difficult-to-treat autoimmune hepatitis. J Hepatol 2013;58(3):529–34.
21. Nedelkopoulou N, Vadamalayan B, Vergani D, et al. Anti-TNFalpha treatment in children and adolescents with combined inflammatory bowel disease and autoimmune liver disease. J Pediatr Gastroenterol Nutr 2018;66(1):100–5.
22. Ricciuto A, Kamath BM, Walters TD, et al. New onset autoimmune hepatitis during anti-tumor necrosis factor-alpha treatment in children. J Pediatr 2017. https://doi.org/10.1016/j.jpeds.2017.10.071.
23. Torisu Y, Nakano M, Takano K, et al. Clinical usefulness of ursodeoxycholic acid for Japanese patients with autoimmune hepatitis. World J Hepatol 2017;9(1):57–63.
24. Di Giorgio A, Sonzogni A, Picciche A, et al. Successful management of acute liver failure in Italian children: a 16-year experience at a referral centre for paediatric liver transplantation. Dig Liver Dis 2017;49(10):1139–45.
25. Ramachandran J, Sajith KG, Pal S, et al. Clinicopathological profile and management of severe autoimmune hepatitis. Trop Gastroenterol 2014;35(1):25–31.
26. Molmenti EP, Netto GJ, Murray NG, et al. Incidence and recurrence of autoimmune/alloimmune hepatitis in liver transplant recipients. Liver Transpl 2002;8(6):519–26.
27. Duclos-Vallee JC, Sebagh M, Rifai K, et al. A 10 year follow up study of patients transplanted for autoimmune hepatitis: histological recurrence precedes clinical and biochemical recurrence. Gut 2003;52(6):893–7.
28. Kerkar N, Hadzic N, Davies ET, et al. De-novo autoimmune hepatitis after liver transplantation. Lancet 1998;351(9100):409–13.
29. Kerkar N, Yanni G. 'De novo' and 'recurrent' autoimmune hepatitis after liver transplantation: a comprehensive review. J Autoimmun 2016;66:17–24.
30. Radhakrishnan KR, Alkhouri N, Worley S, et al. Autoimmune hepatitis in children–impact of cirrhosis at presentation on natural history and long-term outcome. Dig Liver Dis 2010;42(10):724–8.
31. Mieli-Vergani G, Vergani D. Unique features of primary sclerosing cholangitis in children. Curr Opin Gastroenterol 2010;26(3):265–8.
32. Deneau M, Jensen MK, Holmen J, et al. Primary sclerosing cholangitis, autoimmune hepatitis, and overlap in Utah children: epidemiology and natural history. Hepatology 2013;58(4):1392–400.
33. Fagundes EDT, Ferreira AR, Hosken CC, et al. Primary sclerosing cholangitis in children and adolescents. Arq Gastroenterol 2017;54(4):286–91.
34. Bergquist A, Lindberg G, Saarinen S, et al. Increased prevalence of primary sclerosing cholangitis among first-degree relatives. J Hepatol 2005;42(2):252–6.
35. Miloh T, Arnon R, Shneider B, et al. A retrospective single-center review of primary sclerosing cholangitis in children. Clin Gastroenterol Hepatol 2009;7(2):239–45.
36. Deneau MR, El-Matary W, Valentino PL, et al. The natural history of primary sclerosing cholangitis in 781 children: a multicenter, international collaboration. Hepatology 2017;66(2):518–27.
37. Smolka V, Karaskova E, Tkachyk O, et al. Long-term follow-up of children and adolescents with primary sclerosing cholangitis and autoimmune sclerosing cholangitis. Hepatobiliary Pancreat Dis Int 2016;15(4):412–8.
38. Tenca A, Farkkila M, Arola J, et al. Clinical course and prognosis of pediatric-onset primary sclerosing cholangitis. United European Gastroenterol J 2016;4(4):562–9.

39. Saubermann LJ, Deneau M, Falcone RA, et al. Hepatic issues and complications associated with inflammatory bowel disease: a clinical report from the NASP-GHAN inflammatory bowel disease and hepatology committees. J Pediatr Gastroenterol Nutr 2017;64(4):639–52.

40. Lindberg J, Stenling R, Palmqvist R, et al. Early onset of ulcerative colitis: long-term follow-up with special reference to colorectal cancer and primary sclerosing cholangitis. J Pediatr Gastroenterol Nutr 2008;46(5):534–8.

41. Alexopoulou E, Xenophontos PE, Economopoulos N, et al. Investigative MRI cholangiopancreatography for primary sclerosing cholangitis-type lesions in children with IBD. J Pediatr Gastroenterol Nutr 2012;55(3):308–13.

42. Shiau H, Ihekweazu FD, Amin M, et al. Unique inflammatory bowel disease phenotype of pediatric primary sclerosing cholangitis: a single-center study. J Pediatr Gastroenterol Nutr 2017;65(4):404–9.

43. LaRusso NF, Shneider BL, Black D, et al. Primary sclerosing cholangitis: summary of a workshop. Hepatology 2006;44(3):746–64.

44. Hirschfield GM, Karlsen TH, Lindor KD, et al. Primary sclerosing cholangitis. Lancet 2013;382(9904):1587–99.

45. Valentino PL, Wiggins S, Harney S, et al. The natural history of primary sclerosing cholangitis in children: a large single-center longitudinal cohort study. J Pediatr Gastroenterol Nutr 2016;63(6):603–9.

46. Kerkar N, Miloh T. Sclerosing cholangitis: pediatric perspective. Curr Gastroenterol Rep 2010;12(3):195–202.

47. Bjornsson E, Boberg KM, Cullen S, et al. Patients with small duct primary sclerosing cholangitis have a favourable long term prognosis. Gut 2002;51(5):731–5.

48. Jossen J, Annunziato R, Kim HS, et al. Liver transplantation for children with primary sclerosing cholangitis and autoimmune hepatitis: unos database analysis. J Pediatr Gastroenterol Nutr 2017;64(4):e83–7.

49. Modha K, Navaneethan U. Diagnosis and management of primary sclerosing cholangitis-perspectives from a therapeutic endoscopist. World J Hepatol 2015;7(5):799–805.

50. Portmann B, Zen Y. Inflammatory disease of the bile ducts-cholangiopathies: liver biopsy challenge and clinicopathological correlation. Histopathology 2012;60(2):236–48.

51. Chapman R, Fevery J, Kalloo A, et al. Diagnosis and management of primary sclerosing cholangitis. Hepatology 2010;51(2):660–78.

52. Abdalian R, Heathcote EJ. Sclerosing cholangitis: a focus on secondary causes. Hepatology 2006;44(5):1063–74.

53. Shi J, Li Z, Zeng X, et al. Ursodeoxycholic acid in primary sclerosing cholangitis: meta-analysis of randomized controlled trials. Hepatol Res 2009;39(9):865–73.

54. Lindor KD, Kowdley KV, Luketic VA, et al. High-dose ursodeoxycholic acid for the treatment of primary sclerosing cholangitis. Hepatology 2009;50(3):808–14.

55. Wunsch E, Trottier J, Milkiewicz M, et al. Prospective evaluation of ursodeoxycholic acid withdrawal in patients with primary sclerosing cholangitis. Hepatology 2014;60(3):931–40.

56. Davies YK, Cox KM, Abdullah BA, et al. Long-term treatment of primary sclerosing cholangitis in children with oral vancomycin: an immunomodulating antibiotic. J Pediatr Gastroenterol Nutr 2008;47(1):61–7.

57. Hoffmeister B, Ockenga J, Schachschal G, et al. Rapid development of secondary sclerosing cholangitis due to vancomycin-resistant enterococci. J Infect 2007;54(2):e65–8.

58. Miloh T, Anand R, Yin W, et al. Pediatric liver transplantation for primary sclerosing cholangitis. Liver Transpl 2011;17(8):925–33.
59. Bjornsson E, Kilander A, Olsson RCA. 19-9 and CEA are unreliable markers for cholangiocarcinoma in patients with primary sclerosing cholangitis. Liver 1999; 19(6):501–8.
60. Chazouilleres O, Poupon R, Capron JP, et al. Ursodeoxycholic acid for primary sclerosing cholangitis. J Hepatol 1990;11(1):120–3.
61. Gregorio GV, Portmann B, Karani J, et al. Autoimmune hepatitis/sclerosing cholangitis overlap syndrome in childhood: a 16-year prospective study. Hepatology 2001;33(3):544–53.
62. Ferri PM, Simoes ESAC, Torres KCL, et al. Autoimmune hepatitis and autoimmune hepatitis overlap with sclerosing cholangitis: immunophenotype markers in children and adolescents. J Pediatr Gastroenterol Nutr 2018;66(2):204–11.
63. Beuers U, Hubers LM, Doorenspleet M, et al. IgG4-associated cholangitis–a mimic of PSC. Dig Dis 2015;33(Suppl 2):176–80.
64. Mendes F, Couto CA, Levy C. Recurrent and de novo autoimmune liver diseases. Clin Liver Dis 2011;15(4):859–78.

Hepatitis B and C

Krupa R. Mysore, MD, MS, Daniel H. Leung, MD*

KEYWORDS

- Viral • Hepatitis • Children • Monitoring • Treatment

KEY POINTS

- The epidemiology, natural history, and risk of chronic infection with hepatitis B virus (HBV) and hepatitis C virus (HCV) are different in children.
- Children are rarely very symptomatic, hence a detailed family history and risk assessment is essential.
- Current and future therapies for HBV and HCV have rapidly evolved and will reduce social stigma, mortality/morbidity, and future health care costs.

INTRODUCTION

Hepatitis B virus (HBV) and hepatitis C virus (HCV) infections represent a major global public health and economic burden, with an estimated 257 million and 71 million people, respectively, having chronic infection worldwide.[1,2] The natural history of HBV and HCV in children depends on age at time of infection, mode of acquisition, ethnicity, and genotype. Most children infected perinatally or vertically remain asymptomatic but are at uniquely higher risk of developing chronic viral hepatitis, progressing to liver cirrhosis and hepatocellular carcinoma (HCC), hence classifying HBV and HCV as oncoviruses.[3] This article discusses the epidemiology, virology, immunobiology, prevention, clinical manifestations, evaluation, and the advances in treatment of hepatitis B and C in children.

HEPATITIS B
Epidemiology

In the United States, approximately 2 million people are chronically infected with HBV with a higher prevalence of chronic hepatitis B among immigrants from highly endemic areas such as Asia, Africa, and western Pacific regions.[2,4] Most individuals with chronic HBV infection acquired the virus through vertical transmission, highlighting the importance of active and passive immunization for HBV. Since implementation of universal infant vaccination for hepatitis B in 1991, there has been a drastic

Disclosure: The authors have no conflicts of interest to disclose as described by the *Clinics in Liver Disease*.

Division of Gastroenterology, Hepatology and Nutrition, Texas Children's Hospital, Department of Pediatrics, Baylor College of Medicine, 6701 Fannin, Suite 1010, Houston, TX 77030, USA

* Corresponding author.

E-mail address: dhleung@texaschildrens.org

reduction in both acute and chronic HBV rates among children in the United States, which is offset by immigration of patients with chronic HBV from other countries.[5] The incidence of acute hepatitis B in US children (<19 years of age) has decreased from approximately 13.8 cases per 100,000 population (10–19 years of age) in the 1980s to 0.34 cases per 100,000 population in 2002.[6] Even though the prevalence has significantly reduced, children with chronic HBV remain at risk for HCC, with a 100-fold greater incidence compared with the HBV-negative population.[7] Although there is racial disparity in prevalence of HBV in adults in the United States, rates among US-born children showed no racial differences.[8]

Virology and Genotyping: Impact on Prognosis and Treatment

HBV is a DNA virus in the family Hepadnaviridae. It is primarily a hepatotropic, enveloped, coated, double-stranded DNA virus that causes both acute and chronic hepatitis. Important components of the viral particle include hepatitis B surface antigen (HBsAg), hepatitis B core antigen (HBcAg), and hepatitis B e antigen (HBeAg). The virion is 42 nm in diameter and contains the nucleocapsid that encloses the viral DNA. The outer shell is a lipoprotein envelope derived from host cells and contain hepatitis B surface proteins. The nucleocapsid is an icosahedral structure consisting of 240 core protein subunits and is detected as HBcAg. Within the nucleocapsid is both the viral genome and polymerase. HBeAg is a soluble antigen produced from the same open reading frame as HBcAg and is a marker of active viral replication. HBV replicates via DNA polymerase through reverse transcription of an RNA intermediate; the lack of proofreading in this process leads to a high frequency of mutations, which is a barrier to successful treatment of HBV.[9]

Ten HBV genotypes, A through J, have been characterized and multiple subgenotypes have been identified using molecular techniques. Some genotypes have discrete HBV geographic distributions, but identifying HBV genotype is important because it has implications on mutation patterns and, importantly, on clinical outcomes, such as likelihood of seroconversion or viral suppression.[10–13] Mixed genotype infections and intergenotypic recombination create challenges for effective treatment in HBV. For example, genotypes A (western hemisphere) and C (Asian-Pacific) have a high tendency toward recombination of viral strains, as does genotype B in certain areas of southeast Asia.[10,14,15] Further, mutations of the S gene (the gene that codes for HBsAg) in genotype B/C regions have led to breakthrough HBV infection in previously vaccinated children, highlighting the importance of genotyping and evolution of the virus through mutations.[16] About 77% of US-born patients with HBV are infected with genotype A, but other genotype infections are frequently seen in immigrants from different countries.[17] Overall, genotypes C, D, and F are higher risk for disease progression and HCC; patients with genotypes C and D have delayed seroconversion of HBeAg, higher histologic activity, and poor response to interferon (IFN) and nucleoside therapy (**Table 1**).[10,18–20]

Immune Mechanisms in Hepatitis B Virus

The host immune system plays a key role in viral clearance and hepatocellular damage in chronic HBV because the virus is not directly cytopathic. Children have differences in immune tolerance and rate of progression of liver disease compared with adults. Ninety percent of infants infected with HBV develop chronic infection, whereas only 5% of infected adults develop chronic HBV. Even among children, groups less than 5 years of age have vastly different seroconversion rates, rates of chronicity, and response to treatment compared with their adolescent counterparts. Several mechanisms have been proposed that lead to the persistence of HBV with progression to HCC.

Table 1
Genotype distribution and clinical implications

Genotype	Endemic Areas	Clinical Impact
A[117]	Sub-Saharan Africa, India, Northern Europe, United States	Increased risk of chronic infection following acute phase, good response to IFN
B[118]	Asia	Subtype B2 associated with HCC in adolescents and young adults, high rates of perinatal transmission
C[10,19]	Asia, Australia	High rates of perinatal transmission, increased risk of disease progression, high viral loads, increased HCC risk
D[119]	Europe, India, Australia	Increased risk of disease progression and HCC, causes HBeAg-negative chronic infection, high mutation frequency
E	Africa, Saudi Arabia	No data available
F[120]	Central and South America	Intense histologic inflammation with higher HCC incidence than genotypes A and D
G[121]	France, Germany	Detected in coinfection with other genotypes, such as A2
H[122]	Central America	Asymptomatic infection
I[123]	Vietnam and Laos	Rare in children <9 y old, low prevalence
J	Japan	No data available

Virus-specific $CD8^+$ T cells with the help of $CD4^+$ T cells play a vital role in clearing HBV by both cytolysis and noncytolytic effector functions, but these are often evaded in chronic HBV, leading to persistence of viruses.[21] HBV suppresses innate immune cells such as natural killer (NK) cells and type 1 IFN responses, leading to HBV replication.[22] Expression of immunosuppressive mediators and coinhibitors on immune cells of both the innate and adaptive immune system, such as increased regulatory T cells (Tregs), upregulated inhibitory pathways of programmed death-1 and its ligand (PD-1/PD-L1) and cytotoxic T lymphocyte–associated protein 4 (CTLA4), dysfunctional dendritic cells (DCs), and low levels of Toll-Like receptor expression (TLR), lead to defects in mounting an effective immune response against HBV, thereby causing the virus to persist in the host.[23–26] Further, on delivery to the nucleus, the HBV genome forms covalently closed circular DNA (cccDNA), which serves as a hidden harbor and template for viral RNA transcription. This cccDNA is very stable, making it challenging to eradicate the virus either by the host immune system or medications.[21,27]

The inhibitory pathways of T cells and DCs have recently garnered attention as potential targets and have led to the development of cancer immunotherapies that block PD-1 and CTLA4 pathways. Increased expression of these T-cell inhibitors leads to T-cell dysfunction and apoptosis.[26] Checkpoint blockade in mouse models of HBV has shown restoration of T-cell function, and human clinical trials using these strategies in patients are underway.[28–30]

Transmission and Natural History

Perinatal, blood, and sexual transmission are the most important routes of HBV transmission.[31] Without immunoprophylaxis with hepatitis B immunoglobulin (HBIG) and administration of the first HBV vaccine series before newborn discharge, perinatal

HBV infection leads to chronic hepatitis in more than 90% of infected children, increasing mortality risk caused by cirrhosis and HCC later in adulthood.[32] The risk of transmission is highest in infants born to untreated mothers infected with HBV who are both HBsAg and HBeAg positive, with rates ranging from 70% to 100% in Asia and 40% in Africa, likely because of variation in genotypes.[2,33–35] In contrast, transmission rates decrease to 5% to 30% in Asia and 5% in Africa among infants born to mothers who are HBeAg negative.[34] This perinatal infection rate can be further reduced to nearly 0% among infants born to HBeAg-negative mothers by ensuring the initial dose of hepatitis B vaccine is given at birth, although the efficacy of the vaccine is inversely proportional to the viral load ($\geq 10^6$ copies/mL) in the mother.[36,37] For example, immunoprophylaxis failure was 0% for maternal HBV DNA level of less than 10^6 copies/mL but increased to 3.2%, 6.7%, and 7.6% in DNA levels of $10^{6-6.99}$ copies/mL, $10^{7-7.99}$ copies/mL, and greater than 10^8 copies/mL, respectively.[38] Importantly, breastfeeding in infants who received proper immunoprophylaxis at birth does not pose additional risk of transmission compared with bottle-fed infants.[39]

Outside the endemic areas, transmission of HBV still remains high with percutaneous and mucosal exposures to infected blood and body fluids. High-risk groups include intravenous drug users, incarcerated individuals, those with multiple unprotected sexual encounters, and those with risk of occupational exposure (eg, needle stick injury in health care workers).[40,41] HBV is 100-fold more virulent than human immunodeficiency virus (HIV) and can survive outside the body for up to 7 days, during which it can enter a high-risk host and replicate.[42]

Acute infection can present with the classic symptoms of fever, jaundice, abdominal pain, nausea, and vomiting lasting 2 to 3 months. These symptoms are present in about 50% of older children and adolescents but rare to absent in infants.[43] The natural history of chronic HBV in children, defined as persistence of HBsAg for greater than 6 months, depends on age at time of infection, mode of acquisition, ethnicity, and genotype. Most children infected perinatally or vertically develop chronic HBV, although fulminant hepatic failure has been rarely reported.[44] Young adults may present with acute hepatitis but chronicity is rare in this population. Other patient populations, such as those on hemodialysis and coinfected with HIV, also have an increased risk of chronic infection. Chronic HBV progresses in a nonlinear fashion through 4 phases with clinically differentiating hallmarks but with occasional overlap (**Table 2**).[45–47] In most children, liver inflammation is minimal despite high rates of HBV replication; this is known as the immune-tolerant phase, which can last for decades, although many patients transition out of this phase in adolescence. This phase is followed by the immune clearance phase, which is characterized by liver inflammation accompanied by periods of both low and high HBV replication as the immune system tries to clear HBV. Should a child seroconvert (HBeAg negative to HBeAb positive) and clear the virus, the child will enter the inactive chronic carrier state. Although this status is usually considered benign, 20% to 30% of patients may undergo reactivation of HBV in the setting of immunosuppression or HBV mutant.[45,46] In an Italian study of 89 children followed for a mean of 14.5 ± 6.1 years, only 4 (4.5%) reactivated either related to puberty, pregnancy, or drug abuse.[48]

Serial monitoring of HBV DNA levels and alanine transaminase (ALT) is necessary to identify the phase of infection and to characterize the host immune response. In children who transition to the immune clearance phase with (anti–hepatitis B e positive) or without seroconversion, a hepatic flare is expected and liver transaminase levels may increase by 10-fold for as long as 12 months. As long as the child is clinically well without cholestasis or signs of decompensation, a 1-year monitoring period

Table 2
Phases of chronic hepatitis B virus infection: biochemical and histologic characteristics

	Immune Tolerant	Immune Clearance	Inactive Chronic Carrier	Reactivation
HBV DNA Level	Increased, typically >10^8 IU/mL	Increased, >20×10^5 IU/mL	Low or undetectable, <2000 IU/mL	Increased, >2000 IU/mL
ALT	Normal[a]	Increased	Normal	Increased
HBeAg	Positive	Positive	Negative	Negative, but can be positive
Histology on Liver Biopsy	Minimal inflammation, minimal to absent fibrosis	Moderate to severe inflammation	Minimal inflammation but variable fibrosis	Moderate to severe inflammation and/or fibrosis
Duration	Prolonged (years) in perinatally acquired HBV	6–12 mo, less common in children, consider treatment	Variable	Variable duration

Abbreviation: ALT, alanine transaminase.
[a] ALT level less than 19 IU/mL for men, less than 30 IU/mL for women, and less than 30 IU/mL in children.
Modified from Terrault NA, Bzowej NH, Chang KM, et al. AASLD guidelines for treatment of chronic hepatitis B. Hepatology 2016;63(1):262; with permission.

(semiannual laboratory tests) during suspected immune clearance is acceptable because the child may eventually seroconvert and become an inactive chronic carrier. This situation is rare in infants and young children less than 3 years of age, occurring at about 2% per year compared with 8% to 12% in pubertal children and young adults.[46] Further, clearance of HBsAg and development of antibody to HBsAg is the hallmark of fully resolved HBV infection, although it is rare, and reduces future risk of decompensation.

Patients with cirrhosis caused by HBV infection are at high risk for HCC. A large Taiwanese study found that the incidence of HCC was associated with serum HBV DNA levels in a dose-response relationship from less than 300 copies/mL (undetectable) to greater than or equal to 1 million copies/mL.[49] In a Japanese series, 15 out of 548 children developed HCC at a median age of 15 years.[50] However, the 5-year survival rate in children with HCC, despite treatment, is low at 30% or less.[50,51] Global adoption of universal immunization practices has substantially reduced the incidence of HCC associated with HBV.[52,53] A Taiwan HCC registry study showed a significant difference in incidence of HCC of 0.23 and 0.92 per 100,000 people in vaccinated and unvaccinated cohorts, respectively, coinciding with a steady decrease in overall seroprevalence of HBsAg-positive patients.[54,55]

Diagnosis

The diagnosis of chronic HBV requires a thorough assessment of the child's risk factors and medical history because the clinical symptoms and signs can be absent or subtle. All household contacts should be immunized appropriately and screened for HBV. In rare cases, children with compromised liver synthetic function (ie, increased conjugated bilirubin level, prolonged International Normalized Ratio (INR), low albumin level) should be referred to a pediatric liver transplant center for evaluation.[56] The diagnostic algorithm (**Fig. 1**) highlights the importance of a thorough clinical examination including evaluation of other possible coinfections and treatment strategies based on HBV serologies.[46,57] Risk of HCC is generally low and evidence is not clear cut, but it is advisable to monitor alpha fetoprotein (AFP) and hepatic imaging every 6 to 12 months, and every 3 months in children with cirrhosis.[56] Liver biopsy is regarded as the best method to assess inflammation, degree of fibrosis, presence of other causes of liver diseases, and to monitor disease severity after treatment.[46] Inflammation on liver biopsy is minimal in the immune-tolerant phase, whereas the immune clearance phase is characterized by portal inflammation, interface hepatitis, and variable fibrosis.[58]

Noninvasive biomarkers to assess degree of liver fibrosis in HBV is under study, although none of them are routinely recommended mainstream tests at this point. Aspartate aminotransferase (AST)-platelet ratio index and fibrosis-4 index based on platelets, ALT, AST, and age are simple and noninvasive indices shown to be beneficial in children with chronic HBV.[59] Research on novel imaging techniques beyond gray scale ultrasonography, such as transient elastography (TE), shear wave elastography, and acoustic radiation force impulse imaging, which help in assessing liver stiffness and fibrosis, are underway in pediatric liver diseases.[60–62]

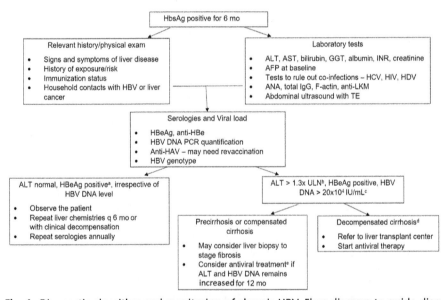

Fig. 1. Diagnostic algorithm and monitoring of chronic HBV. Flow diagram to guide diagnosis and monitoring of children with hepatitis B infection based on initial HBsAg screening. [a] There are no randomized clinical trials in children who are HBeAg negative. [b] HBV clinical trials have used ALT levels of 30 to 45 IU/L as upper limit of normal (ULN).[3] [c] Consider work-up for other causes of liver disease, including a liver biopsy in patients with persistently increased ALT level and less than 20×10^4 IU/mL. Consider treatment if cirrhotic and remainder of work-up is negative. [d] Pegylated IFN treatment is contraindicated in decompensated cirrhosis. [e] Treatment may be indefinite until seroconversion for precirrhosis but likely indefinite for cirrhosis regardless of seroconversion status. ANA, antinuclear antibodies; AST, aspartate aminotransferase; GGT, gamma-glutamyl transferase; HAV, hepatitis A virus; HDV, hepatitis D virus; IgG, immunoglobulin G; LKM, liver-kidney microsome; PCR, polymerase chain reaction; q, every; TE, transient elastography.

Management

Treatment of acute HBV is purely supportive. Most children with chronic HBV are in the immune-tolerant phase marked by high replication of virus with minimal inflammation and normal ALT levels. It is advisable to observe these patients with periodic monitoring without treatment.[20] As mentioned earlier, annual spontaneously clearance rates of HBV in children, although low, are respectable at 12% annually among adolescents, highlighting the importance of carefully selecting patients needing antiviral therapy without unnecessarily inducing resistance to these drugs. Antiviral therapy in children aged 2 years and older with chronic HBV is recommended in HBeAg-positive patients with persistently increased ALT levels for at least 6 months and increased HBV DNA level greater than 10^6 IU/mL (**Table 3**).[46] The goal of therapy and treatment end points in the immune clearance phase is seroconversion from HBeAg to anti–HBe, suppression of viral replication, and normalization of ALT level.[63] At present, entecavir and lamivudine, both oral nucleoside analogues, are approved for treatment of HBV in children older than 2 years, whereas injectable IFN-α-2b is approved for children older than 1 year of age. However, lamivudine given for more than 5 years has a 70% mutation rate, so is not a first-line treatment when entecavir is available. Recently, tenofovir, a nucleotide analogue, was approved for children more than 12 years of age, and newer formulations, such as tenofovir alafenamide, that have an improved safety profile are currently being studied in children. Adefovir is another nucleotide analogue approved for children more than 12 years of age but, because of its renal toxicities and high viral resistance (about 30%), it is not a first-line treatment. Importantly, adefovir conferred no significant benefits compared with placebo in children with HBV younger than 11 years of age.[64] Instead, adefovir is considered as an add-on therapy in adults with lamivudine or entecavir resistance.[65]

The duration of therapy with oral antivirals can be indefinite and may need additional consolidation therapy for 1 year following e antigen seroconversion before discontinuation. Because of its higher rate of seroconversion, particularly among HBV genotypes A and B, IFN remains a reasonable therapy, although its side effects may preclude interest by families. Entecavir and tenofovir are considered first-line therapies in children. They are certainly first-line therapies for patients with cirrhosis and lifelong antiviral treatment may be needed to reduce progression and risk of HCC.[65,66]

Children are monitored at a minimum of every 3 months while on therapy as well as during the first year off therapy with liver biochemistries, HBV serologies, and HBV DNA. If liver transaminase levels remain persistently increased, then a repeat liver biopsy may be considered to rule out other causes of liver disease. At present there are no recommendations for combining oral nucleos(t)ide analogues with IFN.

A recent meta-analysis published by Jonas and colleagues[20] examined 14 studies of antiviral treatment in children with chronic HBV and found that antiviral therapy for HBV yielded improved rates of ALT normalization, HBeAg seroconversion, HBV DNA suppression, and HBsAg loss compared with placebo (relative risk 2.2). The effect of antiviral therapy on HBeAg seroconversion is comparable, at about 26% for IFN, 23% for lamivudine, 26.2% for entecavir, and 21% for tenofovir. Long-term data on antiviral effects on cirrhosis and prevention of HCC in children with chronic HBV are lacking. Further, there are just as few data to inform decisions about treating HBV in children who are HBeAg negative.[67] New immune modulators, such as retinoic acid inducible gene I activators that interfere with viral transcription and packaging while also stimulating IFN production or JNJ-379, which binds to HBV core protein, producing nonfunctional viral particles, are being studied in adult clinical trials. Also in the pipeline are drugs such as REP 2139, a nucleic acid polymer, and ARB-1467, a synthetic small

Table 3
Current antiviral therapies and treatment strategies in children with hepatitis B virus

	Interferon[a]	Lamivudine	Entecavir	Tenofovir
Approved Age (y)	>1	>2	>2	>12
Mechanism of Action	Immunomodulatory, promotes hepatocyte lysis by CD8+ T cells and has mild antiviral effects	Drug is incorporated into viral DNA by HBV polymerase leading to DNA chain termination	Inhibits viral polymerase, blocks reverse transcriptase and viral synthesis	Nucleotide reverse transcriptase inhibitor, inhibits HBV DNA polymerase
Dosage	5–10 million IU/m² 3 times a week, subcutaneous	3 mg/kg daily with maximum of 100 mg[b]	Lower doses for treatment-naive patients[c]	300 mg daily
Duration of Therapy	24 wk	1 y after HBeAg conversion	1 y after HBeAg conversion	1 y after HBeAg conversion
Side Effects	Immune reconstitution, flulike symptoms, fatigue, depression, anorexia, weight loss, bone marrow suppression	Resistance up to 24% after 1 y and 70% at 5 y of treatment, lactic acidosis	Lactic acidosis	Fanconi syndrome, osteomalacia, lactic acidosis
Monitoring on Treatment[d]	CBC, TSH, neuropsychiatric assessment	Lactate	Lactate	Bone density, kidney function

Abbreviations: CBC, complete blood count; TSH, thyroid-stimulating hormone.
[a] Pegylated IFN is not approved for children for HBV, although it has been approved for HCV and is often used in pediatric HBV.
[b] For lamivudine resistance or treatment-experienced children, doses are: 0.30 mg (10–11 kg), 0.4 mg (>11–14 kg), 0.5 mg (>14–17 kg), 0.6 mg (>17–20 kg), 0.7 mg (>20–23 kg), 0.8 mg(>23–26 kg), 0.9 mg (>26–30 kg), and 1.0 mg (>30 kg) daily.
[c] Entecavir doses in treatment-naive children are: 0.15 mg (10–11 kg), 0.2 mg (>11–14 kg), 0.25 mg (>14–17 kg), 0.3 mg (>17–20 kg), 0.35 mg (>20–23 kg), 0.4 mg (>23–26 kg), 0.45 mg (>26–30 kg), and 0.5 mg (>30 kg) daily.
[d] In addition to the standard Chem 7, HBV DNA, liver panel, anti-HBe, and HBeAg, different therapies may warrant specific lab monitoring.
Data from Refs.[20,46,56,124]

RNA, which is being tested in combination with tenofovir and pegylated IFN to evaluate HBsAg clearance (also known as functional cure).

Although viral clearance has traditionally been a marker of successful HBV treatment, achieving complete functional cure (clearance of HBsAg and antibody to hepatitis B surface Ag seroconversion) remains a challenge and a dream for both hepatologists and their patients. Combining antivirals targeting distinct enzymes critical to the HBV viral life cycle with immune boosting regimens in a safe manner to eradicate HBV is the ideal for future research and therapeutics in this field.

Vaccine and Prevention of Hepatitis B Virus

The US Centers for Disease Control and Prevention and the World Health Organization recommend universal immunization of all infants with recombinant HBsAg vaccine within 24 hours of birth followed by 2 doses (at 1 month and 6 months) usually given as a combination with diphtheria, pertussis, and tetanus vaccines. This vaccination schedule provides immunity (anti-HBs >10 mIU/mL) in greater than 95% of children.

Infants born to previously untreated HBsAg-positive mothers can acquire infection and, if the mother is HBeAg positive, the risk of acquiring infection is greater than 70%. In these cases, HBIG is administered at a separate intramuscular site from the vaccine given at birth. Not surprisingly, treatment of HBeAg-positive pregnant mothers with nucleos(t)ide analogues to reduce HBV DNA levels to less than 2×10^5 IU/mL diminishes perinatal transmission even further (relative risk, 0.32 compared with untreated mothers).[2,46,68,69]

Immunogenicity to HBV vaccine in patients who already have cirrhosis varies from response rates of 38% after the first dose to 53% after 2 doses.[70] Monitoring of anti-HBs titers is recommended in patients undergoing hemodialysis, health care workers, patients with HIV infection, and liver transplant recipients. More than two-thirds of pediatric liver transplant recipients who had completed the vaccine series at the recommended intervals were nonimmune at 5.6 years after liver transplant in a large cross-sectional study.[71] The poor response to vaccination is attributed to lower immunogenicity in these patients but the exact immune mechanisms are currently unknown. Future studies on functional cellular and humoral immune responses that examine poor immunogenicity after vaccine will be important in helping clinicians understand some of these mechanisms.

Efforts to educate children, adolescents, and young adults on transmission of HBV through shared razors or needles and unsafe sex practices, along with universal precautions for health care workers and screening of all blood donors, can also reduce transmission of HBV.[72]

Despite advances in therapeutics and continued research for new antiviral and immunotherapies, prevention of perinatal and vertical transmission continues to be the central aspect of controlling chronic HBV. Access to universal immunization of infants, screening of all pregnant mothers, and appropriate treatment of pregnant women can eliminate new HBV infections across the globe.

HEPATITIS C
Epidemiology and Transmission

HCV is found worldwide, with sub-Saharan Africa, eastern Mediterranean, and western Pacific regions having the highest prevalence at 5.3%, 4.6%, and 3.9% respectively.[73] An estimated 5 million children have active infection worldwide.[74] In the United States, approximately 4 million people are chronically infected, with an estimated prevalence in children of 0.2% to 0.4% (6–11 years and 12–19 years old, respectively).[75]

Historically, HCV was acquired in children through transfusion of blood and blood-related products. Since 1992, blood transfusions in the United States have been screened for HCV (rate of transmission is now only 0.01%), making vertical transmission responsible for greater than 60% of pediatric HCV infection, and adding approximately 7200 new cases in the United States.[56,76,77] Mother-to-child transmission occurs in 2% to 7% of mothers infected with HCV, but rates are 2-fold increased with high HCV viral load (HCV RNA 10^6 copies/mL) and/or HIV coinfection.[78,79] Studies have found no differences in transmission of HCV via cesarean section or vaginal delivery, or through breast feeding.[80,81] However, internal fetal monitoring, prolonged rupture of membranes, and episiotomy should be avoided in managing labor in pregnant women with HCV.[82] Unlike HBV, there is no vaccine for HCV and effective strategies to prevent transmission from infected mother to infant are currently lacking.

In adolescents and older children, transmission of HCV can occur through intravenous and intranasal drug use and high-risk sexual behaviors.[83,84]

Virology and Immunology

HCV is an enveloped single-stranded, positive-sense RNA virus of family Flaviviridae with 6 well-known genotypes and multiple subtypes. The most common, genotype 1, is globally distributed and dominates in North America and Europe. Genotypes 2 and 3 are globally distributed as well, whereas genotypes 4, 5, and 6 are found in the Middle East, South Africa, and Asia respectively.[73,85]

There are 3 structural proteins (nucleocapsid forming protein core and envelope glycoproteins E1and E2) and 7 nonstructural proteins (viroporin p7, NS2, NS3, NS4A, NS4B, NS5A, and NS5B), which are the primary targets for drug and vaccine development. The virus is diverse because of the error-prone viral RNA-dependent RNA polymerase (NS5b), which replicates the viral genome. NS4A is a cofactor for NS3. NS4B creates changes in the cellular membrane that allow viral replication. NS5A is essential for regulation of viral replication.[86] In chronically infected patients, more than 10^{10} viral genomes are produced per day, resulting in diversity of the hypervariable region-1 of the virus, with a complex viral population and survival advantage for the virus.[87]

Responses to HCV depend on innate and adaptive immune responses of the host. NK and gamma/delta T cells may play a role at the level of the placenta to prevent transmission of HCV to the infant.[88] The gene IL28B codes for IFN lambda 3, which has potent antiviral activity.[89] Patients with polymorphisms in this gene are known to have differences in spontaneous resolution of acute HCV infection. For example, the single nucleotide polymorphism (SNP) on chromosome 19, rs12979860, is significantly associated with up to 2-fold increased spontaneous HCV clearance with C/C genotype compared with T/T genotype.[90–92] Similarly, SNPs on human leukocyte antigen class II DQB1*03:01 are associated with increased spontaneous clearance of HCV, highlighting the importance of host adaptive immune responses in combating this virus. Adaptive T-cell responses to HCV can be detected as early as 1 to 2 weeks, which often coincides with increased transaminase levels. Polyfunctional virus-specific memory CD4$^+$ and CD8$^+$ T-cell responses in both the liver microenvironment and peripheral blood correlate with protection and clearance of virus.[93,94] In contrast, downregulation of virus-specific CD8$^+$ T-cell responses caused by functional exhaustion and eventual apoptosis of virus-specific T cells leads to persistence of HCV.[25] Based on these factors, T-cell response and envelope glycoprotein–based therapies are now in phase II development.[95]

Natural History

Symptomatic acute HCV is rare in childhood but can present with lethargy, fever, and myalgia. Acute HCV should be monitored for 6 to 8 weeks for spontaneous resolution.[81] Antibodies to HCV appear 20 to 150 days after exposure. Similarly, HCV RNA (detected by nucleic acid amplification technology [NAT]) levels are maximal by 8 to 10 days and reach a plateau by 46 to 68 days after exposure.[96] High HCV RNA levels during the first month of infection predict spontaneous viral clearance. About 20% to 25% of acute HCV infections can be spontaneously cleared. In contrast with hepatitis B, by 3 years of age, infants who acquired HCV perinatally show 25% to 40% spontaneous resolution.[97]

In contrast, children who do not clear HCV spontaneously develop chronic HCV that progresses slowly with limited liver disease in the initial 10 to 15 years following infection.[98] Up to 10% to 20% of children infected with HCV may have persistent increase of aminotransferase levels and 1% may develop cirrhosis.[99] Patients with HIV/HCV co-infection, obesity, and a history of childhood cancer have lower rates of spontaneous clearance of HCV and are more commonly viremic and likely to develop progressive fibrosis and cirrhosis.[100,101] There are very few cases of HCC reported in children with HCV.[102] Thus, the duration of chronic HCV infection, presence of coinfection with HIV and HBV, and age of the patient are determinants of morbidity and mortality.[98,103]

Diagnosis and Monitoring

Screening of all high-risk individuals, including pregnant women, is currently recommended. Initial screening with anti-HCV is recommended and, if positive, confirmed by HCV RNA and genotyping. The American Academy of Pediatrics (AAP), Infectious Diseases Society of America (IDSA), and American Association for the Study of Liver Diseases (AASLD) recommend testing of all children born to pregnant mothers infected with HCV no earlier than 18 months of age because of persistence of maternal antibodies (immunoglobulin G) before that time. However, infants of high-risk families with HCV and unreliable follow-up may merit earlier testing. If indicated, testing platforms using NAT to detect HCV RNA in a quantitative manner should be used. If, at 18 months, HCV antibody is positive, then confirmatory HCV RNA testing is essential. Up to 50% of infected infants spontaneously resolve HCV infection by 3 years of age and hence no intervention is recommended for children less than 3 years of age.[81]

Similar to HBV, the diagnosis of chronic HCV requires a careful history and thorough assessment of high-risk features because the clinical symptoms and signs can be absent or subtle. In immunocompromised hosts, antibody conversion is unreliable and may not be detected. When HCV RNA is positive, accurate genotyping of chronic HCV is obtained using molecular sequencing data and is important in determining choice of antivirals and duration of therapy.[104–106] The diagnostic algorithm (**Fig. 2**) highlights initial evaluation in high-risk children and testing in maternal transmission of HCV. Liver biopsy is not routinely indicated for diagnosis but may be considered in patients with suspected overlapping causes advanced disease, before antiviral therapy. Histologic features are generally absent or mild but there are rare reports of cirrhosis in about 2% of young children and teenagers.[107] Risk of HCC is low and evidence is inconclusive, but it is advisable to monitor AFP levels and hepatic imaging every 6 to 12 months, especially in children with cirrhosis.[77,108] In untreated cirrhotic children, baseline endoscopy to detect varices is recommended, with follow-up screening every year.

Parents and children with HCV should be counseled regarding modes and risk of transmission of virus. Children should be allowed to freely participate in all childhood

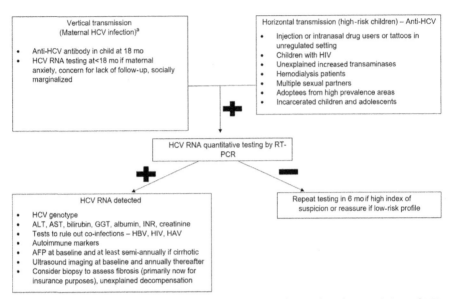

Fig. 2. Diagnostic algorithm for hepatitis C, highlighting the modes of transmission of HCV, risk factors, and diagnosis. [a] Circulating maternal antibodies may be present up to 18 months of age. RT-PCR, reverse transcriptase PCR.

activities while following universal precautions, such as avoiding sharing sharps, hepatotoxic medications, alcohol, and high-risk behaviors.[106] All children should be updated on vaccination and tested for hepatitis B and hepatitis A immune status.

Management

Rapid development of direct-acting antiviral (DAA) therapies for HCV infection has drastically changed both clinical outcome and patient tolerability because continual advances in therapy are approaching 100% cure in as short as 8 weeks in select populations. Use of DAAs is currently limited because of under diagnosis of HCV, the cost of treatment, and barriers posed by insurance companies.[109] Although DAAs are expensive (ranges from US$70,000–90,000), treatment on a large-scale basis could reduce HCV prevalence by 94% and liver-related mortality by 75% in areas such as Egypt with a high density of infection and hence overall is cost-effective for health care.[110,111] In a recent database analysis, rates of HCC and liver transplantation caused by HCV are decreasing because of effective screening and treatment options, whereas nonalcoholic steatohepatitis leading to cirrhosis and liver transplant are exponentially increasing.[112]

Treatment should be recommended in children greater than 12 years of age where DAAs are available commercially; currently the combination of sofosbuvir and ledipasvir has been approved by the US Food and Drug Administration (FDA) for children more than 12 years old. Other combination regimens are likely not far behind, and an indication for the younger cohort of children down to 3 years of age is expected. Importantly, treatment is not recommended for children less than 3 years of age because of high rates of spontaneous resolution. In children aged 3 to 11 years, treatment should be sought through open-label DAA clinical trials. Interferon-containing regimens are no longer advised because of multiple side effects, including headaches, pyrexia, gastrointestinal symptoms, alopecia, weight loss, depression, anemia, and neutropenia. In addition, IFN-based regimens have limited success in genotypes 1 and 4 infection.

The goals of treatment are to reduce mortality, progression of cirrhosis/decompensation and to achieve sustained virological response (SVR), defined as undetectable HCV RNA 12 weeks after cessation of therapy with oral DAA therapy. Response to antivirals is variable based on genotype. Pegylated IFN given in combination with ribavirin achieves 50% SVR in genotype 1 (48-week therapy) and 80% to 93% in children with genotypes 2 and 3 (24-week therapy).[113] Even with DAA therapy, knowing the genotype, treatment history (naive vs experienced) and cirrhosis status (none vs compensated) is very important to guide treatment selection and duration.

At present, a few regimens (sofosbuvir with ledipasvir and sofosbuvir with ribavirin) are approved for children older than 12 years of age, whereas current clinical trials in the same age group and for children 3 to 11 years of age are ongoing. Sofosbuvir (inhibits HCV NS5B, RNA polymerase essential for viral replication) has been viewed as a potential backbone for HCV therapy. Sofosbuvir with ledipasvir (NS5A inhibitor) was approved in 2014 after the success from the ION trials and is a potent combination, with a >95% SVR with 12 weeks of therapy for HCV genotypes 1 and 4 in adults. The same has been shown in pediatric clinical trials.[114,115] The combination of sofosbuvir and ribavirin is approved in both adults and adolescents for genotype 2 (12 weeks) and genotype 3 (24 weeks) with SVR rates greater than 95%.[116] **Table 4** highlights the current approved antiviral regimens for children aged 12 years and older with chronic HCV.

The treatment of hepatitis C is ever changing and evolving with newer combination medications being approved by the FDA. Several drugs are in the pipeline with pediatric clinical trials in progress. The triple-drug combination of ombitasvir (N5SA), paritaprevir (NS3/NS4A), ritonavir (CYP3A inhibitor that boosts paritaprevir), and dasabuvir (NS5B) with or without ribavirin are under phase III study in pediatric patients with genotypes 1 and 4. Twelve-week pan-genotypic medications such as sofosbuvir (NS5B) with velpatasvir (NS5A) and glecaprevir (NS3/4A) with pibrentasvir

Table 4
Recommended regimens for adolescents greater than or equal to 12 years of age or greater than or equal to 35 kg without cirrhosis or with compensated cirrhosis

Genotype	Regimen	· Duration (wk)
1	Ledipasvir (90 mg) with sofosbuvir (400 mg) for treatment naive without cirrhosis or with compensated cirrhosis, or treatment experienced[a] without cirrhosis	12
	Ledipasvir (90 mg) with sofosbuvir (400 mg) for treatment experienced with compensated cirrhosis	24
2	Sofosbuvir (400 mg) with ribavirin[b] for treatment naive/experienced with compensated cirrhosis or without cirrhosis	12
3	Sofosbuvir (400 mg) with ribavirin[b] for treatment naive/experienced with compensated cirrhosis or without cirrhosis	24
4, 5 or 6	Ledipasvir (90 mg) with sofosbuvir (400 mg) for treatment naive or treatment experienced without cirrhosis or with compensated cirrhosis	12

[a] Treatment experienced: patients who have failed IFN-based therapy.
[b] Ribavirin dosages (in 2 divided doses): less than 47 kg, 15 mg/kg/d; 47 to 49 kg, 600 mg/d; 50 to 65 kg, 800 mg/d; 66 to 80 kg, 1000 mg/d; greater than 80 kg, 1200 mg/d.

(NS5A) were approved by the FDA in 2016 and 2017, respectively, for adults with HCV without decompensated cirrhosis and are now in phase 2 and 2/3 study, respectively in children with HCV. The promise of a once-daily, patient-tailored (ie, HIV coinfection, renal insufficiency, with or without cirrhosis), single-pill treatment with a 95% cure and minimal side effects for children seems to be very much within reach.

SUMMARY

Our understanding of the pathobiology and immunology of hepatitis B and C is unprecedented. As new antiviral therapies are being developed for the pediatric population, the differences in management and monitoring between children and adults with HBV and HCV are beginning to narrow but still important. Soon to be available DAA's for HCV will be curative in children as young as 3 years of age, changing the natural history of HCV and prevalence of hepatocellular carcinoma over the next several decades for the better. Advances in new rapid diagnostic testing and montioring for HBV have also arrived, however current nucleos(t)ide analogues for the treatment of HBV are unable to eradicate the hepatocyte pool of cccDNA, which plays a key role in HBV persistence and reactivation. New anti-viral approaches that destroy or silence cccDNA as well as those that block viral protein production, expression, and release are in the pipeline. Importantly, novel immune modulators are also in preclinical or early clinical development, with the goal of achieving functional cure of HBV infection. The biggest hurdle for pediatric gastroenterologists and hepatologists to overcome at present and in years to come will be access and approval of these costly therapies by insurance companies to treat or cure children with these deadly oncogenic viruses while they still show very little signs of disease.

REFERENCES

1. Schweitzer A, Horn J, Mikolajczyk RT, et al. Estimations of worldwide prevalence of chronic hepatitis B virus infection: a systematic review of data published between 1965 and 2013. Lancet 2015;386(10003):1546–55.
2. World Health Organization. Global hepatitis report. Geneva: World Health Organization; 2017.
3. Mui UN, Haley CT, Tyring SK. Viral oncology: molecular biology and pathogenesis. J Clin Med 2017;6(12) [pii:E111].
4. Kowdley KV, Wang CC, Welch S, et al. Prevalence of chronic hepatitis B among foreign-born persons living in the United States by country of origin. Hepatology 2012;56(2):422–33.
5. Roberts H, Kruszon-Moran D, Ly KN, et al. Prevalence of chronic hepatitis B virus (HBV) infection in U.S. Households: National Health and Nutrition Examination Survey (NHANES), 1988-2012. Hepatology 2016;63(2):388–97.
6. Acute hepatitis B among children and adolescents–United States, 1990-2002. MMWR Morb Mortal Wkly Rep 2004;53(43):1015–8.
7. Hall AJ, Winter PD, Wright R. Mortality of hepatitis B positive blood donors in England and Wales. Lancet 1985;1(8420):91–3.
8. Wasley A, Kruszon-Moran D, Kuhnert W, et al. The prevalence of hepatitis B virus infection in the United States in the era of vaccination. J Infect Dis 2010; 202(2):192–201.
9. Schinzari V, Barnaba V, Piconese S. Chronic hepatitis B virus and hepatitis C virus infections and cancer: synergy between viral and host factors. Clin Microbiol Infect 2015;21(11):969–74.

10. Lin CL, Kao JH. Natural history of acute and chronic hepatitis B: the role of HBV genotypes and mutants. Best Pract Res Clin Gastroenterol 2017;31(3):249–55.
11. Lin CL, Kao JH. Hepatitis B viral factors and treatment responses in chronic hepatitis B. J Formos Med Assoc 2013;112(6):302–11.
12. Kao JH, Chen PJ, Lai MY, et al. Genotypes and clinical phenotypes of hepatitis B virus in patients with chronic hepatitis B virus infection. J Clin Microbiol 2002; 40(4):1207–9.
13. Chotiyaputta W, Lok AS. Hepatitis B virus variants. Nat Rev Gastroenterol Hepatol 2009;6(8):453–62.
14. Yang J, Xing K, Deng R, et al. Identification of Hepatitis B virus putative intergenotype recombinants by using fragment typing. J Gen Virol 2006;87(Pt 8): 2203–15.
15. Munshi SU, Tran TTT, Vo TNT, et al. Molecular characterization of hepatitis B virus in Bangladesh reveals a highly recombinant population. PLoS One 2017; 12(12):e0188944.
16. Chang MH. Breakthrough HBV infection in vaccinated children in Taiwan: surveillance for HBV mutants. Antivir Ther 2010;15(3 Pt B):463–9.
17. Swenson PD, Van Geyt C, Alexander ER, et al. Hepatitis B virus genotypes and HBsAg subtypes in refugees and injection drug users in the United States determined by LiPA and monoclonal EIA. J Med Virol 2001;64(3):305–11.
18. Sunbul M. Hepatitis B virus genotypes: global distribution and clinical importance. World J Gastroenterol 2014;20(18):5427–34.
19. Lin S, Liu C, Shang H, et al. HBV serum markers of 49164 patients and their relationships to HBV genotype in Fujian Province of China. J Clin Lab Anal 2013; 27(2):130–6.
20. Jonas MM, Lok AS, McMahon BJ, et al. Antiviral therapy in management of chronic hepatitis B viral infection in children: a systematic review and meta-analysis. Hepatology 2016;63(1):307–18.
21. Guidotti LG, Chisari FV. Immunobiology and pathogenesis of viral hepatitis. Annu Rev Pathol 2006;1:23–61.
22. Tsai KN, Kuo CF, Ou JJ. Mechanisms of hepatitis B virus persistence. Trends Microbiol 2018;26(1):33–42.
23. Zhang Z, Zhang JY, Wang LF, et al. Immunopathogenesis and prognostic immune markers of chronic hepatitis B virus infection. J Gastroenterol Hepatol 2012;27(2):223–30.
24. Li W, Han J, Wu H. Regulatory T-cells promote hepatitis B virus infection and hepatocellular carcinoma progression. Chronic Dis Transl Med 2016;2(2):67–80.
25. Knolle PA, Thimme R. Hepatic immune regulation and its involvement in viral hepatitis infection. Gastroenterology 2014;146(5):1193–207.
26. Schurich A, Khanna P, Lopes AR, et al. Role of the coinhibitory receptor cytotoxic T lymphocyte antigen-4 on apoptosis-Prone CD8 T cells in persistent hepatitis B virus infection. Hepatology 2011;53(5):1494–503.
27. Shin EC, Sung PS, Park SH. Immune responses and immunopathology in acute and chronic viral hepatitis. Nat Rev Immunol 2016;16(8):509–23.
28. El-Khoueiry AB, Sangro B, Yau T, et al. Nivolumab in patients with advanced hepatocellular carcinoma (CheckMate 040): an open-label, non-comparative, phase 1/2 dose escalation and expansion trial. Lancet 2017;389(10088): 2492–502.
29. Zhang E, Zhang X, Liu J, et al. The expression of PD-1 ligands and their involvement in regulation of T cell functions in acute and chronic woodchuck hepatitis virus infection. PLoS One 2011;6(10):e26196.

30. Gane E, Gaggar A, Nguyen AH, et al. A phase1 study evaluating anti-PD-1 treatment with or without GS-4774 in HBeAg negative chronic hepatitis B patients. J Hepatol 2017;66(1):S26–7.
31. Hou J, Liu Z, Gu F. Epidemiology and prevention of hepatitis B virus infection. Int J Med Sci 2005;2(1):50–7.
32. McMahon BJ, Alward WL, Hall DB, et al. Acute hepatitis B virus infection: relation of age to the clinical expression of disease and subsequent development of the carrier state. J Infect Dis 1985;151(4):599–603.
33. Okada K, Kamiyama I, Inomata M, et al. e antigen and anti-e in the serum of asymptomatic carrier mothers as indicators of positive and negative transmission of hepatitis B virus to their infants. N Engl J Med 1976;294(14):746–9.
34. Keane E, Funk AL, Shimakawa Y. Systematic review with meta-analysis: the risk of mother-to-child transmission of hepatitis B virus infection in sub-Saharan Africa. Aliment Pharmacol Ther 2016;44(10):1005–17.
35. Zhang WL, Zhao J, Li W. Influencing factors of mother-infant vertical transmission of hepatitis B virus. Zhongguo Dang Dai Er Ke Za Zhi 2011;13(8):644–6 [in Chinese].
36. Machaira M, Papaevangelou V, Vouloumanou EK, et al. Hepatitis B vaccine alone or with hepatitis B immunoglobulin in neonates of HBsAg+/HBeAg- mothers: a systematic review and meta-analysis. J Antimicrob Chemother 2015;70(2):396–404.
37. Li Z, Xie Z, Ni H, et al. Mother-to-child transmission of hepatitis B virus: evolution of hepatocellular carcinoma-related viral mutations in the post-immunization era. J Clin Virol 2014;61(1):47–54.
38. Zou H, Chen Y, Duan Z, et al. Virologic factors associated with failure to passive-active immunoprophylaxis in infants born to HBsAg-positive mothers. J Viral Hepat 2012;19(2):e18–25.
39. Wang JS, Zhu QR, Wang XH. Breastfeeding does not pose any additional risk of immunoprophylaxis failure on infants of HBV Carrier mothers. Int J Clin Pract 2003;57(2):100–2.
40. Goldstein ST, Alter MJ, Williams IT, et al. Incidence and risk factors for acute hepatitis B in the United States, 1982-1998: implications for vaccination programs. J Infect Dis 2002;185(6):713–9.
41. Khan AJ, Simard EP, Bower WA, et al. Ongoing transmission of hepatitis B virus infection among inmates at a state correctional facility. Am J Public Health 2005; 95(10):1793–9.
42. Kidd-Ljunggren K, Holmberg A, Blackberg J, et al. High levels of hepatitis B virus DNA in body fluids from chronic carriers. J Hosp Infect 2006;64(4):352–7.
43. Bortolotti F. Chronic viral hepatitis in childhood. Baillieres Clin Gastroenterol 1996;10(2):185–206.
44. Chen HL, Chang CJ, Kong MS, et al. Pediatric fulminant hepatic failure in endemic areas of hepatitis B infection: 15 years after universal hepatitis B vaccination. Hepatology 2004;39(1):58–63.
45. EASL Jury. EASL International Consensus Conference on Hepatitis B. 13-14 September, 2002: Geneva, Switzerland. Consensus statement (short version). J Hepatol 2003;38(4):533–40.
46. Terrault NA, Bzowej NH, Chang KM, et al. AASLD guidelines for treatment of chronic hepatitis B. Hepatology 2016;63(1):261–83.
47. Karnsakul W, Schwarz KB. Hepatitis B and C. Pediatr Clin North Am 2017;64(3): 641–58.

48. Bortolotti F, Guido M, Bartolacci S, et al. Chronic hepatitis B in children after e antigen seroclearance: final report of a 29-year longitudinal study. Hepatology 2006;43(3):556–62.
49. Chen CJ, Yang HI. Natural history of chronic hepatitis B REVEALed. J Gastroenterol Hepatol 2011;26(4):628–38.
50. Tajiri H, Takano T, Tanaka H, et al. Hepatocellular carcinoma in children and young patients with chronic HBV infection and the usefulness of alpha-fetoprotein assessment. Cancer Med 2016;5(11):3102–10.
51. Zhang XF, Liu XM, Wei T, et al. Clinical characteristics and outcome of hepatocellular carcinoma in children and adolescents. Pediatr Surg Int 2013;29(8):763–70.
52. McMahon BJ, Bulkow LR, Singleton RJ, et al. Elimination of hepatocellular carcinoma and acute hepatitis B in children 25 years after a hepatitis B newborn and catch-up immunization program. Hepatology 2011;54(3):801–7.
53. Chang MH, Chen CJ, Lai MS, et al. Universal hepatitis B vaccination in Taiwan and the incidence of hepatocellular carcinoma in children. Taiwan Childhood Hepatoma Study Group. N Engl J Med 1997;336(26):1855–9.
54. Chang MH, You SL, Chen CJ, et al. Long-term effects of hepatitis B immunization of infants in preventing liver cancer. Gastroenterology 2016;151(3): 472–80.e1.
55. Chien YC, Jan CF, Kuo HS, et al. Nationwide hepatitis B vaccination program in Taiwan: effectiveness in the 20 years after it was launched. Epidemiol Rev 2006; 28:126–35.
56. Hsu EK, Murray KF. Hepatitis B and C in children. Nat Clin Pract Gastroenterol Hepatol 2008;5(6):311–20.
57. Schwarz KB, Cloonan YK, Ling SC, et al. Children with chronic hepatitis B in the United States and Canada. J Pediatr 2015;167(6):1287–94.e2.
58. Andreani T, Serfaty L, Mohand D, et al. Chronic hepatitis B virus carriers in the immunotolerant phase of infection: histologic findings and outcome. Clin Gastroenterol Hepatol 2007;5(5):636–41.
59. McGoogan KE, Smith PB, Choi SS, et al. Performance of the AST-to-platelet ratio index as a noninvasive marker of fibrosis in pediatric patients with chronic viral hepatitis. J Pediatr Gastroenterol Nutr 2010;50(3):344–6.
60. Hanquinet S, Rougemont AL, Courvoisier D, et al. Acoustic radiation force impulse (ARFI) elastography for the noninvasive diagnosis of liver fibrosis in children. Pediatr Radiol 2013;43(5):545–51.
61. Wang X, Qian L, Jia L, et al. Utility of shear wave elastography for differentiating biliary atresia from infantile hepatitis syndrome. J Ultrasound Med 2016;35(7): 1475–9.
62. Talwalkar JA, Kurtz DM, Schoenleber SJ, et al. Ultrasound-based transient elastography for the detection of hepatic fibrosis: systematic review and meta-analysis. Clin Gastroenterol Hepatol 2007;5(10):1214–20.
63. Lok AS, McMahon BJ. Chronic hepatitis B: update of recommendations. Hepatology 2004;39(3):857–61.
64. Jonas MM, Kelly D, Pollack H, et al. Safety, efficacy, and pharmacokinetics of adefovir dipivoxil in children and adolescents (age 2 to <18 years) with chronic hepatitis B. Hepatology 2008;47(6):1863–71.
65. Sarin SK, Kumar M, Lau GK, et al. Asian-Pacific clinical practice guidelines on the management of hepatitis B: a 2015 update. Hepatol Int 2016;10(1):1–98.
66. Su TH, Hu TH, Chen CY, et al. Four-year entecavir therapy reduces hepatocellular carcinoma, cirrhotic events and mortality in chronic hepatitis B patients. Liver Int 2016;36(12):1755–64.

67. Wu JF, Chiu YC, Chang KC, et al. Predictors of hepatitis B e antigen-negative hepatitis in chronic hepatitis B virus-infected patients from childhood to adulthood. Hepatology 2016;63(1):74–82.
68. Lee C, Gong Y, Brok J, et al. Hepatitis B immunisation for newborn infants of hepatitis B surface antigen-positive mothers. Cochrane database Syst Rev 2006;(2):CD004790.
69. Brown RS Jr, McMahon BJ, Lok AS, et al. Antiviral therapy in chronic hepatitis B viral infection during pregnancy: a systematic review and meta-analysis. Hepatology 2016;63(1):319–33.
70. Aggeletopoulou I, Davoulou P, Konstantakis C, et al. Response to hepatitis B vaccination in patients with liver cirrhosis. Rev Med Virol 2017;27(6). https://doi.org/10.1002/rmv.1942.
71. Leung DH, Ton-That M, Economides JM, et al. High prevalence of hepatitis B nonimmunity in vaccinated pediatric liver transplant recipients. Am J Transplant 2015;15(2):535–40.
72. Terrault NA, Lok AS, McMahon BJ, et al. Update on prevention, diagnosis, and treatment and of chronic hepatitis B: AASLD 2018 hepatitis B guidance. Hepatology 2018;67(4):1560–99.
73. El-Shabrawi MH, Kamal NM. Burden of pediatric hepatitis C. World J Gastroenterol 2013;19(44):7880–8.
74. Gower E, Estes C, Blach S, et al. Global epidemiology and genotype distribution of the hepatitis C virus infection. J Hepatol 2014;61(1 Suppl):S45–57.
75. Denniston MM, Jiles RB, Drobeniuc J, et al. Chronic hepatitis C virus infection in the United States, National Health and Nutrition Examination Survey 2003 to 2010. Ann Intern Med 2014;160(5):293–300.
76. Jhaveri R, Grant W, Kauf TL, et al. The burden of hepatitis C virus infection in children: estimated direct medical costs over a 10-year period. J Pediatr 2006;148(3):353–8.
77. Pham YH, Rosenthal P. Chronic hepatitis C infection in children. Adv Pediatr 2016;63(1):173–94.
78. Prasad MR, Honegger JR. Hepatitis C virus in pregnancy. Am J Perinatol 2013; 30(2):149–59.
79. Benova L, Mohamoud YA, Calvert C, et al. Vertical transmission of hepatitis C virus: systematic review and meta-analysis. Clin Infect Dis 2014;59(6):765–73.
80. Cottrell EB, Chou R, Wasson N, et al. Reducing risk for mother-to-infant transmission of hepatitis C virus: a systematic review for the U.S. Preventive Services Task Force. Ann Intern Med 2013;158(2):109–13.
81. Mast EE, Hwang LY, Seto DS, et al. Risk factors for perinatal transmission of hepatitis C virus (HCV) and the natural history of HCV infection acquired in infancy. J Infect Dis 2005;192(11):1880–9.
82. Hughes BL, Page CM, Kuller JA. Hepatitis C in pregnancy: screening, treatment, and management. Am J Obstet Gynecol 2017;217(5):B2–12.
83. van de Laar TJ, Matthews GV, Prins M, et al. Acute hepatitis C in HIV-infected men who have sex with men: an emerging sexually transmitted infection. AIDS 2010;24(12):1799–812.
84. Shiffman ML. The next wave of hepatitis C virus: the epidemic of intravenous drug use. Liver Int 2018;38(Suppl 1):34–9.
85. Global surveillance and control of hepatitis C. Report of a WHO consultation organized in collaboration with the Viral Hepatitis Prevention Board, Antwerp, Belgium. J Viral Hepat 1999;6(1):35–47.

86. Bell TW. Drugs for hepatitis C: unlocking a new mechanism of action. Chem-MedChem 2010;5(10):1663–5.
87. Gerotto M, Resti M, Dal Pero F, et al. Evolution of hepatitis C virus quasispecies in children with chronic hepatitis C. Infection 2006;34(2):62–5.
88. Hurtado CW, Golden-Mason L, Brocato M, et al. Innate immune function in placenta and cord blood of hepatitis C–seropositive mother-infant dyads. PLoS One 2010;5(8):e12232.
89. Marcello T, Grakoui A, Barba-Spaeth G, et al. Interferons alpha and lambda inhibit hepatitis C virus replication with distinct signal transduction and gene regulation kinetics. Gastroenterology 2006;131(6):1887–98.
90. Duggal P, Thio CL, Wojcik GL, et al. Genome-wide association study of spontaneous resolution of hepatitis C virus infection: data from multiple cohorts. Ann Intern Med 2013;158(4):235–45.
91. Ge D, Fellay J, Thompson AJ, et al. Genetic variation in IL28B predicts hepatitis C treatment-induced viral clearance. Nature 2009;461(7262):399–401.
92. Thomas DL, Thio CL, Martin MP, et al. Genetic variation in IL28B and spontaneous clearance of hepatitis C virus. Nature 2009;461(7265):798–801.
93. Grakoui A, Shoukry NH, Woollard DJ, et al. HCV persistence and immune evasion in the absence of memory T cell help. Science 2003;302(5645):659–62.
94. Lauer GM, Barnes E, Lucas M, et al. High resolution analysis of cellular immune responses in resolved and persistent hepatitis C virus infection. Gastroenterology 2004;127(3):924–36.
95. Ghasemi F, Rostami S, Meshkat Z. Progress in the development of vaccines for hepatitis C virus infection. World J Gastroenterol 2015;21(42):11984–2002.
96. Glynn SA, Wright DJ, Kleinman SH, et al. Dynamics of viremia in early hepatitis C virus infection. Transfusion 2005;45(6):994–1002.
97. A significant sex–but not elective cesarean section–effect on mother-to-child transmission of hepatitis C virus infection. J Infect Dis 2005;192(11):1872–9.
98. Seeff LB. Natural history of chronic hepatitis C. Hepatology 2002;36(5 Suppl 1):S35–46.
99. Alter HJ, Seeff LB. Recovery, persistence, and sequelae in hepatitis C virus infection: a perspective on long-term outcome. Semin Liver Dis 2000;20(1):17–35.
100. Indolfi G, Bartolini E, Serranti D, et al. Hepatitis C in children co-infected with human immunodeficiency virus. J Pediatr Gastroenterol Nutr 2015;61(4):393–9.
101. Delgado-Borrego A, Healey D, Negre B, et al. Influence of body mass index on outcome of pediatric chronic hepatitis C virus infection. J Pediatr Gastroenterol Nutr 2010;51(2):191–7.
102. Gonzalez-Peralta RP, Langham MR Jr, Andres JM, et al. Hepatocellular carcinoma in 2 young adolescents with chronic hepatitis C. J Pediatr Gastroenterol Nutr 2009;48(5):630–5.
103. Hajarizadeh B, Grebely J, Dore GJ. Epidemiology and natural history of HCV infection. Nat Rev Gastroenterol Hepatol 2013;10(9):553–62.
104. Avo AP, Agua-Doce I, Andrade A, et al. Hepatitis C virus subtyping based on sequencing of the C/E1 and NS5B genomic regions in comparison to a commercially available line probe assay. J Med Virol 2013;85(5):815–22.
105. Ciotti M, D'Agostini C, Marrone A. Advances in the diagnosis and monitoring of hepatitis C virus infection. Gastroenterology Res 2013;6(5):161–70.
106. Mack CL, Gonzalez-Peralta RP, Gupta N, et al. NASPGHAN practice guidelines: diagnosis and management of hepatitis C infection in infants, children, and adolescents. J Pediatr Gastroenterol Nutr 2012;54(6):838–55.

107. Rumbo C, Fawaz RL, Emre SH, et al. Hepatitis C in children: a quaternary referral center perspective. J Pediatr Gastroenterol Nutr 2006;43(2):209–16.
108. Bruix J, Sherman M. Management of hepatocellular carcinoma: an update. Hepatology 2011;53(3):1020–2.
109. Thomas DL. Curing hepatitis C with pills: a step toward global control. Lancet 2010;376(9751):1441–2.
110. Estes C, Abdel-Kareem M, Abdel-Razek W, et al. Economic burden of hepatitis C in Egypt: the future impact of highly effective therapies. Aliment Pharmacol Ther 2015;42(6):696–706.
111. Wittenborn J, Brady J, Dougherty M, et al. Potential epidemiologic, economic, and budgetary impacts of current rates of hepatitis C treatment in Medicare and non-Medicare populations. Hepatol Commun 2017;1(2):99–109.
112. Goldberg D, Ditah IC, Saeian K, et al. Changes in the prevalence of hepatitis C virus infection, nonalcoholic steatohepatitis, and alcoholic liver disease among patients with cirrhosis or liver failure on the waitlist for liver transplantation. Gastroenterology 2017;152(5):1090–9.e1.
113. Schwarz KB, Gonzalez-Peralta RP, Murray KF, et al. The combination of ribavirin and peginterferon is superior to peginterferon and placebo for children and adolescents with chronic hepatitis C. Gastroenterology 2011;140(2):450–8.e1.
114. Afdhal N, Zeuzem S, Kwo P, et al. Ledipasvir and sofosbuvir for untreated HCV genotype 1 infection. N Engl J Med 2014;370(20):1889–98.
115. Balistreri WF, Murray KF, Rosenthal P, et al. The safety and effectiveness of ledipasvir-sofosbuvir in adolescents 12-17 years old with hepatitis C virus genotype 1 infection. Hepatology 2017;66(2):371–8.
116. Wirth S, Rosenthal P, Gonzalez-Peralta RP, et al. Sofosbuvir and ribavirin in adolescents 12-17 years old with hepatitis C virus genotype 2 or 3 infection. Hepatology 2017;66(4):1102–10.
117. Suzuki Y, Kobayashi M, Ikeda K, et al. Persistence of acute infection with hepatitis B virus genotype A and treatment in Japan. J Med Virol 2005;76(1):33–9.
118. Ni YH, Chang MH, Wang KJ, et al. Clinical relevance of hepatitis B virus genotype in children with chronic infection and hepatocellular carcinoma. Gastroenterology 2004;127(6):1733–8.
119. Ghosh S, Mondal RK, Banerjee P, et al. Tracking the naturally occurring mutations across the full-length genome of hepatitis B virus of genotype D in different phases of chronic e-antigen-negative infection. Clin Microbiol Infect 2012;18(10):E412–8.
120. Pezzano SC, Torres C, Fainboim HA, et al. Hepatitis B virus in Buenos Aires, Argentina: genotypes, virological characteristics and clinical outcomes. Clin Microbiol Infect 2011;17(2):223–31.
121. Sakamoto T, Tanaka Y, Watanabe T, et al. Mechanism of the dependence of hepatitis B virus genotype G on co-infection with other genotypes for viral replication. J Viral Hepat 2013;20(4):e27–36.
122. Panduro A, Maldonado-Gonzalez M, Fierro NA, et al. Distribution of HBV genotypes F and H in Mexico and Central America. Antivir Ther 2013;18(3 Pt B):475–84.
123. Li GJ, Hue S, Harrison TJ, et al. Hepatitis B virus candidate subgenotype I1 varies in distribution throughout Guangxi, China and may have originated in Long An county, Guangxi. J Med Virol 2013;85(5):799–807.
124. Sokal EM, Paganelli M, Wirth S, et al. Management of chronic hepatitis B in childhood: ESPGHAN clinical practice guidelines: consensus of an expert panel on behalf of the European Society of Pediatric Gastroenterology, Hepatology and Nutrition. J Hepatol 2013;59(4):814–29.

Nonalcoholic Liver Disease in Children and Adolescents

Sara Kathryn Smith, MD*, Emily R. Perito, MD

KEYWORDS

- NAFLD • NASH • Pediatric • Steatohepatitis • Fatty liver disease

KEY POINTS

- Pediatric nonalcoholic fatty liver disease (NAFLD) is the most common cause of liver disease in children.
- The spectrum of NAFLD ranges from steatosis to nonalcoholic steatohepatitis (NASH) to fibrosis. Obesity rates in children continue to rise and, as a result, NAFLD in children is becoming more prevalent.
- The pathophysiology, natural history, and progression of disease are still being elucidated but NAFLD/NASH in children may represent a more severe phenotype that will benefit from early identification and management.

DEFINITIONS

Pediatric nonalcoholic fatty liver disease (NAFLD) is chronic hepatic steatosis in children, ages 18 years or younger, that cannot be attributed to a genetic or metabolic disorder, infection, steatogenic medications, ethanol, or malnutrition. NAFLD can further be divided into NAFL and nonalcoholic steatohepatitis (NASH), based on histology. NAFL is characterized by bland steatosis whereas NASH is characterized by steatosis with lobular inflammation and hepatocellular injury. Fibrosis, when present, may indicate a more severe disease phenotype, even in the absence of NASH. Pediatric NAFLD is most often diagnosed in children between the ages of 12 and 13; however, it has been reported in children as young as 2 years, with NASH-related cirrhosis noted as early as 8 years of age (**Table 1**).[1]

EPIDEMIOLOGY

Estimating the prevalence of NAFLD in pediatric populations is difficult due to differences in screening laboratory tests and imaging studies, thresholds for detection,

Disclosure Statement: Neither author has any direct financial interest in subject matter or materials discussed in article or with a company making a competing product.
Department of Pediatric Gastroenterology, Hepatology, and Nutrition, University of California, San Francisco, 550 16th Street, 5th Floor, Mail Code 0136, San Francisco, CA 94143, USA
* Corresponding author.
E-mail address: Kathryn.Smith@ucsf.edu

Clin Liver Dis 22 (2018) 723–733
https://doi.org/10.1016/j.cld.2018.07.001
1089-3261/18/Published by Elsevier Inc.

liver.theclinics.com

Table 1
Nonalcoholic fatty liver disease definitions and phenotypes in children

Phenotype	Definition
NAFLD	Encompasses the full spectrum of disease from NAFL to NASH, without evidence of significant alcohol consumption, genetic or metabolic diseases, infection, or steatogenic medications
NAFL	Presence of ≥5% hepatic steatosis without evidence of hepatocellular injury
NASH	Presence of ≥5% of hepatic steatosis with inflammation, with or without ballooning injury to hepatocytes and fibrosis
NAFLD with fibrosis	NAFL or NASH with periportal, portal, sinusoidal, or bridging fibrosis
NAFLD with cirrhosis	Cirrhosis in the setting of diagnosed NAFLD

From Vos MB, Abrams SH, Barlow SE, et al. NASPGHAN clinical practice guideline for the diagnosis and treatment of nonalcoholic fatty liver disease in children: Recommendations from the Expert Committee on NAFLD (ECON) and the North American Society of Pediatric Gastroenterology, Hepatology, and Nutrition (NASPGHAN). J Pediatr Gastroenterol Nutr 2017;64(2):319-34; with permission.

and demographics of the region being sampled. A 2015 meta-analysis determined the pooled mean prevalence of NAFLD to be 7.6% in the general US pediatric population and 34.2% in studies based in pediatric obesity clinics.[2] A study of liver histology obtained at autopsy in 742 children ages 2 years to 19 years found an NAFLD prevalence of 9.6% after adjusting for age, gender, race, and ethnicity.[3]

This variation by race and ethnicity suggests that genetic factors likely play a large role in the pathogenesis and progression of NAFLD.[1] Hispanic adolescents have a 4-fold increased risk of developing hepatic steatosis compared with non-Hispanic adolescents ages 11 years old to 22 years old.[4] White and Asian children and adolescents also have high prevalence compared with African American children. NAFLD is also more prevalent in male children than female children.[1,5,6] Finally, prevalence is higher in obese children compared with those with normal weight; however, not all children with NAFLD are obese. NAFLD can occur in up to 5% of children with a normal body mass index (BMI).[1]

A single nucleotide polymorphism common variant allele in PNPLA3 has been associated with increased susceptibility to NAFLD.[7] Adult studies have demonstrated this variant allele associated with increased hepatic fat and histologic severity. Studies have been conflicting, however, regarding PNPLA3 association with histology of NAFLD in children.[8,9]

RISK FACTORS AND COMORBIDITIES

NAFLD is more common in children with metabolic syndrome.[10] Studies have shown that children with biopsy-proved NASH have increased risk for multiple cardiovascular factors, including high cholesterol, low-density lipoprotein, triglycerides, and systolic blood pressure compared with obese children.[11–13] Elevated ALT is more common in Hispanic children newly diagnosed with type 2 diabetes mellitus compared with African American children.[14]

NAFLD has been associated with obstructive sleep apnea. Hypoxia and oxidative stress from apnea are believed to contribute to progression of steatohepatitis and fibrosis because of ischemia-reperfusion injury. Two pediatric studies have shown an association of obstructive sleep apnea with the presence of NASH, independent of BMI and standard metabolic risk factors.[15] Studies have shown an association be-tween obstructive sleep apnea prevalence and severity with NASH and fibrosis stage.[16–18]

As in adult studies, pediatric patients with panhypopituitarism have an increased risk of NAFLD, NASH, and even cirrhosis.[19,20]

ASSOCIATED MORBIDITY

NAFLD seems to be asymptomatic in most children, but symptoms reported by NAFLD patients include irritability, fatigue, headache, trouble concentrating, and mus-cle aches or cramps.[21] Studies have shown a higher rate of depression in adolescents with NAFLD compared with obese controls.[22] Quality-of-life scores are also lower with many endorsing fatigue, trouble sleeping, and sadness.[21]

NAFLD increases the risk of hepatocellular carcinoma in adults; hepatocellular car-cinoma in pediatric NAFLD is extremely rare. Longitudinal studies are lacking, but it is likely that NAFLD in children predicts a more severe phenotype in adulthood and may represent an important risk factor for the development of hepatocellular carcinoma as an adult.

NATURAL HISTORY AND PROGRESSION OF DISEASE

The pathogenesis of NAFLD is not completely understood. Current research suggests that NAFLD represents "lipotoxic" liver injury resulting when excess dietary carbohy-drates and fatty acids mobilized from adipose tissue are converted into free fatty acids in the liver. Some of these fatty acids are packaged into triglyceride droplets, mani-fested as simple hepatic steatosis. Excess fatty acids may induce irreversible cell damage and trigger proinflammatory signaling pathways. Excess free fatty acids are then metabolized to toxic intermediates, leading to chronic inflammation, the hallmark of NASH, and eventually fibrosis. Findings suggest that increased hepatic triglyceride synthesis may play a protective role against free fatty acid–mediated cell toxicity.[23]

Longitudinal studies in adults have shown that patients with NAFLD have increased mortality compared with matched control populations.[24] Fibrosis stage at baseline has been shown predictive of future liver disease–related mortality.[25] Some studies suggest that children diagnosed with NAFLD have increased morbidity and mortality in adulthood.[26] One study shows that 15% of children with NAFLD have stage 3 fibrosis or higher at diagnosis.[12] In adult studies, presence of fibrosis has proved more predictive of clinical outcome compared with the presence of NASH.[27,28] In rare cases, children can have rapid progression of disease, leading to cirrhosis and life-threatening complications that may require liver transplant.[29]

SCREENING AND DIAGNOSIS

The purpose of screening for NAFLD in children and adolescents is to prevent irrevers-ible, end-stage liver disease. Unfortunately, NAFLD is still underdiagnosed in children due to lack of recognition, screening, and underappreciation of associated risk fac-tors. In 1 study, fewer than one-third of children with obesity were screened for NAFLD.[30] ALT is the currently recommended screening laboratory test, because it is widely available, inexpensive to obtain, and sensitive. Although the assay is stan-dardized among laboratories, the reporting of normal values is not. Gender-specific cutoffs, 22 U/L for girls and 26 U/L for boys, have been designated in the United States using nationally derived data and have been validated in a diverse cohort.[1,31] Aspar-tate aminotransferase (AST) and γ-glutamyl transferase (GGT) have not been independently tested as screening tests for NAFLD in children; however, in the context of elevated ALT, higher AST and GGT are associated with worse histology.[32]

Although imaging has been used as a screening tool for NAFLD, routine ultrasonography is not sensitive or specific for the detection of steatosis in children, especially in children with steatosis occupying less than 33% of hepatocytes.[33] Using ultrasonography in addition to ALT as a screening tool can lead to confusion, because patients with NAFLD can have ALT less than 40 U/L despite steatosis on ultrasound.[32] Routine ultrasound is not recommended as a screening test for NAFLD in children.[34] Although ultrasonography has not been proved accurate for the detection of hepatic steatosis due to low sensitivity and specificity, it can be performed to exclude other causes of elevated ALT, such as hepatic masses, cysts, or gallbladder pathology.[33,35]

MRI and magnetic resonance spectroscopy are accurate for detection and quantification of hepatic steatosis in children, but magnetic resonance (MR)–based methods are not widely used for screening due to cost, availability, and validation. CT scans can also detect steatosis but are not used for pediatric screening given radiation risks. If hepatic steatosis is identified on imaging studies, further diagnostic work-up is required to determine the etiology of steatosis. ALT remains the preferred first-line screening tool for NALFD in children due to expense, availability, and validation.[34]

WHO TO SCREEN

Children with features of metabolic syndrome, such as obesity, hypertension, insulin resistance, diabetes, prediabetes, central adiposity, and dyslipidemia, are at higher risk for NAFLD. Certain races and ethnicities are also at risk. Children with features of metabolic syndrome, even if they are not overweight, are at risk for NAFLD. Overweight siblings and parents of patients with NAFLD also are at increased risk for development of NAFLD.[36]

The optimal age to begin screening for NAFLD has not been determined. Current recommendations include screening in children beginning between ages 9 years old and 11 years old if obese (BMI ≥95th percentile for age and gender) or if overweight (BMI ≥85th percentile and <94th percentile) with additional risk factors (central adiposity, insulin resistance, prediabetes or diabetes, dyslipidemia, sleep apnea, and family history of NAFLD/NASH).[34] Younger patients with severe obesity, those with a family history of NASH/NAFLD, and those with hypopituitarism should also be screened. Interpretation of ALT should be based on gender-specific upper limits of normal and not individual laboratory upper limits of normal (discussed previously).

DIAGNOSIS

When diagnosing NAFLD in children, the use of 2-times the upper limit of normal in overweight and obese children ages 10 and older (ALT ≥50 U/L for boys and ALT ≥44 U/L for girls) has sensitivity and specificity of 88% and 26%, respectively.[32] In Canada, recommendations are to use 30 U/L in children 1 year of age to 12 years of age and 24 U/L in children between 13 years of age and 19 years of age as cutoffs for further evaluation.[3]

NASH is more common in children with ALT greater than or equal to 80 U/L than in children with ALT less than or equal to 80 U/L (41% vs 21%).[32] ALT elevation greater than 2-times the upper limit of normal, persisting for 3 months or longer, requires evaluation for NAFLD and other causes of hepatitis. ALT greater than 80 U/L is concerning for significant liver disease and requires more urgent evaluation and work-up. In cases of the initial screening ALT normal, recent clinical guidelines recommend repeat ALT every 2 years to 3 years if risk factors remain unchanged. In patients in whom clinical risk factors increase in severity or number, consider repeat screening earlier.[34]

INITIAL EVALUATION

Any child presenting with chronically elevated ALT should not be assumed to have NAFLD. A complete evaluation should be performed to rule out other causes of hepatic steatosis and/or elevated ALT (**Table 2**). Until a specific test is developed to identify pediatric NAFLD, it remains a diagnosis of exclusion. Some conditions causing pediatric hepatic steatosis require specific treatments distinct from those used to manage NAFLD, which, if not pursued, could lead to poor outcomes.

Several scoring systems, such as the NAFLD liver fat score, fatty liver index, hepatic steatosis index, and pediatric prediction score, have been developed to predict steatosis; however, none of these has demonstrated accuracy compared with the use of hepatic histology. They are not clinically useful at this time.[37]

It is important to identify patients with NAFLD and NASH who have fibrosis because these children are more likely to progress to cirrhosis.[27] Unfortunately, at this time, clinical parameters, such as severity of obesity and/or metabolic syndrome, cannot distinguish patients with NASH from those with NAFL.[38] Although ALT is used in children as a screening tool (discussed previously), it is not sensitive enough on its own to predict NAFLD phenotype or severity. Children with ALT greater than or equal to 80 U/L are more likely to have NASH compared with those with ALT less than or equal to 80 U/L.[32]

Liver biopsy remains the current standard to diagnose NAFLD and to determine its severity, including the presence of NASH, and to rule out alternative diagnoses. Biopsy allows for staging of disease and thus identification of patients who are more likely to progress and require more intensive management and treatment. In addition, it allows for diagnosis of other diseases that may be contributing to or causing hepatomegaly and elevated ALT. Liver biopsy has several limitations, however, when it comes to staging NAFLD, including the small sample size

Table 2
Differential diagnosis for hepatic steatosis in children and adolescents

Genetic/Metabolic Disorders	Medications	Dietary Causes	Infections
NAFLD	Amiodarone	Protein-energy	Hepatitis C
Fatty acid oxidation,	Corticosteroids	malnutrition	(genotype 3)
mitochondrial disorders	Methotrexate	(kwashiorkor)	
Citrin deficiency	Certain antipsychotics	Alcohol abuse	
Wilson disease	Certain	Rapid surgical	
Uncontrolled diabetes	antidepressants	weight loss	
Lipodystrophies	Highly active ART	Parenteral	
Lysosomal acid lipase deficiency	Valproic acid	nutrition	
Familial combined hyperlipidemia			
Abetalipoproteinemia/			
hypobetalipoproteinemia			

From Vos MB, Abrams SH, Barlow SE, et al. NASPGHAN clinical practice guideline for the diagnosis and treatment of nonalcoholic fatty liver disease in children: Recommendations from the Expert Committee on NAFLD (ECON) and the North American Society of Pediatric Gastroenterology, Hepatology, and Nutrition (NASPGHAN). J Pediatr Gastroenterol Nutr 2017;64(2):319–34; with permission.

obtained. Sample length greater than or equal to 2 cm with adequate width reduces the risk of misclassification.

Liver biopsy has been proved safe in children, including in children who are obese.[39] Children with severe obesity, defined as BMI greater than or equal to 120% of the 95th percentile for age and gender or BMI greater than 35 kg/m^2, may require referral to interventional radiology for liver biopsy, due to challenges assessing the position of the liver and increased depth of subcutaneous adipose tissue layer.[34] When it comes to timing of liver biopsy, a standard clinical practice has not been established. The decision to proceed with liver biopsy should be made after a thorough discussion of benefits and risks with patient and caregivers.

Current guidelines recommend screening children with NAFLD for diabetes at diagnosis and annually thereafter, using either fasting serum glucose level or glycosylated hemoglobin A_{1C} level. A glucose tolerance test is indicated in patients with fasting glucose or hemoglobin A_{1C} level in the prediabetic range.[34]

HISTOLOGY

At least 3 patterns of NAFLD histology have been demonstrated in children. Histology with the presence of steatosis and relatively mild features overall, those with portal centered steatosis (zone 1), and those with venule centered steatosis (Zone 3). Zone 1 steatosis, inflammation, and fibrosis are more common in children compared with the zone 3 predominance of lesions in adults. Children with zone 1 steatosis (portal predominant) with ballooning are more likely to present with fibrosis compared to children with zone 3 steatosis (venule centered) often without ballooning.[40]

MANAGEMENT

Longitudinal studies of NAFLD/NASH in children are lacking, so much management is extrapolated from adult studies.

LIFESTYLE CHANGES

The primary treatment of NAFLD/NASH centers on lifestyle changes, including adherence to a healthy diet and daily routine physical activity. Because the progression of disease in children is difficult to predict, all children who are diagnosed with NAFLD/NASH should be offered lifestyle intervention counseling. Ideally, management should include consultation with a registered dietician to assess quality of diet and caloric intake. Available data do not support any specific diet for NAFLD, although 2 large randomized pediatric trials showed that reduction of sugar sweetened beverages decrease central adiposity in children and may benefit overweight children with NAFLD.[41,42] Trials have also demonstrated that aerobic and resistance exercise can reduce hepatic steatosis.[43] One of the goals of treatment is to address dyslipidemia, insulin resistance, high blood pressure, and central adiposity, all of which are closely associated with NAFLD. At this time, it is not known how much weight loss is necessary for improvement in NAFLD in children. Adult studies have shown that weight loss greater than or equal to 10% of baseline weight was associated with greater than or equal to 90% resolution of NASH.[34]

PHARMACOTHERAPY

Various medications and supplements have been studied for use in the management of pediatric NAFLD, including metformin, vitamin E, ursodeoxycholic acid, and delayed-release cysteamine. The most commonly studied agents include metformin or vitamin E.[44–47] The TONIC trial was a 2-year randomized control trial comparing vitamin E or metformin to placebo in the management of pediatric NAFLD, with liver biopsies obtained at baseline and at 2 years' follow-up.[48] All patients received lifestyle counseling. The primary endpoint, sustained reduction in ALT, was not different between drug and placebo; however, vitamin E treatment led to statistically significant improvements in histology, as demonstrated by a lower NAFLD activity score (NAS). The use of long-term high-dose vitamin E in adults has raised concern for increased mortality and increased cardiovascular events and cancer based on meta-analyses.[49] The same study found that metformin had no effect on ALT improvement or NAS score compared with placebo.

Delayed-release cysteamine was compared with placebo in another large, randomized controlled trial. The primary outcome of reduction in NAS score of 2 or more did not reach statistical significance. A secondary outcome comparing reduction in serum ALT between treatment and placebo did reach significance.[50] This medication is not currently available, however, for treatment of pediatric NAFLD in clinical practice.

Omega-3 fatty acids and fish oil have been considered for treatment of NAFLD in children. A small RCT trial showed no improvement in ALT when docosahexaenoic acid (DHA) was compared with placebo in pediatric NAFLD; however, there was a decrease in visceral fat and liver fat and improvement in metabolic abnormalities.[51] It is known that vitamin D insufficiency is common in pediatric NAFLD. In a recent randomized trial, 41 children with NAFLD and vitamin D deficiency were placed on vitamin D supplementation and DHA versus placebo. DHA plus vitamin D treatment improved insulin resistance, lipid profile, ALT, and NAFLD activity score compared with placebo alone.[52]

SURGERY

Bariatric surgery, or weight loss surgery, is considered for adolescent patients with severe obesity, defined as BMI greater than or equal to 35 kg/m^2, with noncirrhotic NAFLD or other serious comorbidities (type 2 diabetes mellitus, severe sleep apnea, and idiopathic intracranial hypertension). There are few studies examining the progression of NAFLD/NASH after weight loss surgery in adolescents, with only 1 including histologic evaluation of NAFLD. In adult studies examining indications and outcomes after bariatric surgery, the proportion of patients with severe NASH undergoing bariatric surgery are low.[53,54] A recent study demonstrated that laparoscopic sleeve gastrectomy was more effective than lifestyle intervention for reducing NASH and liver fibrosis in obese adolescents with resolution of NASH in all patients and resolution of hepatic fibrosis in 90% of patients after sleeve gastrectomy.[58]

The main outcome indicating regression of NAFLD is demonstration of decrease in steatosis, inflammation, and/or fibrosis. Due to the invasive nature of liver biopsy, a decrease in ALT often is used as a surrogate marker for improvement in histology.[48] Because ultrasound has not been proved to reliably detect steatosis, it is not used in assessment of progression or regression of disease. Other imaging studies, such as MRI and CT, have not been adequately studied in children and, therefore, do not have a role in assessing treatment success. Despite the risk associated with liver biopsy, it remains the clinical standard for defining interval change in liver histology after treatment. Frequency and timing of repeat biopsy have not been established.

FUTURE RESEARCH

Long-term studies demonstrating clinical outcomes in pediatric NAFLD will require follow-up of patients into adulthood. Unfortunately, children are now seen with earlier-onset and more severe obesity, with increased rates of insulin resistance, and extrapolation from current adult studies will not be sufficient. In addition, pharmacologic treatments to aid in the treatment of NAFLD/NASH are still lacking; additional trials are needed.

REFERENCES

1. Schwimmer JB, Deutsch R, Kahen T, et al. Prevalence of fatty liver disease in children and adolescents. Pediatrics 2006;118:1388–93.
2. Anderson EL, Howe LD, Jones HE, et al. The prevalence of nonalcoholic fatty liver disease in children and adolescents: a systematic review and meta-analysis. PLoS One 2015;10(10):eD140908.
3. Schwimmer JB, Behlong C, Newbury R, et al. Histopathology of pediatric nonalcoholic fatty liver disease. Hepatology 2005;42:641–9.
4. Rehm JL, Connor EL, Wolfgram PM, et al. Predicting hepatic steatosis in a racially and ethnically diverse cohort of adolescent girls. J Pediatr 2014;165:319–25.e1.
5. Wiegand S, Keller KM, Robl M, et al. Obese boys at increased risk for nonalcoholic fatty liver disease evaluation of 16,390 overweight or obese children and adolescents. Int J Obes 2010;34:1468–74.
6. Malespin M, Sleesman B, Lau A, et al. Prevalence and correlates of suspected nonalcoholic fatty liver disease in Chinese American children. J Clin Gastroenterol 2015;49:345–9.
7. Viitasalo A, Pihlajamaki J, Lindi V, et al. Associations of I148M variant in PNPLA3 gene with plasma ALT levels during 2 year follow-up in normal weight and overweight/obese Mexican children. Gene 2013;520(2):185–8.
8. Santoro N, Kursawe R, D'Adamo E, et al. A common variant in the patatin-like phospholipase 3 gene (PNPLA3) is associated with fatty liver disease in obese children and adolescents. Hepatology 2010;52(4):1281–90.
9. Romeo S, Sentinelli F, Cambuli VM, et al. The 148M allele of the PNPPLA3 gene is associated with indices of liver damage early in life. J Hepatol 2010;53(2):335–8.
10. Schwimmer JB, Pardee PE, Lavine JE, et al. Cardiovascular risk factors and the metabolic syndrome in a pediatric nonalcoholic fatty liver disease. Circulation 2008;118(3):69–90.
11. Sartorio A, Del Col A, Agosti F, et al. Predictors of non alcoholic fatty liver disease in obese children. Eur J Clin Nutr 2007;61(7):877–83.
12. Schwimmer JB, Zepeda A, Newton KP, et al. Longitudinal assessment of high blood pressure in children with nonalcoholic fatty liver disease. PLoS One 2014;9(11):e112569.
13. Cali AM, Zern TL, Taksali SE, et al. Intrahepatic fat accumulation and alterations in lipoprotein composition in obese adolescents: a perfect proatherogenic state. Diabetes Care 2007;30(12):3093–8.
14. Hudson OD, Nunez M, Shaibi GQ. Ethnicity and elevated liver transaminases among newly diagnosed children with type 2 diabetes. BMC Pediatr 2012;12:174.
15. Nobili V, Cutrera R, Liccardo D, et al. Obstructive sleep apnea syndrome affects liver histology and inflammatory cell activation in pediatric nonalcoholic fatty liver disease, regardless of obesity/insulin resistance. Am J Respir Crit Care Med 2014;189:66–76.

16. Mathurin P, Durand F, Ganne N, et al. Ischemic hepatitis due to obstructive sleep apnea. Gastroenterology 1995;109(5):1682–4.

17. Henrion J, Colin L, Schapira M, et al. Hypoxic hepatitis caused by severe hypoxemia from obstructive sleep apnea. J Clin Gastroenterol 1997;24(4):245–9.

18. Sundaram SS, Sokol RJ, Capocelli KE, et al. Obstructive sleep apnea and hypoxemia are associated with advanced liver histology in pediatric nonalcoholic fatty liver disease. J Pediatr 2014;164(4):699–706.e1.

19. Adams LA, Feldstein A, Lindor KD, et al. Nonalcoholic fatty liver disease among patients with hypothalamic and pituitary dysfunction. Hepatology 2004;39: 909–14.

20. Nakajima K, Hashimoto E, Kaneda H, et al. Pediatric nonalcoholic steatohepatitis associated with hypopituitarism. J Gastroenterol 2005;40:312–5.

21. Kistler KD, Molleston J, Unalp A, et al. Symptoms and quality of life in obese children and adolescents with non alcoholic fatty liver disease. Aliment Pharmacol Ther 2010;31(3):396–406.

22. Kerkar N, D'Urso C, Van Nostrand K, et al. Psychosocial outcomes for children with nonalcoholic fatty liver disease over time and compared to obese controls. J Pediatr Gastroenterol Nutr 2012;56(1):77–82.

23. Bass NM. Lipidomic dissection of non alcoholic steatohepatitis: moving beyond foie gras to fat traffic. Hepatology 2009;51:4–7.

24. Ekstedt M, Franzen LE, Mathiesen UL, et al. Long-term follow-up of patients with NAFLD and elevated liver enzymes. Hepatology 2006;44:865–73.

25. Ekstedt M, Hagstrom H, Nasr P, et al. Fibrosis stage is the strongest predictor for disease-specific mortality in NAFLD after up to 33 years of follow-up. Hepatology 2015;61:1547–54.

26. Feldstein AE, Charatcharoenwitthaya P, Treeprasertsuk S, et al. The natural history of non-alcoholic fatty liver disease in children: a follow-up study for up to 20 years. Gut 2009;58:1538.

27. Loomba R, Chalasani N. The hierarchical model of NAFLD: prognostic significance of histologic features in NASH. Gastroenterology 2015;149:278–81.

28. Angulo P, Kleiner DE, Dam-Larsen S, et al. Liver fibrosis but no other histologic features, is associated with long-term outcomes of patients with nonalcoholic fatty liver disease. Gastroenterology 2015;149:389–97.e10.

29. Holterman AX, Guzman G, Fatuzzi G, et al. Nonalcoholic fatty liver disease in severely obese adolescent and adult pateints. Obesity (Silver Spring) 2013;21: 591–7.

30. Riley MR, Bass NM, Rosenthal P, et al. Underdiagnosis of pediatric obesity and underscreening for fatty liver disease and metabolic syndrome by pediatricians and pediatric subspecialists. J Pediatr 2005;147:839–42.

31. Lavine JE, Schwimmer JB, Molleston JP, et al. Treatment of nonalcoholic fatty liver disease in children: TONIC trial design. Contemp Clin Trials 2010;31:62–70.

32. Schwimmer JB, Newton KP, Awai HI, et al. Pediatric gastroenterology evaluation of overweight and obese children referred from primary care for suspected nonalcoholic fatty liver disease. Aliment Pharmacol Ther 2013;38:1267–77.

33. Awai HI, Newton KP, Sirlin CB, et al. Evidence and recommendations for imaging liver fat in children, based on systematic review. Clin Gastroenterol Hepatol 2014; 12:765–73.

34. Vos MB, Abrams SH, Barlow SE, et al. NASPHGAN clinical practice guideline for the diagnosis and treatment of nonalcoholic fatty liver disease in children: recommendations from the expert committee on NAFLD (ECON) and the North

American Society of Pediatric Gastroenterology, Hepatology, and Nutrition (NASPGHAN). J Pediatr Gastroenterol Nutr 2017;64(2):319–34.

35. El-Koofy N, El-Karaksy H, El-Akel W, et al. Ultrasonography as a non-invasive tool for detection of nonalcoholic fatty liver disease in overweight/obese Egyptian children. Eur J Radiol 2012;81:3210–3.

36. Schwimmer JB, Celedon MA, Lavine JE, et al. Heritability of nonalcoholic fatty liver disease. Gastroenterology 2009;136:1585–92.

37. Koot BG, Van der Baan-Slootweg OH, Bohte AE, et al. Accuracy of prediction scores and novel biomarkers for predicting nonalcoholic fatty liver disease in obese children. Obesity (Silver Spring) 2012;21:583–90.

38. Singh DK, Sakhuja P, Malhotra V, et al. Independent predictors of steatohepatitis and fibrosis in Asian Indian patients with nonalcoholic steatohepatitis. Dig Dis Sci 2008;53:1967–76.

39. Harwood J, Bishop P, Liu H, et al. Safety of blind percutaneous liver biopsy in obese children: a retrospective analysis. J Clin Gastroenterol 2010;44:e253–5.

40. Africa JA, Behling CA, Brunt EM, et al. Children with nonalcoholic fatty liver disease, zone 1 steatosis is associated with advanced fibrosis. Clin Gastroenterol Hepatol 2018;16(3):438–46.e1.

41. De Ruyter JC, Olthof MR, Seidell JC, et al. A trial of sugar free or sugar sweetened beverages and body weight in children. N Engl J Med 2012;367:1397–406.

42. Ebbeling CB, Feldman HA, Chomitz VR, et al. A randomized trial of sugar sweetened beverages and adolescent body weight. N Engl J Med 2012;367:1407–16.

43. Lee S, Bacha F, Hannon T, et al. Effects of aerobic versus resistance exercise without caloric restriction on abdominal fat, intrahepatic lipid, and insulin sensitivity in obese adolescent boys: a randomized, controlled clinical trial. Diabetes 2012;61:2787–95.

44. Schwimmer JB, Middleton MS, Deutsch R, et al. A phase 2 clinical trial of metformin as a treatment for non-diabetic pediatric nonalcoholic steatohepatitis. Aliment Pharmacol Ther 2005;21:871–9.

45. Nadeu KJ, Ehlers LB, Zeitler PS, et al. Treatment of nonalcoholic fatty liver disease with metformin versus lifestyle intervention in insulin-resistant adolescents. Pediatr Diabetes 2009;10:5–13.

46. Lavine JE. Vitamin E treatment of nonalcoholic steatohepatitis in children: a pilot study. J Pediatr 2000;136:734–8.

47. Vajro P, Mandato C, Franzese A, et al. Vitamin E treatment in pediatric obesity-related liver disease: a randomized study. J Pediatr Gastroenterol Nutr 2004; 38:48–55.

48. Lavine JE, Schwimmer JB, Van Natta ML, et al. Effect of vitamin E or metformin for treatment of nonalcoholic fatty liver disease in children and adolescents: the TONIC randomized controlled trial. JAMA 2011;305:1659–68.

49. Bjelakovic G, Nikolova D, Gluud C. Meta-regression analyses, metaanalyses, and trial sequential analyses of the effects of supplementation with beta-caroten, vitamin A, and vitamin E singly or in different combinations on all-cause mortality: do we have evidence for lack of harm? PLoS One 2013;8:e74558.

50. Schwimmer JB, Lavine JE, Wilson LA, et al. In children with nonalcoholic fatty liver disease, cysteamine bitartrate delayed release improves liver enzymes but does not reduce disease activity scores. Gastroenterology 2016;151:1141–54.

51. Pacifico L, Bonci E, Di Martino M, et al. A double-blind, placebo-controlled randomized trial to evaluate the efficacy of docosahexaenoic acid supplementation on hepatic fat and associate cardiovascular risk factors in overweight children

with nonalcoholic fatty liver disease. Nutr Metab Cardiovasc Dis 2015;25(8): 734–41.

52. Della Corte C, Carpino G, De Vito R, et al. Docosahexanoic acid plus vitamin D treatment improves features of NAFLD in children with serum vitamin D deficiency: results from a single center trial. PLoS One 2016;11(12):e0168216.

53. Holterman AX, Holterman M, Browne A, et al. Patterns of surgical weight loss and resolution of metabolic abnormalities in superobese bariatric adolescents. J Pediatr Surg 2012;47:1633–9.

54. Manco M, Mosca A, De Peppo F, et al. The benefit of sleeve gastrectomy in obese adolescents on nonalcoholic steatohepatitis and hepatic fibrosis. J Pediatr 2017;180:31–7.

Cirrhosis and Portal Hypertension in the Pediatric Population

Catherine A. Chapin, MD, Lee M. Bass, MD*

KEYWORDS

- Cirrhosis • Portal hypertension • Esophageal varices • Ascites • Biliary atresia
- Children

KEY POINTS

- Cirrhosis is a complex diffuse process whereby the architecture of the liver has been replaced by structurally abnormal nodules due to fibrosis.
- Portal hypertension is characterized by a hepatic venous pressure gradient (HVPG) greater than 5 mm Hg with complications, such as ascites and varices, occurring at an HVPG greater than 10 mm Hg.
- Common causes of portal hypertension in children include extrahepatic portal vein obstruction, biliary atresia, alpha 1 antitrypsin deficiency, and autoimmune hepatitis, among others.
- Gastrointestinal bleeding secondary to esophageal or gastric varices may present as hematemesis or melena. Vasoactive drug therapy should be initiated as soon as possible before endoscopic treatment.
- Surgical shunt procedures or transjugular intrahepatic portosystemic shunt may be useful therapeutic options in patients with refractory portal hypertension.

INTRODUCTION

Cirrhosis is defined by the World Health Organization as a diffuse process whereby the architecture of the liver has been replaced by structurally abnormal nodules due to fibrosis.[1] Cirrhosis is a common outcome of a wide spectrum of disease processes (**Table 1**). The pathophysiology of cirrhosis is complex and involves a dynamic interplay between hepatocyte injury, cellular response to injury, and regeneration.[2] Fibrosis

---

Conflict of Interest Statement: Neither Dr L.M. Bass nor Dr C.A. Chapin have any financial conflicts pertaining to the subject matter of this article.
Division of Pediatric Gastroenterology, Hepatology and Nutrition, Ann & Robert H. Lurie Children's Hospital of Chicago, Northwestern University Feinberg School of Medicine, 225 East Chicago Avenue, Box #65, Chicago, IL 60611, USA
* Corresponding author.
E-mail address: lbass@luriechildrens.org

Table 1
Causes of cirrhosis and/or portal hypertension in children

Type	Disorders
Genetic-metabolic disorders	α1-Antitrypsin deficiency *Amyloidosis* Bile acid synthesis defects Cystic fibrosis Galactosemia Gaucher disease Glycogen storage disease type III and IV Hepatic porphyrias Hereditary fructose intolerance Hereditary hemochromatosis Indian childhood cirrhosis Langerhans cell histiocytosis Mitochondrial hepatopathies Niemann-Pick disease type C *Sarcoidosis* Tyrosinemia type I Wilson disease Wolman disease (lysosomal acid lipase deficiency)
Infectious diseases	Ascending cholangitis Chronic hepatitis B ± delta virus Chronic hepatitis C Cytomegalovirus Hepatitis E Herpes simplex virus Recurrent neonatal sepsis Rubella *Schistosomiasis* *Tuberculosis*
Inflammatory diseases	Autoimmune hepatitis Primary sclerosing cholangitis
Cholestatic diseases and biliary malformations	Alagille syndrome and nonsyndromic bile duct paucity Bile duct stenosis Biliary atresia Choledochal cyst Congenital hepatic fibrosis Caroli disease (intrahepatic cystic biliary dilatation) Progressive familial intrahepatic cholestasis
Vascular lesions	*Arteriovenous fistula* Budd-Chiari syndrome Congenital cardiomyopathy *Congenital stenosis or extrinsic compression of the portal vein* Congestive heart failure Constrictive pericarditis *Nodular regenerative hyperplasia* *Portal vein thrombosis* Sinusoidal obstructive syndrome *Splenic vein thrombosis* Venocaval web/inferior vena cava obstruction
Drugs and toxins	Hepatotoxic drugs (isoniazid, methotrexate) Hypervitaminosis A Natural toxins (eg, mushrooms) Organic solvents *Peliosis hepatis* (anabolic steroids, azathioprine) Total parenteral nutrition

(continued on next page)

Table 1 *(continued)*	
Type	**Disorders**
Other	Fatty liver disease
	Hepatocellular carcinoma
	Idiopathic neonatal hepatitis
	Idiopathic or noncirrhotic portal hypertension
	Liver infiltration in hematologic diseases
	Zellweger (cerebrohepatorenal) syndrome

Disorders in bold/italic are causes of isolated portal hypertension.

is a common response to liver injury characterized by accumulation of extracellular matrix (ECM). Prolonged or sustained liver injury leads to chronic inflammation, excessive ECM deposition, and development of scar tissue. Alterations in sinusoidal structure and the formation of bands of connective tissue between portal areas results in poor blood flow and further injury with attempts at compensatory regeneration (nodule formation). Sinusoidal endothelial cells lose the ability to secrete and respond to vasodilators (such as nitric oxide), and levels of vasoconstrictors (such as endothelin-1) are increased.

Hepatic fibrosis may be staged by the degree of severity, from portal expansion to cirrhosis. METAVIR and Ishak are the most commonly used pathologic staging systems (**Table 2**).[3] More often cirrhosis is classified based on clinical outcomes. Patients with compensated cirrhosis have preserved liver synthetic function, with or without varices. Patients with decompensated cirrhosis on the other hand have loss of liver synthetic ability and development of jaundice or complications of portal hypertension including variceal hemorrhage, ascites, and hepatic encephalopathy. In adults the Child-Pugh classification has been widely used to assess the degree of hepatic dysfunction and the relative risk of mortality among patients with cirrhosis.[4] Similarly, the model for end-stage liver disease and pediatric end-stage liver disease scores, including age less than 1 year, serum albumin, serum bilirubin, international normalized ratio, and growth failure, can be used to predict short-term survival for adults and children with chronic liver disease.[5]

Portal hypertension occurs when there is an increase in portal blood flow, an increase in portal resistance to blood flow, or both. A basic paradigm of the pathophysiology of portal hypertension is in **Fig. 1**. Normally the portal venous system

Table 2 METAVIR fibrosis and activity score			
Fibrosis Score		**Activity Score**	
No fibrosis	F0	No activity	A0
Portal fibrosis without septa	F1	Mild activity	A1
Portal fibrosis with few septa	F2	Moderate activity	A2
Portal fibrosis with numerous septa without cirrhosis	F3	Severe activity	A3
Cirrhosis	F4	—	—

From Intraobserver and interobserver variations in liver biopsy interpretation in patients with chronic hepatitis C. The French METAVIR Cooperative Study Group. Hepatology 1994;20(1 Pt 1):15–20; with permission.

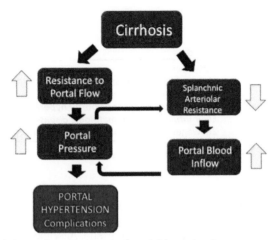

Fig. 1. Pathophysiology of development of portal hypertension.

has a low pressure with a hepatic venous pressure gradient (HVPG) of 1 to 4 mm Hg (the difference between the wedged hepatic venous pressure and the free hepatic venous pressure). Portal hypertension is defined as HVPG greater than 5 mm Hg. An HVPG greater than 10 mm Hg is associated with the development of esophageal varices, and greater than 12 mm Hg is associated with variceal bleeding and ascites. Decreased portal blood flow leads to an increase in systemic vascular resistance and marked splanchnic arterial vasodilation. This increase results in several systemic hemodynamic alterations. A state of low effective circulating blood volume activates the renin-angiotensin-aldosterone system, with a subsequent increase in antidiuretic hormone and sodium and free water retention. Low effective circulating blood volume leads to splanchnic vasodilation and the development of a hyperdynamic circulatory state with increased cardiac output and heart rate. Excess sodium and water retention leads to increased portal blood flow, increased portal pressure, and further exacerbates portosystemic shunting.

Portal hypertension can result from several disorders, including but not exclusive to conditions that also may lead to cirrhosis (see **Table 1**). In children, extrahepatic portal vein thrombosis (EHPVO) is the most common cause of portal hypertension, followed by biliary atresia (BA).[6]

Clinical and Physical Examination Findings and Evaluation

The clinical and physical examination manifestations of cirrhosis and portal hypertension vary depending on the underlying cause and degree of hepatocellular dysfunction and fibrosis (**Table 3**). Signs of portal hypertension include splenomegaly, ascites, and thrombocytopenia. Children frequently exhibit nonspecific signs of systemic illness, including fatigue, muscle weakness, anorexia, nausea, vomiting, and growth failure. Evaluation of patients with suspected cirrhosis and/or portal hypertension should focus on determining the cause of the liver dysfunction, the stage of fibrosis, and the presence and severity of extrahepatic complications. Some of the many diagnostic tests that may be considered are listed in **Table 4**. In addition, all patients should have an abdominal ultrasound with Doppler to evaluate the hepatic echotexture and determine the presence of any structural or vascular anomalies.

Table 3
Findings on clinical history and physical examination that may be seen in patients with cirrhosis and/or portal hypertension

General	Fatigue, anorexia, poor growth, malnutrition, decreased exercise tolerance, fever, nausea
HEENT	Easy bruising or bleeding (nose, gums)
Skin and extremities	Jaundice, pruritus, digital clubbing, cyanosis, flushing or pallor, palmar erythema, spider angiomata, xanthoma, telangiectasia
Msk	Muscle wasting, bone pain or fractures, peripheral edema
Abdomen	Caput medusa, ascites, abdominal distention, abdominal pain, hepatomegaly or a firm small nodular liver, splenomegaly, rectal varices
GU	Delayed puberty, testicular atrophy, gynecomastia
CNS	Asterixis, positive Babinski reflex, hyperreflexia, mental status changes, reversal of sleep-wake cycle, emotional lability

Abbreviations: CNS, central nervous system; GU, genitourinary; HEENT, head, eyes, ears, nose, throat; Msk, Musculoskeletal.

Complications of Portal Hypertension

Ascites

Ascites frequently develops in pediatric patients with cirrhosis and portal hypertension. Ascites occurs when osmotic and hydrostatic pressure within hepatic and mesenteric capillaries exceeds the drainage capacity of lymphatics and excess fluid

Table 4
Diagnostic tests in cirrhosis and/or portal hypertension

Disorder	Diagnostic Tests
Hepatitis B	Hepatitis B surface antigen
Hepatitis C	Hepatitis C antibody
Cytomegalovirus	Serology and/or viral DNA with PCR
Epstein-Barr virus	Serology and/or viral DNA with PCR
Autoimmune hepatitis	Antinuclear antibodies, anti–smooth muscle antibody, anti-liver-kidney-microsomal antibody, and total IgG level
α1-Antitrypsin deficiency	Serum α1-antitrypsin level and α1-antitrypsin phenotype
Glycogen storage disease	Lactic acid, fasting lipid panel, fasting glucose level, uric acid, genetic testing
Galactosemia	Urinary reducing substances, red blood cell galactose-1-phosphate uridyltransferase level
Tyrosinemia	Urine succinylacetone, serum amino acids
Gestational alloimmune liver disease; neonatal hemochromatosis	Buccal biopsy, MRI pancreas, ferritin, alpha-fetoprotein
Cystic fibrosis	Newborn screen, sweat chloride test, genetic testing
Wilson disease	Serum ceruloplasmin, urine 24-h copper, slit-lamp examination, liver copper quantification, genetic testing

Abbreviations: IgG, immunoglobulin G; PCR, polymerase chain reaction.

accumulates in the peritoneal space.[7] Clinically, this may manifest as weight gain, abdominal distention, a fluid wave, ballotable spleen, or shifting dullness on physical examination. Hypoalbuminemia worsens ascites formation, as albumin helps to retain fluid in the capillary lumen. Performance of a diagnostic paracentesis and calculation of the serum-to-ascites albumin gradient (SAAG) helps to differentiate ascites due to portal hypertension (SAAG $\geq$1.1 g/dL) from ascites due to other causes.[8,9] Initial treatment of ascites includes sodium restriction ($\leq$2 mEq/kg/d) as well as diuretic therapy. Fluid restriction is recommended in the setting of severe hyponatremia with serum sodium levels less than 125 mEq/L.[10] Spironolactone, which targets the hyperaldosteronism of portal hypertension, is typically the first-line diuretic, with hydrochlorothiazide and furosemide used as secondary agents. Intermittent therapeutic paracentesis can be performed for symptomatic ascites (abdominal discomfort or respiratory compromise), and in severe cases transjugular intrahepatic portosystemic shunt (TIPS) may be considered.[11] Any patient with ascites who presents with fever and abdominal pain should have a diagnostic paracentesis performed to evaluate for spontaneous bacterial peritonitis (SBP), which is defined as a positive ascitic fluid culture or absolute polymorphonuclear cell count greater than 250 cells per microliter. SBP is usually monomicrobial secondary to gram-negative enteric organisms, most commonly *Escherichia coli*, *Klebsiella pneumoniae*, and *Streptococcal pneumoniae*.[12] Cefotaxime or a similar third-generation cephalosporin is the initial treatment of choice for a 5- to 10-day course.[13] As the risk of recurrence is high, secondary antibiotic prophylaxis with oral norfloxacin, ciprofloxacin, or trimethoprim/sulfamethoxazole is typically recommended.[14,15]

Gastrointestinal bleeding

Gastrointestinal (GI) bleeding secondary to esophageal or gastric varices, presenting as hematemesis and melena, may be the initial manifestation of portal hypertension. Variceal bleeding is associated with an HVPG of greater than 12 mm Hg. There are several grading systems looking at the size of varices; however, few of them have been validated for interobserver reliability[16,17] (**Box 1**). Describing esophageal varices as small or large may be more reproducible among different endoscopists and better correspond to treatment and surveillance recommendations based on variceal size.[18,19] Gastric varices are typically supplied by the short gastric veins and develop in 4 basic patterns. Primary gastric varices generally refer to the presence of gastric varices at initial examination in someone who has never had treatment of esophageal varices. Secondary gastric varices refer to the development of gastric varices after

---

Box 1
Classification of esophageal and gastric varices

Esophageal varices, designed from the Japanese Research Society for Portal Hypertension.[16,17]
- Grade I varices are flattened by insufflation.
- Grade II varices are not flattened by insufflation and are separated by areas of healthy mucosa.
- Grade III varices are confluent and not flattened by insufflation.

Sarin classification of gastric varices
- GOV1 extend 2 to 5 cm below gastroesophageal junction and are in continuity with esophageal veins.
- GOV2 are in cardia/fundus and in continuity with esophageal varices.
- IGV1 are varices that occur in fundus in absence of esophageal varices.
- IGV2 are varices that occur in gastric body, antrum or pylorus.

endoscopic therapy for esophageal varices. Gastric varices in continuity with esophageal varices may regress following treatment of esophageal varices. Additionally, varices may be noted in the small intestine[20] or gall bladder[21] or may present as symptomatic hemorrhoids in the rectum.[22]

Portal hypertensive gastropathy (PHG) is characterized by dilation of the mucosal and submucosal vessels of the stomach and visually appears as discrete cherry-red spots in a lacy mosaic pattern. Bleeding from PHG is usually chronic and should be suspected in cirrhotic patients with persistent iron-deficiency anemia. A high rate of PHG has been demonstrated in pediatric patients with end-stage liver disease.[23] In addition, patients with portal hypertension are at an increased risk of bleeding from other lesions not secondary to portal hypertension, such as gastric or duodenal ulcers and gastritis.

The incidence of gastroesophageal varices in children is disease dependent, as is the risk of bleeding. Large varices, elevated prothrombin time, ascites, increased total bilirubin, the presence of variceal red markings, and the presence of gastric varices are associated with an increased risk of bleeding.[24,25] One long-term study of children with BA demonstrated that the risk of bleeding is 27%.[26] A cross-sectional study of children with BA demonstrated 19% had experienced GI bleeding with 7% having had multiple episodes.[27] In a single-center study evaluating liver transplant in alpha 1 antitrypsin deficiency, 35% of patients presented with liver failure with variceal bleeding.[28] Most patients with cystic fibrosis–related liver disease (CFLD) have splenomegaly and varices,[29] and 10-year cumulative variceal bleeding has been demonstrated to be 6.6%.[30] Age at bleeding also depends on the underlying cause of cirrhosis, with patients who have surgically corrected but progressive BA bleeding for the first time at a mean age of 3 years and those with cystic fibrosis at a mean age of 11.5 years.[31]

Prophylaxis of variceal hemorrhage
Prevention of variceal hemorrhage is categorized by strategy. *Primary prophylaxis* refers to approaches to prevent the first episode of bleeding from established varices and *secondary prophylaxis* targets varices that have already bled.

Primary prophylaxis
In adults with cirrhosis and esophageal varices, the 1-year risk of a variceal hemorrhage is approximately 12%[32]; primary prophylaxis to prevent bleeding is recommended. Although there are no clear pediatric guidelines, surveillance of varices may identify children with cirrhosis and portal hypertension who have an increased risk of bleeding.

Surveillance approaches Most gastroenterologists use clinical features that suggest a child is likely to have varices to decide which patients should undergo primary prophylaxis surveillance. Although more prospective studies are needed to determine the full utility of noninvasive parameters, the clinical predictive rule, albumin level, platelet count, and spleen size may be used for triaging children for endoscopic evaluation.[17,33,34] Less invasive modalities that may be used to screen for varices include esophageal capsule endoscopy, transnasal endoscopy, and small bowel capsule endoscopy. In patients with BA and CFLD, measuring liver stiffness by transient elastography has also been used to screen for varices.[35–37] A pilot study found that measurement of liver and spleen stiffness by acoustic radiation force impulse identified children with high-risk varices.[38]

Most centers perform primary prophylaxis[39] as studies have shown that there is an increased risk of morbidity and mortality even with a first variceal bleed.[40,41] A recent study of screening endoscopy in children with BA and portal hypertension found that 28% of patients who had endoscopy before 2 years of age had grade II and III varices. GI bleeding occurred in 20% of patients, with 6% having a bleeding episode that preceded the first endoscopy.[24] Serial endoscopy in patients who initially have small varices reveals an increase in size over time.[42] However, the utility of primary prophylaxis in the pediatric population remains in question.[43] In the current era with widespread use of vasoactive drugs, such as octreotide, and with liver transplantation options, such as living donation, it is unclear if there is a true mortality risk. The Baveno VI pediatric conference on portal hypertension was unable to come to a conclusion about the benefit of primary prophylaxis in the pediatric population.[44] At this time, decisions regarding primary prophylaxis in children are considered on an individual basis and take into account the specific circumstances of patients, including their proximity to adequate medical care.

Beta-blockade

Beta-blockers reduce portal venous flow by unopposed α-receptor–mediated splanchnic vasoconstriction, thus, decreasing portal pressure. Beta-blockade also decreases cardiac output and reduces the norepinephrine-induced constriction of intrahepatic myofibroblasts, activated stellate cells, and vascular smooth muscle cells.[32,45] Meta-analysis of nonselective beta-blockade (NSBB) as the primary prophylaxis in adults with cirrhosis demonstrated a decrease in the rate of first variceal bleed and mortality over a median 2-year follow-up.[46] The beta-blocker dose is titrated to achieve a reduction in the heart rate of 25% or the maximally tolerated dose.

Potential side effects of NSBB, which may impact the pediatric population, include a lack of response to bronchodilators in patients with reactive airway disease or asthma, exacerbation of peripheral artery disease, blunted response to hypoglycemia, depression, fatigue, and weight gain. Beta-blockade may also inhibit the ability to mount a compensatory increase in heart rate in the setting of hypovolemia, thereby worsening the outcome from a variceal bleed, especially in young infants.[45,47] This concern has limited the use of NSBB in younger children. Although, some clinicians use NSBB as the primary prophylaxis in older children, based on results from adult trials, clear recommendations for this approach await additional evidence.[17]

In children, both endoscopic variceal ligation (EVL) and sclerotherapy have been studied for primary prophylaxis. Duche and colleagues[48] used both techniques for primary prophylaxis in children with BA and major endoscopic risk factors for variceal bleeding and found that 11% went on to have a GI bleed. Approaches for primary prophylaxis of gastric varices in both adults and children are based on bleeding risk, and surgical options or TIPS should be considered.[49]

Secondary prophylaxis

Because of the high recurrence rate of variceal hemorrhage once a first bleed has occurred, secondary prophylaxis is indicated.[17] In children, esophageal variceal obliteration by either EVL or sclerotherapy is recommended to decrease the risk of rebleeding. Treatment sessions should occur every 2 to 4 weeks until varices are eradicated.[18]

Therapy for acute variceal hemorrhage

GI bleeding is the major cause of morbidity in patients with portal hypertension. However, as previously discussed, the risk of mortality has improved over the last few decades with improved medical management[32,50]; mortality rates in children are lower than in adults.

The treatment of patients with portal hypertension and an acute GI hemorrhage is summarized in **Box 2**. The first steps to be taken include protecting the airway, assuring that patients are breathing, and maintaining circulation. A nasogastric tube should be placed to monitor ongoing bleed and remove blood from the GI tract, which can predispose patients with cirrhosis to encephalopathy. Prophylactic antibiotics are recommended in the setting of acute esophageal variceal hemorrhage; all patients should have vasoactive drug therapy, such as octreotide, initiated as soon as possible.[17,51] These drugs work by decreasing splanchnic blood flow, reducing portal venous inflow, and reducing portal pressure. Octreotide can be given as a bolus (1 μg/kg) followed by continuous infusion (1–5 μg/kg/h) or as subcutaneous injections 3 times daily and has been shown to safely slow the rate of GI bleeding in children with varices.[52]

Endoscopy should be performed as soon as possible once patients are stable to determine the source of bleeding. Recent guidelines recommend the administration of erythromycin 3 mg/kg intravenously over 30 minutes before endoscopy to enhance emptying of the stomach and improve visualization on endoscopy.[53,54] Patients failing to respond to fluids, vasoactive medications, and correction of coagulopathy may require emergent endoscopy and rarely placement of a balloon tamponade device, emergent surgical intervention, or TIPS.[17] Endoscopic variceal ligation has largely supplanted endoscopic sclerotherapy for treatment of esophageal varices in both adults and children with good success.[48,55] In pediatrics, sclerotherapy is currently used only in infants and small children (<10 kg) in whom the band ligation device is too large to pass through the upper esophageal sphincter. When sclerotherapy is performed, injections may be either intravariceal, inducing thrombus formation within the vessel, or paravariceal, causing local inflammation that compresses the vessel. Sclerotherapy is effective in the treatment of variceal bleeding but is associated with a higher rate of complications than EVL, including aspiration pneumonia and esophageal stricture.[56] EVL causes thrombosis of the varix and the band and varix subsequently slough off together in about 5 to 7 days. Long-term administration of proton pump inhibitors should be considered to reduce the risk of treatment failure after EVL.[57]

Box 2
Therapy for acute variceal hemorrhage

- Secure the airway

- Intravenous placement with volume resuscitation with blood, crystalloid, or colloid to achieve hemodynamic stability

- Nasogastric tube placement to evaluate ongoing bleed and remove blood from the stomach

- Blood transfuse to a goal of approximately 7 to 8 g/dL

- Octreotide 1 mcg/kg bolus plus 1 mcg/kg/h infusion

- Measurement of platelets and prothrombin time/international normalized ratio

- Vitamin K administration

- Antibiotics: ceftriaxone or norfloxacin

- Consider urgent/emergent endoscopy if ongoing bleeding or hemodynamic instability

- Urgent elective endoscopy if controlled with octreotide and volume expansion

From Shneider BL, Bosch J, de Franchis R, et al. Portal hypertension in children: expert pediatric opinion on the report of the Baveno v consensus workshop on methodology of diagnosis and therapy in portal hypertension. Pediatr Transplant 2012;16(5):426–37; with permission.

The approach to bleeding gastric varices is similar to that of esophageal varices, including initiation of medical therapy with vasoactive agents. Some gastric varices may regress following thrombosis of associated esophageal varices. Injection of varices with tissue adhesives, such as n-butyl-2-cyanoacrylate, has been successful in halting gastric variceal bleeding in children[58,59]; but complications, including pyrexia and abdominal pain, have been described.[60] Balloon-occluded retrograde transvenous obliteration (BRTO) is an interventional radiology technique that obliterates gastric fundal varices[61] and has been used safely in children.[62] Although both BRTO and cyanoacrylate injection may be considered in children with gastric varices, TIPS or portosystemic shunting may be associated with better long-term resolution and outcome.[17]

Surgical therapy and transjugular intrahepatic portosystemic shunt

In patients who fail endoscopic therapy or in whom there are additional problems, such as refractory ascites, shunt surgery, or TIPS, may be considered. In many cases, children with progressive liver disease who fail endoscopic therapies are best treated with liver transplantation. In patients with stable liver disease who are not likely to progress to transplantation soon, surgical shunting may be an excellent option.

Surgical shunting is used to treat complications resulting from noncirrhotic portal hypertension, including idiopathic portal hypertension, congenital hepatic fibrosis, and EHPVO. In the long-term, surgical shunts control bleeding from esophageal or gastric varices in more than 90% of patients[63] and overall outcomes are very good.[64–66] The type of shunt selected depends on the underlying etiology and the vascular anatomy. Meso rex shunt is the recommended option for patients with EHPVO[44] but requires normal liver architecture to ensure long-term patency. The distal splenorenal shunt selectively decompresses esophageal and gastric varices through the splenic vein to the left renal vein.

Creation of a TIPS effectively reduces portal pressure by creating a communication between the hepatic and portal vein. The shunt can be placed by an interventional radiologist and is technically feasible in children.[67] Indications for TIPS in pediatric patients with portal hypertension include recurrent variceal bleeding not responsive to more conservative therapy, hypersplenism, refractory ascites, hepatorenal syndrome, and hepatopulmonary syndrome.[68] Complications include portal vein leakage, encephalopathy, perforation, hemolysis, infection, and restenosis; but overall mortality from the procedure is low.[69] Studies of children with severe portal hypertensive and refractory variceal bleeding or ascites demonstrate a high degree of resolution of symptoms with TIPS.[70,71]

Extrahepatic Manifestations of Portal Hypertension

Cardiopulmonary

Patients with cirrhosis are at an increased risk of cardiopulmonary complications. Hepatopulmonary syndrome (HPS) and portopulmonary hypertension (POPH) are associated with increased mortality.[72] HPS is due to intrapulmonary vasodilation and the development of arteriovenous shunting with resultant hypoxemia. Increased circulating levels of endothelin-1 and nitric oxide as well as pulmonary vascular angiogenesis are thought to play a role.[73] The disorder typically manifests as dyspnea on exertion, but patients may also have digital clubbing, cough, decreased oxygen saturation, and shortness of breath or hypoxemia that worsens with sitting up (platypnea and orthodeoxia, respectively).[74] Liver transplantation is the preferred treatment of HPS with a significant improvement in 5-year survival.[75] POPH is due to increased pulmonary vascular resistance resulting in elevated mean pulmonary artery pressure and is diagnosed by right heart catheterization. POPH typically responds to vasodilators and may improve with liver transplantation but carries a higher risk of cardiopulmonary mortality. Patients with cirrhosis and portal hypertension may also develop cirrhotic cardiomyopathy, which is characterized by impaired contractile response to stress, diastolic dysfunction, and electromechanical abnormalities.[76]

Endocrine and hematologic

Endocrine abnormalities including increased circulating levels of estrogen and other sex hormones may lead to gynecomastia, testicular atrophy, spider angiomata, palmar erythema, and delayed puberty.[77] Hyperinsulinemia or diabetes mellitus and hypothyroidism are also more common in cirrhosis, and patients with end-stage liver disease have relative adrenal insufficiency.[78] Patients with cirrhosis and portal hypertension frequently have anemia, which is multifactorial due to GI blood loss, hemolysis from hypersplenism, micronutrient deficiency secondary to malabsorption and malnutrition, and a dilutional effect from sodium and water retention. Decreased synthesis of liver-derived clotting factors (prothrombin, factor VII and IX) and increased consumption of clotting factors through fibrinolysis and disseminated intravascular coagulation contributes to coagulopathy in cirrhosis, which may be exacerbated by vitamin K deficiency. As anticoagulant and procoagulant factors are decreased to a similar degree, cirrhotic patients are often in a state of homeostasis.[79] However, with any perturbation in this balance, they are at an increased risk of both bleeding and thrombosis. Thrombocytopenia due to splenic sequestration from portal hypertension is common. In addition, patients with cirrhosis are immunocompromised and at an increased risk of infection, most commonly from SBP, urinary tract infections, and pneumonia.[80]

Renal

Hepatorenal syndrome (HRS) is a condition that occurs in patients with cirrhosis and portal hypertension and is associated with increased mortality. Renal vasoconstriction leads to poor renal perfusion, decreased glomerular filtration rate, and a decreased ability to excrete sodium and free water.[81] Type 1 HRS is characterized by the rapid onset of progressive kidney failure and a high mortality versus type 2 HRS, which is more slowly progressive and has a better prognosis.[82] In adults, albumin infusion has been shown to prevent HRS in the setting of SBP.[83,84] Management includes the treatment of reversible causes of renal failure, including hypovolemia, discontinuation of diuretics, and avoidance of nephrotoxic drugs. Vasoconstrictor therapy with terlipressin, octreotide and midodrine, or norepinephrine, with or without albumin, has been shown to be effective in adults and reduce mortality.[85] Renal replacement therapy is often used in patients with azotemia, fluid overload, or electrolyte abnormalities. Liver transplantation can be a treatment of HRS, but some patients continue to require hemodialysis for some interval after transplant.

Growth and nutrition

Malnutrition is a common problem in cirrhosis because of anorexia and inadequate intake, increased metabolic demand, malabsorption, steatorrhea, and fat-soluble vitamin deficiency. Most children with cirrhosis will require fat-soluble vitamin supplementation as well as an increase in total fat and calories. If unable to meet these requirements orally, there should be a low threshold to initiate nasogastric tube feedings; if this fails, begin parenteral nutrition. Stunting secondary to chronic malnutrition is often seen in children with cirrhosis and is associated with poor outcomes.[86] Because of vitamin D deficiency and other factors, cirrhotic patients often have liver-associated bone disease putting them at an increased risk of fractures, which should be screened for with dual energy x-ray absorptiometry scans.[87]

Neurologic

Hepatic encephalopathy (HE) encompasses several reversible neuropsychiatric abnormalities that can be seen in patients with cirrhosis and/or portosystemic shunting. Effects are thought to be secondary to increased levels of potentially neurotoxic substances, such as ammonia, in the systemic circulation and crossing the blood-brain barrier. Manifestations range from mild to severe and are grouped into stages **(Table 5)**.[88] In children, HE is associated with cerebral atrophy and impaired cognitive function that may persist even after liver transplantation.[89] Patients with HE are at risk of cerebral edema secondary to astrocyte swelling from ammonia metabolism. However, in patients with cirrhosis who have chronically elevated ammonia levels, brain osmoregulatory mechanisms are often able to compensate.[90] Minimal HE (MHE) is the mildest form of HE in which patients have no overt symptoms but may have subtle motor and cognitive defects and impairment on neuropsychological tests. Studies suggest that up to 50% of children with chronic liver disease have MHE, which negatively impacts brain function and school performance.[91,92] In most patients, HE is triggered by some precipitating event, such as infection, GI bleeding, or renal failure; initial treatment should focus on identifying and treating these complications. More

Table 5				
Stages of hepatic encephalopathy				
Stage	**Clinical Manifestations**	**Asterixis/ Reflexes**	**Neurologic Signs**	**EEG Changes**
Subclinical	None	Absent/normal	Abnormalities on psychometric testing and proton magnetic spectroscopy in older patients	Usually absent
I	Confused, mood changes, altered sleep habits, loss of spatial orientation, forgetfulness	Absent/normal	Tremor, apraxia, impaired handwriting	May be absent or diffuse, slowing to theta rhythm, triphasic waves
II	Drowsy, inappropriate behavior, decreased inhibitions	Present/ hyperreflexive	Dysarthria, ataxia	Abnormal, generalized slowing, triphasic waves
III	Child is stuporous but obeys simple commands; infant is sleeping but arousable	Present/ hyperreflexive with positive Babinski sign	Muscle rigidity	Abnormal, generalized slowing, triphasic waves
IV	Child is comatose but arousable by painful stimuli (IVa) or does not respond to stimuli (IVb)	Absent	Decerebrate or decorticate	Abnormal, very slow delta activity

Abbreviation: EEC, electroencephalography.

Data from Rogers EL. Hepatic encephalopathy. Crit Care Clin 1985;1(2):313–25; and Devictor D, Tahiri C, Lanchier C, et al. Flumazenil in the treatment of hepatic encephalopathy in children with fulminant liver failure. Intensive Care Med 1995;21(3):253–6.

long-term therapeutic options include nonabsorbable disaccharides (such as lactulose or lactitol) that acidify the stool and trap ammonia as the less absorbable ammonium and nonabsorbable antibiotics (such as rifaximin), which decrease ammonia production from gut bacteria.[93]

SUMMARY

Portal hypertension remains a significant cause of morbidity and mortality in pediatric patients with cirrhosis. The natural history of portal hypertension in pediatrics still requires further elucidation. As we develop a better understanding of the underlying mechanisms of this disease, more treatment options for portal hypertension may arise.

REFERENCES

1. Garcia-Tsao G, Friedman S, Iredale J, et al. Now there are many (stages) where before there was one: in search of a pathophysiological classification of cirrhosis. Hepatology 2010;51:1445–9.
2. Schuppan D, Afdhal NH. Liver cirrhosis. Lancet 2008;371:838–51.
3. Intraobserver and interobserver variations in liver biopsy interpretation in patients with chronic hepatitis C. The French METAVIR cooperative study group. Hepatology 1994;20:15–20.
4. Pugh RN, Murray-Lyon IM, Dawson JL, et al. Transection of the oesophagus for bleeding oesophageal varices. Br J Surg 1973;60:646–9.
5. McDiarmid SV, Anand R, Lindblad AS. Development of a pediatric end-stage liver disease score to predict poor outcome in children awaiting liver transplantation. Transplantation 2002;74:173–81.
6. Weiss B, Shteyer E, Vivante A, et al. Etiology and long-term outcome of extrahepatic portal vein obstruction in children. World J Gastroenterol 2010;16:4968–72.
7. Giefer MJ, Murray KF, Colletti RB. Pathophysiology, diagnosis, and management of pediatric ascites. J Pediatr Gastroenterol Nutr 2011;52:503–13.
8. Runyon BA, Montano AA, Akriviadis EA, et al. The serum-ascites albumin gradient is superior to the exudate-transudate concept in the differential diagnosis of ascites. Ann Intern Med 1992;117:215–20.
9. European Association for the Study of the Liver. EASL clinical practice guidelines on the management of ascites, spontaneous bacterial peritonitis, and hepatorenal syndrome in cirrhosis. J Hepatol 2010;53:397–417.
10. Suchy FJ, Sokol RJ, Balistreri WF, editors. Liver disease in children. 4th edition. New York: Cambridge University Press; 2014.
11. Lane ER, Hsu EK, Murray KF. Management of ascites in children. Expert Rev Gastroenterol Hepatol 2015;9:1281–92.
12. Caruntu FA, Benea L. Spontaneous bacterial peritonitis: pathogenesis, diagnosis, treatment. J Gastrointest Liver Dis 2006;15:51–6.
13. Runyon BA, McHutchison JG, Antillon MR, et al. Short-course versus long-course antibiotic treatment of spontaneous bacterial peritonitis. A randomized controlled study of 100 patients. Gastroenterology 1991;100:1737–42.
14. Gines P, Rimola A, Planas R, et al. Norfloxacin prevents spontaneous bacterial peritonitis recurrence in cirrhosis: results of a double-blind, placebo-controlled trial. Hepatology 1990;12:716–24.
15. Singh N, Gayowski T, Yu VL, et al. Trimethoprim-sulfamethoxazole for the prevention of spontaneous bacterial peritonitis in cirrhosis: a randomized trial. Ann Intern Med 1995;122:595–8.

16. Beppu K, Inokuchi K, Koyanagi N, et al. Prediction of variceal hemorrhage by esophageal endoscopy. Gastrointest Endosc 1981;27:213–8.

17. Shneider BL, Bosch J, de Franchis R, et al. Portal hypertension in children: expert pediatric opinion on the report of the Baveno v consensus workshop on methodology of diagnosis and therapy in portal hypertension. Pediatr Transplant 2012; 16:426–37.

18. D'Antiga L. Medical management of esophageal varices and portal hypertension in children. Semin Pediatr Surg 2012;21:211–8.

19. D'Antiga L, Betalli P, De Angelis P, et al. Interobserver agreement on endoscopic classification of oesophageal varices in children. J Pediatr Gastroenterol Nutr 2015;61:176–81.

20. Bass LM, Kim S, Superina R, et al. Jejunal varices diagnosed by capsule endoscopy in patients with post-liver transplant portal hypertension. Pediatr Transplant 2017;21. https://doi.org/10.1111/petr.12818.

21. Yamada RM, Hessel G. Ultrasonographic assessment of the gallbladder in 21 children with portal vein thrombosis. Pediatr Radiol 2005;35:290–4.

22. Heaton ND, Davenport M, Howard ER. Symptomatic hemorrhoids and anorectal varices in children with portal hypertension. J Pediatr Surg 1992;27:833–5.

23. Ng NB, Karthik SV, Aw MM, et al. Endoscopic evaluation in children with end-stage liver disease-associated portal hypertension awaiting liver transplant. J Pediatr Gastroenterol Nutr 2016;63:365–9.

24. Duche M, Ducot B, Tournay E, et al. Prognostic value of endoscopy in children with biliary atresia at risk for early development of varices and bleeding. Gastroenterology 2010;139:1952–60.

25. Duche M, Ducot B, Ackermann O, et al. Portal hypertension in children: high-risk varices, primary prophylaxis and consequences of bleeding. J Hepatol 2017;66:320–7.

26. Lampela H, Kosola S, Koivusalo A, et al. Endoscopic surveillance and primary prophylaxis sclerotherapy of esophageal varices in biliary atresia. J Pediatr Gastroenterol Nutr 2012;55:574–9.

27. Shneider BL, Abel B, Haber B, et al. Portal hypertension in children and young adults with biliary atresia. J Pediatr Gastroenterol Nutr 2012;55:567–73.

28. Bakula A, Pawlowska J, Niewiadomska O, et al. Liver transplantation in Polish children with alpha1-antitrypsin deficiency: a single-center experience. Transplant Proc 2016;48:3323–7.

29. Stonebraker JR, Ooi CY, Pace RG, et al. Features of severe liver disease with portal hypertension in patients with cystic fibrosis. Clin Gastroenterol Hepatol 2016; 14:1207–15.e3.

30. Ye W, Narkewicz MR, Leung DH, et al. Variceal hemorrhage and adverse liver outcomes in patients with cystic fibrosis cirrhosis. J Pediatr Gastroenterol Nutr 2017. https://doi.org/10.1097/MPG.0000000000001728.

31. Debray D, Lykavieris P, Gauthier F, et al. Outcome of cystic fibrosis-associated liver cirrhosis: management of portal hypertension. J Hepatol 1999;31:77–83.

32. Garcia-Tsao G, Bosch J. Management of varices and variceal hemorrhage in cirrhosis. N Engl J Med 2010;362:823–32.

33. Colli A, Gana JC, Yap J, et al. Platelet count, spleen length, and platelet count-to-spleen length ratio for the diagnosis of oesophageal varices in people with chronic liver disease or portal vein thrombosis. Cochrane Database Syst Rev 2017;(4):CD008759.

34. Witters P, Hughes D, Karthikeyan P, et al. King's variceal prediction score: a novel noninvasive marker of portal hypertension in pediatric chronic liver disease. J Pediatr Gastroenterol Nutr 2017;64:518–23.

35. Chang HK, Park YJ, Koh H, et al. Hepatic fibrosis scan for liver stiffness score measurement: a useful preendoscopic screening test for the detection of varices in postoperative patients with biliary atresia. J Pediatr Gastroenterol Nutr 2009; 49:323–8.

36. Colecchia A, Di Biase AR, Scaioli E, et al. Non-invasive methods can predict oesophageal varices in patients with biliary atresia after a Kasai procedure. Dig Liver Dis 2011;43:659–63.

37. Malbrunot-Wagner AC, Bridoux L, Nousbaum JB, et al. Transient elastography and portal hypertension in pediatric patients with cystic fibrosis Transient elastography and cystic fibrosis. J Cyst Fibros 2011;10:338–42.

38. Tomita H, Ohkuma K, Masugi Y, et al. Diagnosing native liver fibrosis and esophageal varices using liver and spleen stiffness measurements in biliary atresia: a pilot study. Pediatr Radiol 2016;46:1409–17.

39. Jeanniard-Malet O, Duche M, Fabre A. Survey on clinical practice of primary prophylaxis in portal hypertension in children. J Pediatr Gastroenterol Nutr 2017;64: 524–7.

40. Ling SC. Advances in the evaluation and management of children with portal hypertension. Semin Liver Dis 2012;32:288–97.

41. van Heurn LW, Saing H, Tam PK. Portoenterostomy for biliary atresia: long-term survival and prognosis after esophageal variceal bleeding. J Pediatr Surg 2004;39:6–9.

42. Duche M, Ducot B, Ackermann O, et al. Progression to high-risk gastroesophageal varices in children with biliary atresia with low-risk signs at first endoscopy. J Pediatr Gastroenterol Nutr 2015;60:664–8.

43. Bozic MA, Puri K, Molleston JP. Screening and prophylaxis for varices in children with liver disease. Curr Gastroenterol Rep 2015;17:27.

44. Shneider BL, de Ville de Goyet J, Leung DH, et al. Primary prophylaxis of variceal bleeding in children and the role of MesoRex Bypass: summary of the Baveno VI pediatric satellite symposium. Hepatology 2016;63:1368–80.

45. Ling SC, Walters T, McKiernan PJ, et al. Primary prophylaxis of variceal hemorrhage in children with portal hypertension: a framework for future research. J Pediatr Gastroenterol Nutr 2011;52:254–61.

46. D'Amico G, Pagliaro L, Bosch J. The treatment of portal hypertension: a meta-analytic review. Hepatology 1995;22:332–54.

47. Ling SC. Should children with esophageal varices receive beta-blockers for the primary prevention of variceal hemorrhage? Can J Gastroenterol 2005;19:661–6.

48. Duche M, Ducot B, Ackermann O, et al. Experience with endoscopic management of high-risk gastroesophageal varices, with and without bleeding, in children with biliary atresia. Gastroenterology 2013;145:801–7.

49. Maruyama H, Sanyal A. Portal hypertension: non-surgical and surgical management. In: Maddrey WS, Eugene R, Sorrell MF, editors. Schiff's diseases of the liver. 11th edition. Hoboken (NJ): Wiley; 2011.

50. Carbonell N, Pauwels A, Serfaty L, et al. Improved survival after variceal bleeding in patients with cirrhosis over the past two decades. Hepatology 2004;40:652–9.

51. de Franchis R. Revising consensus in portal hypertension: report of the Baveno V consensus workshop on methodology of diagnosis and therapy in portal hypertension. J Hepatol 2010;53:762–8.

52. Eroglu Y, Emerick KM, Whitingon PF, et al. Octreotide therapy for control of acute gastrointestinal bleeding in children. J Pediatr Gastroenterol Nutr 2004;38:41–7.
53. Altraif I, Handoo FA, Aljumah A, et al. Effect of erythromycin before endoscopy in patients presenting with variceal bleeding: a prospective, randomized, double-blind, placebo-controlled trial. Gastrointest Endosc 2011;73:245–50.
54. Barkun AN, Bardou M, Martel M, et al. Prokinetics in acute upper GI bleeding: a meta-analysis. Gastrointest Endosc 2010;72:1138–45.
55. dos Santos JM, Ferreira AR, Fagundes ED, et al. Endoscopic and pharmacological secondary prophylaxis in children and adolescents with esophageal varices. J Pediatr Gastroenterol Nutr 2013;56:93–8.
56. Abd El-Hamid N, Taylor RM, Marinello D, et al. Aetiology and management of extrahepatic portal vein obstruction in children: King's College Hospital experience. J Pediatr Gastroenterol Nutr 2008;47:630–4.
57. Hidaka H, Nakazawa T, Wang G, et al. Long-term administration of PPI reduces treatment failures after esophageal variceal band ligation: a randomized, controlled trial. J Gastroenterol 2012;47:118–26.
58. Rivet C, Robles-Medranda C, Dumortier J, et al. Endoscopic treatment of gastroesophageal varices in young infants with cyanoacrylate glue: a pilot study. Gastrointest Endosc 2009;69:1034–8.
59. Fuster S, Costaguta A, Tobacco O. Treatment of bleeding gastric varices with tissue adhesive (Histoacryl) in children. Endoscopy 1998;30:S39–40.
60. Turler A, Wolff M, Dorlars D, et al. Embolic and septic complications after sclerotherapy of fundic varices with cyanoacrylate. Gastrointest Endosc 2001;53: 228–30.
61. Kumamoto M, Toyonaga A, Inoue H, et al. Long-term results of balloon-occluded retrograde transvenous obliteration for gastric fundal varices: hepatic deterioration links to portosystemic shunt syndrome. J Gastroenterol Hepatol 2010;25: 1129–35.
62. Hisamatsu C, Kawasaki R, Yasufuku M, et al. Efficacy and safety of balloon-occluded retrograde transvenous obliteration for gastric fundal varices in children. Pediatr Surg Int 2008;24:1141–4.
63. de Ville de Goyet J, D'Ambrosio G, Grimaldi C. Surgical management of portal hypertension in children. Semin Pediatr Surg 2012;21:219–32.
64. Emre S, Dugan C, Frankenberg T, et al. Surgical portosystemic shunts and the Rex bypass in children: a single-centre experience. HPB (Oxford) 2009;11: 252–7.
65. Lillegard JB, Hanna AM, McKenzie TJ, et al. A single-institution review of portosystemic shunts in children: an ongoing discussion. HPB Surg 2010;2010: 964597.
66. Scholz S, Sharif K. Surgery for portal hypertension in children. Curr Gastroenterol Rep 2011;13:279–85.
67. Lorenz JM. Placement of transjugular intrahepatic portosystemic shunts in children. Tech Vasc Interv Radiol 2008;11:235–40.
68. Paramesh AS, Husain SZ, Shneider B, et al. Improvement of hepatopulmonary syndrome after transjugular intrahepatic portasystemic shunting: case report and review of literature. Pediatr Transplant 2003;7:157–62.
69. Gazzera C, Righi D, Doriguzzi Breatta A, et al. Emergency transjugular intrahepatic portosystemic shunt (TIPS): results, complications and predictors of mortality in the first month of follow-up. Radiol Med 2012;117:46–53.

70. Di Giorgio A, Agazzi R, Alberti D, et al. Feasibility and efficacy of transjugular in-trahepatic portosystemic shunt (TIPS) in children. J Pediatr Gastroenterol Nutr 2012;54:594–600.

71. Heyman MB, LaBerge JM, Somberg KA, et al. Transjugular intrahepatic portosys-temic shunts (TIPS) in children. J Pediatr 1997;131:914–9.

72. Hoeper MM, Krowka MJ, Strassburg CP. Portopulmonary hypertension and hep-atopulmonary syndrome. Lancet 2004;363:1461–8.

73. Sussman NL, Kochar R, Fallon MB. Pulmonary complications in cirrhosis. Curr Opin Organ Transplant 2011;16:281–8.

74. Sari S, Oguz D, Sucak T, et al. Hepatopulmonary syndrome in children with cirrhotic and non-cirrhotic portal hypertension: a single-center experience. Dig Dis Sci 2012;57:175–81.

75. Swanson KL, Wiesner RH, Krowka MJ. Natural history of hepatopulmonary syn-drome: impact of liver transplantation. Hepatology 2005;41:1122–9.

76. Wiese S, Hove JD, Bendtsen F, et al. Cirrhotic cardiomyopathy: pathogenesis and clinical relevance. Nat Rev Gastroenterol Hepatol 2014;11:177–86.

77. Maheshwari A, Thuluvath PJ. Endocrine diseases and the liver. Clin Liver Dis 2011;15:55–67.

78. Kim G, Huh JH, Lee KJ, et al. Relative adrenal insufficiency in patients with cirrhosis: a systematic review and meta-analysis. Dig Dis Sci 2017;62:1067–79.

79. Zakeri N, Tsochatzis EA. Bleeding risk with invasive procedures in patients with cirrhosis and coagulopathy. Curr Gastroenterol Rep 2017;19:45.

80. Bonnel AR, Bunchorntavakul C, Reddy KR. Immune dysfunction and infections in patients with cirrhosis. Clin Gastroenterol Hepatol 2011;9:727–38.

81. Arroyo V, Fernandez J, Gines P. Pathogenesis and treatment of hepatorenal syn-drome. Semin Liver Dis 2008;28:81–95.

82. Salerno F, Gerbes A, Gines P, et al. Diagnosis, prevention and treatment of hep-atorenal syndrome in cirrhosis. Gut 2007;56:1310–8.

83. Sort P, Navasa M, Arroyo V, et al. Effect of intravenous albumin on renal impair-ment and mortality in patients with cirrhosis and spontaneous bacterial peritonitis. N Engl J Med 1999;341:403–9.

84. Sigal SH, Stanca CM, Fernandez J, et al. Restricted use of albumin for sponta-neous bacterial peritonitis. Gut 2007;56:597–9.

85. Gluud LL, Christensen K, Christensen E, et al. Systematic review of randomized trials on vasoconstrictor drugs for hepatorenal syndrome. Hepatology 2010;51: 576–84.

86. Utterson EC, Shepherd RW, Sokol RJ, et al. Biliary atresia: clinical profiles, risk factors, and outcomes of 755 patients listed for liver transplantation. J Pediatr 2005;147:180–5.

87. Lopez-Larramona G, Lucendo AJ, Gonzalez-Castillo S, et al. Hepatic osteodys-trophy: an important matter for consideration in chronic liver disease. World J Hepatol 2011;3:300–7.

88. Wijdicks EF. Hepatic encephalopathy. N Engl J Med 2016;375:1660–70.

89. Garcia-Martinez R, Rovira A, Alonso J, et al. Hepatic encephalopathy is associ-ated with posttransplant cognitive function and brain volume. Liver Transpl 2011;17:38–46.

90. Mas A. Hepatic encephalopathy: from pathophysiology to treatment. Digestion 2006;73(Suppl 1):86–93.

91. Srivastava A, Chaturvedi S, Gupta RK, et al. Minimal hepatic encephalopathy in children with chronic liver disease: prevalence, pathogenesis and magnetic resonance-based diagnosis. J Hepatol 2017;66:528–36.

92. Mack CL, Zelko FA, Lokar J, et al. Surgically restoring portal blood flow to the liver in children with primary extrahepatic portal vein thrombosis improves fluid neuro-cognitive ability. Pediatrics 2006;117:e405–12.

93. Elwir S, Rahimi RS. Hepatic encephalopathy: an update on the pathophysiology and therapeutic options. J Clin Transl Hepatol 2017;5:142–51.

Pediatric Liver Tumors

Kenneth Ng, DO, Douglas B. Mogul, MD, MPH*

KEYWORDS

- Liver • Tumor • Pediatrics • Evaluation • Diagnosis • Management

KEY POINTS

- Although liver tumors are rare in the pediatric population, they are common in the setting of children with specific risk factors requiring increased awareness and, in some instances, screening.
- The evaluation of a liver mass in children is largely driven by the age at diagnosis, the presence of any medical comorbidities, and initial testing with alpha fetoprotein and imaging.
- Specific guidelines for the management of different tumors have been implemented in recent years such that a multidisciplinary approach is ideal and care should be provided by centers with experience in their management.

INTRODUCTION

Liver tumors in childhood are rare. Approximately two-thirds of all pediatric liver tumors are malignant, including hepatoblastoma (HB; 37%), hepatocellular carcinoma (HCC; 21%), and sarcoma (8%), and these cancers comprise approximately 1% of all childhood tumors reported to the Surveillance, Epidemiology, and End Results (SEER) registry.[1–3] Benign tumors (vascular lesions such as hemangiomas and hemangioendotheliomas [15%], focal nodular hyperplasia [5%], mesenchymal hamartomas [7%]) can also be clinically challenging if they are large enough to compress neighboring organs and replace normal-functioning hepatic tissue.

Although uncommon, it is important that general pediatricians as well as subspecialists in pediatric gastroenterology and hepatology continue to be aware of the epidemiology, clinical presentation, and the initial approach to the diagnosis of these diseases. First, these tumors may be more frequently seen in specific subgroups, such as in individuals with genetic conditions associated with increased cancer risk as well as children with specific risk factors such as prematurity (**Table 1**).[4,5] Furthermore, evidence exists that the incidence of HB is increasing, with a doubling of the rate from 0.6

Disclosure: The authors have nothing to disclose, and no commercial or financial conflicts of interest.
Department of Pediatrics, Johns Hopkins School of Medicine, 600 North Wolfe Street, CMSC 2-117, Baltimore, MD 21287, USA
* Corresponding author.
E-mail address: dmogul1@jhmi.edu

Table 1
Risk factors for hepatoblastoma and hepatocellular carcinoma in children

Risk Factor	HB	HCC
Extreme prematurity and low birthweight	X	—
Total parenteral nutrition	—	X
Infections		
Hepatitis B virus	—	X
Hepatitis C virus	—	X
Tumor syndromes		
Familial adenomatous polyposis and Gardner syndrome	X	X
Beckwith-Wiedemann	X	—
Neurofibromatosis	—	X
Li-Fraumeni	X	—
Glycogen storage disease (type I and III)	X	X
Hereditary tyrosinemia	—	X
Congenital cholestasis		
Biliary atresia	—	X
Progressive familial intrahepatic cholestasis type 2	—	X
Alagille syndrome	—	X
α-1-antitrypsin deficiency	—	X
Other Genetic Diseases		
Trisomy 21	X	—
Ataxia telangiectasia	—	X
Fanconi anemia	—	X
Medications		
Methotrexate	—	X
Oral contraceptives	—	X
Anabolic steroids	—	X
Underlying Liver Disease		
Congenital hepatic fibrosis	—	X
Congenital portosystemic shunt	X	X
Hepatic adenoma	—	X

cases per million between 1973 and 1977 to 1.2 cases per million between 1993 and 1997, and this can likely be attributed to the increased survival of premature infants.[1,6] Third, the increasing use of computed tomography (CT) and ultrasonography scanning for the routine evaluation of children in the emergency room and other settings has led to a corresponding increase in the identification of incidental findings of hepatic lesions in children.[7] Pediatricians may therefore see increasing numbers of these masses over time.

CLINICAL PRESENTATION

Most liver masses are asymptomatic and are detected through palpation by either a parent or a physician.[5,8] In rare instances, children present with complications stemming from obstruction of major bile ducts by the mass, leading to jaundice and pruritus, as well as fever (ie, cholangitis) and biliary colic. Compression of hepatic vasculature can lead to portal hypertension with resultant ascites and gastrointestinal bleeding. HCC and sarcoma may also present with advanced stages of liver disease, including ascites, malnutrition, and anorexia, as well as additional complications of liver failure, including hepatic encephalopathy and multiorgan failure; metastatic disease to the lungs is rare but may occur.[5]

Specific sequelae can be seen with individual tumors, including fever and thrombocytosis in HB.[9] Precocious puberty may occur with tumors that produce human chorionic gonadotropin (HCG) or testosterone, such as germ cell tumors. Hemangiomas may be associated with lesions in the skin, and may also present with symptoms of hypothyroidism and congestive heart failure.[10,11]

INITIAL APPROACH

The differential diagnosis of hepatic tumors is largely driven by the age of presentation (**Table 2**). Ninety percent of children less than 5 years of age with a malignant hepatic mass have HB.[1] Among older children, HCC is the most common malignancy, whereas HB is extremely rare.[1,9] A different spectrum of hepatic masses may exist for neonates, with a single-center review identifying hemangiomas (60%) as the most frequent tumors in infants less than 2 months old, followed by mesenchymal hamartomas (23%) and HB (17%).[12]

Alpha fetoprotein (AFP) is the most important tumor marker in the evaluation of hepatic masses. AFP level is increased in 90% of children with HB and 50% of children with HCC. Normal AFP level in the setting of HB has been generally shown to correlate with a worse prognosis, although some subtypes of HB (eg, well-differentiated, fetal-type HB) may have normal/low AFP level and favorable prognosis.[5,13,14] In healthy neonates, AFP levels are extremely high (eg, 500,000 ng/mL) but decrease over the course of infancy before reaching adult levels by around the eighth month of life.[15] Consequently, given the wide ranges for normal levels during the first several months of life, this can obfuscate the clinician's ability to determine whether an individual's level is excessive and suggests an AFP-producing tumor. Similarly, increased AFP level has been reported in individuals with benign tumors, such as infantile hemangiomas and mesenchymal hamartomas, such that this marker by itself cannot be used to confirm HB or HCC. Nonetheless, AFP is an important test in the initial work-up of children with a hepatic tumor, and in risk stratification for children with HB.

In addition to routine bloodwork (blood count, albumin, transaminases, bilirubin, alkaline phosphatase, gamma-glutamyl transferase, and coagulation studies), several additional tests can aid in the diagnosis.[9] Second-line studies to be considered include hepatitis B and C, given their known association with HCC, as well as Epstein Barr Virus, which can cause lymphoma. Levels of other markers may be increased in

Table 2		
Pediatric liver tumors according to age at presentation		
Age	**Malignant**	**Benign**
Infants and toddlers	Hepatoblastoma Rhabdoid Malignant germ cell	Hemangioma/vascular Mesenchymal hamartoma Teratoma
School age and adolescents	Hepatocellular carcinoma Embryonal (undifferentiated) sarcoma Angiosarcoma	Adenoma Focal nodular hyperplasia

tumors of the liver and should be checked, including β-HCG (germ cell tumors), ferritin (HCC and metastatic neuroblastoma), carcinoembryonic antigen (HCC and metastatic colon cancer), lactate dehydrogenase (many tumors), and catecholamines (metastatic neuroblastoma).

Ultrasonography is frequently used in the initial assessment of a hepatic mass that has been detected on physical examination.[16] This technique can provide screening information regarding size, echogenicity, focality, and demarcation. Doppler can also be used to better understand whether there is vascular involvement or presence of thrombi. Given that ultrasonography is nonradiating, and can be performed quickly and without anesthesia, this modality can be especially useful in following up benign lesions such as hemangiomas, hamartomas, and adenomas. Ultimately, most masses require additional cross-sectional imaging such as CT or MRI, which more accurately describe the properties of the mass, the degree of demarcation, and the extent of invasion into vessels or other organs.

MALIGNANT TUMORS
Staging

No system of staging applies to all pediatric liver tumors or is universally accepted by all oncology groups. In Europe, the Liver Tumor Strategy Group of the Societe Internationale d'Oncologie Pediatrique (SIOPEL) developed the PRETEXT (pretreatment extent of disease) classification, based on the number of contiguous sections that are tumor free on cross-sectional imaging, to define the extent of disease and guide treatment, and this has been adopted by the Children's Oncology Group (COG) (**Fig. 1**).

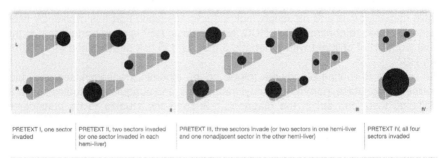

PRETEXT Pretreatment Extent of Disease
POSTTEXT Posttreatment Extent of Disease (i.e., extent of liver involvement after pre-operative chemotherapy)

The tumor is classified into one of the following four stages depending on the number of liver sectors that are invaded by the tumor.

| PRETEXT I, one sector invaded | PRETEXT II, two sectors invaded (or one sector invaded in each hemi-liver) | PRETEXT III, three sectors invade (or two sectors in one hemi-liver and one nonadjacent sector in the other hemi-liver) | PRETEXT IV, all four sectors invaded |

Additional Criteria
(annotation factors):

V	Involvement of the inferior vena cava and/or hepatic veins	R	Tumor rupture or Intraperitonealhaemorrhage
P	Involvement of the portal vein	N	Lymph node metastases
E	Extrahepatic abdominal disease	C	Caudate lobe involvement
F	Tumor focality	M	Distant metastases

Fig. 1. PRETEXT/POSTTEXT groups I, II, III, and IV, with annotation. (*Courtesy of* J. Skeele, Baltimore, MD.)

Patients should also have a chest CT scan as part of the work-up to evaluate for metastases. Additional modifiers are given to further describe the mass:

- (V) inferior vena cava and/or hepatic veins involvement
- (P) portal vein involvement
- (E) extrahepatic disease
- (C) caudate lobe involvement
- (R) tumor rupture or intraperitoneal bleed
- (N) lymph node metastases
- (F) multifocal tumor
- (M) presence of distant metastases[17]

The POSTTEXT (posttreatment extent of disease after chemotherapy but before surgery) classification is used to downstage tumors after neoadjuvant chemotherapy. For HB, COG assigns patients into treatment strata based on a combination of PRETEXT/POSTTEXT staging, history, AFP values, and elements of the Evans staging system:

1. Complete resection at diagnosis
2. Resection at diagnosis with residual microscopic disease
3. Biopsy without resection at diagnosis
4. Distant metastases

For HCC, PRETEXT or the Evans staging system are used. In contrast with the surgical staging system in the United States, Europeans adhere to a risk stratification system to stage patients and guide chemotherapy for all patients before surgery, as discussed later.

Hepatoblastoma

Epidemiology and genetics
Approximately two-thirds of all malignant liver tumors in children are HB, and 90% of patients present before 5 years of age.[1] Although data from 1999 identified an estimated 100 cases per year, the incidence has increased approximately 4% per year between 1992 and 2004, which is greater than other childhood cancers.[18,19] Part of the shift in epidemiology may largely be caused by emerging evidence that prematurity and very low birth weight are associated with development of HB.[19] This finding has been reported consistently in several studies using diverse cohorts throughout the world, further strengthening the likely causal association. Odds of developing HB given prematurity have been reported to range from 9.5 to 69, and are likely influenced by the degree of birth weight reduction, with most studies investigating infants less than 1500 g, rather than gestational age. The mechanism leading to increased risk of HB is unknown but oxygen, other medications (eg. diuretics and total parenteral nutrition), radiation, and plasticizers that are present in the neonatal intensive care unit are possible factors.

Clinical factors may confer increased risk in infants. Preeclampsia, polyhydramnios/oligohydramnios, and high pregnancy weight may be associated with HB.[19] Infertility and its treatment may also be independently associated with HB, whereas increased maternal or paternal age do not seem to increase risk.

Several environmental factors have been explored as potential causes of HB. Studies have put forth a risk of smoking in either parent, and more strongly if both parents smoke, such that the International Agency for Research on Cancer has declared parental tobacco exposure a carcinogen to the liver.[19,20] Parental exposure to metal and petroleum products has been suggested as being associated with increased occurrence of HB and a recent study of paternal paint exposure was also independently associated with HB development.[21,22]

In addition to prematurity and environmental exposures, the strong association with genetic syndromes (see **Table 1**) has facilitated the identification of some of the genetic underpinnings, including gene mutations in the *Wnt/β*-catenin signaling pathway, which is well-known to influence oncogenesis as well as embryonal development.[23] One Japanese study showed that most patients with HB had an abnormality in the pathway, such as accumulation of β-catenin, and upregulation of genes including *cyclin, D1, survivin,* and *MYC,* as well as *TERT,* which regulates the expression of telomerase, which is involved in cell death.[24] These specific mutations seem to be associated with specific tumor histology as well as treatment response.

Pathology

HB is an embryonal tumor that is derived from hepatic precursor cells in various stages of maturation and that frequently contains heterogeneous cell types. Most tumors are composed entirely of epithelial cells and can be categorized further as well-differentiated fetal, mixed embryonal/fetal, macrotrabecular, small cell undifferentiated, or cholangioblastic (**Box 1**).[25] The well-differentiated fetal subtype can be divided further as showing low mitotic activity or being mitotically active with crowding. Although systematic assessments of HB invariably are based on small cohorts of patients, a recent international symposium organized by COG found that more than half of the patients with pure epithelial tumors had well-differentiated fetal histology. The macrotrabecular subtype is largely distinguished by its growth in cords, with a subtype that also contains fetal/embryonal elements and another type that looks more hepatocellular and may be confused with HCC. Individuals with the small cell undifferentiated subtype usually have low to normal serum AFP levels and,

---

Box 1
International consensus classification for hepatoblastoma

Epithelial variants

Pure fetal with low mitotic activity

Fetal, mitotically active

Pleomorphic, poorly differentiated

Embryonal

Small cell undifferentiated
   Integrase interactor 1 (INI1) negative
   INI1 positive

Epithelial mixed (any/all above)

Cholangioblastic

Epithelial macrotrabecular pattern

Mixed epithelial and mesenchymal variants

Without teratoid features

With teratoid features

Adapted from López-Terrada D, Alaggio R, de Dávila MT, et al. Towards an international pediatric liver tumor consensus classification: proceedings of the Los Angeles COG liver tumors symposium. Mod Pathol 2014;27(3):474; with permission.

---

correspondingly, are associated with poorer prognosis. These tumors may share several characteristics with malignant rhabdoid tumors, including lack of integrase interactor 1 (INI1) expression, and therefore may respond to a different treatment algorithm including chemotherapeutic agents directed toward malignant rhabdoid tumors.

In addition to epithelial elements, approximately 20% to 30% of cases of HB have mesenchymal derivatives, including spindle cells, osteoid, skeletal muscle, and cartilage.[26] If these mesenchymal cells are derived from endoderm, neuroectoderm, or melanin-containing elements, then the tumor can be classified as containing teratoid features.

Given variable risk associated with tumor subtype, it is recommended that all patients undergo a biopsy. Specimens may be collected using percutaneous, laparoscopic core needle or wedge biopsy, or open core needle or wedge biopsy; fine-needle aspiration should not be used to avoid inadequate sampling.[26] If core needles are used, it is recommended that 5 to 10 samples are taken, each 1×0.3 cm. Biopsies should be taken before chemotherapy is started and should ideally be fresh samples. Care should be taken to avoid seeding, close communication between surgeon and radiologist is paramount, and the tract should be one that will be incorporated into the surgical resection. If possible, adjacent, nontumor should be biopsied to better characterize the tumor and to assess the liver for evidence of chronic liver disease.

Risk stratification

Several factors have been shown to correlate with prognosis as reported by the recently formed Children's Hepatic Tumors International Collaboration (CHIC); this consortium with members of COG, SIOPEL, the German Society for Pediatric Oncology and Hematology (GPOH), and the Japanese Study Group for Pediatric Liver Tumors (JPLT) pooled data and experience in order to more thoroughly address prognostic risk factors in HB and help individualize therapy.[27]

Pooled data from CHIC identified several important prognostic variables in HB. Age at start of treatment less than 1 year was associated with favorable response, whereas greater than 8 years was associated with worse outcomes; prematurity or birth weight were not independently associated with worse prognosis, nor was a diagnosis of Beckwith-Wiedemann syndrome. AFP levels less than 1000 ng/mL and greater than 1×10^6 ng/mL were associated with poorer outcomes. Better prognosis was seen in PRETEXT I and II, and worse in PRETEXT IV or any tumors that had metastasis at diagnosis, unresectable vessel involvement, extrahepatic tumor extension, multifocal tumors, or tumor rupture at diagnosis. Notably, this consortium did not examine tissue histology as a determinant of outcomes, even though COG studies have shown that the well-differentiated or fetal subtype has favorable prognosis because it is not recognized by the other groups and a clear definition does not presently exist. Likewise, evidence exists that the small cell undifferentiated subtype has a worse prognosis but was not directly addressed by CHIC.[28] Posttreatment factors are likely to inform outcomes, including response to chemotherapy, surgical margins and resectability, and tumor relapse.

Although these variables provide independent assessment of an individual's prognosis, different organizations still have different approaches to risk stratification. COG stratifies individuals based primarily on PRETEXT staging. PRETEXT I or II tumors with pure fetal histology are considered very low risk, whereas PRETEXT I or II tumors with other histologies (excluding small cell undifferentiated) are considered low/standard risk (**Table 3**).[29–32] PRETEXT III/IV tumors or tumors with small cell undifferentiated histology represent intermediate risk, whereas any tumors with metastatic disease

Table 3
Risk stratification in hepatoblastoma

	Very Low Risk	Low/Standard Risk	Intermediate Risk	High Risk
COG	PRETEXT I/II, pure fetal histology, primary resection	PRETEXT I/II, any histology, primary resection	PRETEXT III/IV; unresectable at diagnosis; V/P/E+; SCUD histology	Any PRETEXT but M+; AFP<100 ng/mL
SIOPEL/ GPOH	—	PRETEXT I–III, AFP>100 ng/	—	PRETEXT IV; PRETEXT I–III but P/V/E/H/M/N+; AFP<100 ng/mL; SCUD histology
JPLT	—	PRETEXT I–III	PRETEXT IV; tumor rupture; N1, P2, P2aV3, and V3a multifocal	Any PRETEXT M1N2, AFP<100 ng/mL

Abbreviation: SCUD, small cell undifferentiated.

or AFP level less than 100 ng/mL are classified as high risk. SIOPEL defines a standard risk for PRETEXT I to III with normal AFP level, or high risk if the individual is PRETEXT IV or PRETEXT III but with additional factors (eg, portal vein invasion, AFP level <100 ng/mL, or small cell undifferentiated histology).

Treatment

Complete surgical resection is the goal of all therapies, but different organizations vary in their approach to management.[33] COG, having defined a very low risk category (ie, well-differentiated fetal histology with PRETEXT I/II), recommends upfront resection with no chemotherapy. Resection at diagnosis is recommended for patients with PRETEXT I or II tumors with 1-cm radiographic margins from the middle hepatic vein, the retrohepatic inferior vena cava, and the portal bifurcation.[34] Low-risk patients receive upfront resection and then adjuvant chemotherapy. Intermediate-risk and high-risk individuals receive neoadjuvant therapy followed by resection and adjuvant chemotherapy. This approach is in distinction to SIOPEL/GPOH, which uses chemotherapy up front for all tumors irrespective of risk.

Cisplatin is the cornerstone of all chemotherapeutic regimens and is typically combined with 5-fluorouracil, with COG recommending the addition of vincristine for low-risk individuals (C5V) and the further addition of doxorubicin (C5VD) for intermediate-risk and high-risk individuals.[34] In a 2009 COG protocol, AHEP0731, the combination of vincristine, irinotecan, and temsirolimus, was explored as adjunct chemotherapeutic agents for high-risk disease. Drug resistance can occur in HB, so surgical resection should take place before prolonged exposure to chemotherapy. Cross-sectional imaging is typically repeated before the third round of chemotherapy and before surgery to downstage the tumor (POSTTEXT). Study have shown that most of the chemotherapeutic effects take place during the first 2 rounds of chemotherapy and most of the tumor shrinkage occurs during this period.[35] Patients with tumors that remain unresectable after the second round of chemotherapy should be referred to a center with expertise in liver transplant.[36]

Indications for transplant

Unresectable HB with disease isolated to the liver should be considered for liver transplant. POSTTEXT scans should be used to identify patients who should be referred to a liver transplant center with expertise in liver tumors. Referral to these centers should be considered early in subsets of patients with either PRETEXT IV disease or if tumor location is very close to both the portal veins and/or all 3 hepatic veins at diagnosis. Current COG guidelines recommend liver transplant after 4 cycles of cisplatin-based chemotherapy. Prolonged chemotherapy in hopes of achieving sufficient margins for resection have been shown to be ineffective and may induce drug resistance.[34] Findings from the upcoming CHIC trial may reshape surgical guidelines.

Transplant is appropriate for individuals with metastatic disease provided there is radiographic evidence of tumor clearance following chemotherapy and/or metastases resection. Notably, primary transplant for individuals with unresectable HB produced better survival than rescue transplant for individuals after tumor resection.[37] At the same time, a retrospective review had similar overall outcomes for individuals who received a transplant compared with complex resection, although randomized trials are lacking.

Adjunct therapies
Transarterial chemoembolization (TACE) and radiofrequency ablation have been trialed in pediatric patients with cancer.[38,39] Both techniques provide localized therapy and may aid in tumor shrinkage. Although these tools are currently not part of COG guidelines, they may be considered in patients who are unable to tolerate systemic chemotherapy.

Hepatocellular Carcinoma

Epidemiology
HCC is a rare tumor in children, with less than 1% of all cases occurring in individuals less than 20 years of age. HCC is more common in male patients than in female patients (3:1).[40] Among children, it is more typically found in adolescents, although it has been reported in school-aged children as well. Factors that are associated with HCC in adults, such as hepatitis B and hepatitis C, have been implicated in childhood HCC, but certain populations of children are also at risk for HCC in the setting of genetic diseases, such as those with tyrosinemia, glycogen storage disease, alpha1-antitrypsin deficiency, Alagille syndrome, and progressive intrahepatic familial cholestasis type 2. HCC has also been reported in diseases that lack a clear genetic cause but is more typically associated with childhood liver disease, including biliary atresia and parenteral nutrition–associated liver disease. Other diseases associated with HCC include autoimmune hepatitis, hemochromatosis, and primary sclerosing cholangitis.[41] Despite these predisposing risk factors and the potential for children with underlying disease to be identified through screening, children are more likely than adults to be identified with advanced disease, including distant metastases and large tumors.[42] Similar to adults, cirrhosis from any cause increases risk but it is not necessary in the pathogenesis of HCC, such that only 20% to 35% of children with HCC have complications of chronic liver disease. Fibrolamellar HCC represents 10% to 25% of HCC in adolescents and is not associated with cirrhosis.[17,40] Children are more likely than adults to present with the fibrolamellar type, although when HCC presents at less than 5 years of age it is more likely to be nonfibrolamellar.[42,43]

Clinical presentation and evaluation
As with most tumors, individuals present with nonspecific symptoms, most commonly abdominal pain, weight loss, or an appreciable abdominal mass, whereas symptoms associated with cirrhosis are less common. AFP levels are increased in only 50% to 70% of patients, and typically exceed 200 ng/mL.[3,44] HCC is readily seen on imaging, with magnetic resonance being the preferred modality.[45] Both CT and MRI have

characteristic enhancement during the arterial phase and hypoenhancement during the portal venous phase. Masses can be either solitary or multifocal, and can be either well defined or infiltrating. Chest CT is recommended to evaluate for metastatic disease. Image-guided needle biopsy should be performed by a skilled biopsy service, with the following precautions: (1) approach through a segment that is unaffected but will be removed during surgery; (2) use of coaxial system that allows for multiple cores from a single puncture; and (3) placement of some form of plug, such as foam.

Histology

HCC is generally divided into 2 histopathologic types: (1) fibrolamellar, which is largely well circumscribed and solitary; and (2) nonfibrolamellar, which is more typically multicentric. The fibrolamellar variant is composed of large cells with copious eosinophilic oncocytic cytoplasm (from mitochondrial accumulation) in a lamellated or hyalinized stroma.[40] In addition, a transitional tumor variant, also referred to as hepatocellular neoplasm not otherwise specified, has been described that has cells that have features of hepatoblasts and mature hepatocytes.[17]

Prognosis and management

HCC is largely chemoresistant so prognosis depends heavily on surgical resectability. Like HB, the PRETEXT system has been used to surgically stage HCC and, given that surgical resectability is integral to survival, may be the best prognostic predictor, with improved 5-year survival in PRETEXT I through III ranging from 100% to 93%, compared with PRETEXT IV at 40%.[17] Other determinants include lymphovascular invasion, extrahepatic disease, and metastatic disease. However, most children present with more advanced disease, with only 20% of children likely to have resectable tumor at diagnosis.[46] Because of chemoresistance, either surgical resectability or transplant should be considered at the earliest possible opportunity. Adults with HCC who require transplant are evaluated according to the Milan criteria. Some clinicians argue that this system may not be applicable to children with HCC because of biological differences between pediatric and adult HCC.[17] Presence of extrahepatic tumor is a contraindication to transplant. Fibrolamellar HCC has better 1-year and 5-year overall survival (OS) compared with nonfibrolamellar HCC, but this observation may be caused by its earlier stage at diagnosis or more favorable opportunities for surgical resectability.[43] Hepatocellular neoplasm not otherwise specified is more challenging to manage, and liver transplant centers may incorporate chemotherapy as part of the treatment plan. As with adults, TACE has been shown to benefit patients who are either awaiting transplant or to increase the potential for resectability. There is some debate as to whether pediatric HCC is more chemosensitive than in adults, with more than one-third responding to platinum-based and doxorubicin-based therapy.[47] More recently, antiangiogenesis drugs such as sorafenib have shown promise in adults and are being explored for use in children.[48,49] Despite these multiple modalities for treatment, treatment of HCC is estimated to be around 20% to 30%.[47]

Other Malignancies

Undifferentiated embryonal sarcoma of the liver

Undifferentiated embryonal sarcoma of the liver (UESL) is derived from the mesenchyme and, as such, shares features with mesenchymal hamartoma. UESL accounts for 9% to 15% of pediatric liver cancers and is the third most common pediatric liver malignancy. Peak incidence occurs between the ages of 6 and 10 years. Just like HB and HCC, patients typically present with abdominal symptoms, including a palpable mass, pain, nausea, and feeding intolerance. Serum AFP level is not usually increased. There have been reports of germline p53 mutations in some patients with UESL.[50] The tumor is usually unifocal and large (ie, >10 cm) but well demarcated from the liver. The mass appears as a hypodense mixture of cystic and solid components on cross-sectional imaging. UESL can present at diagnosis with metastases to the lungs or lymph nodes. Liver biopsy can be difficult given its cystic nature. The tumor consists of spindle-shaped or stellate-shaped cells in a myxoid matrix with multinucleated giant cells and eosinophilic globules. Negative myogenin staining differentiates UESL from rhabdomyosarcomas.

Treatment requires complete surgical resection and typically chemotherapy.[51] There is no standardized chemotherapy protocol for UESL, and centers have used agents used to treat other soft tissue sarcomas or rhabdomyosarcoma in patients with UESL. Unresectable UESL localized to the liver benefits from liver transplant. Shi and colleagues[51] looked at OS in 103 children less than 18 years of age with UESL in the National Cancer Database between 1998 and 2012 and found that the 5-year OS was 86%. Five-year OS in children who underwent combination therapy (chemotherapy and surgery) was 92%. Ten of 103 patients received orthotopic liver transplant and all survived to 5 years. Tumor size greater than or equal to greater than or equal to 15 cm and combination therapy were independent prognostic factors.

Biliary rhabdomyosarcoma

Biliary rhabdomyosarcoma (BR) is another mesenchymal cancer that may present as an intraluminal biliary mass or cluster of grapelike masses.[52] Median age of presentation is 3 years and children may present with abdominal pain, abdominal distension, vomiting, or jaundice.[53] Patients may have markedly increased conjugated bilirubin levels. Ultrasonography is usually used during the initial stages of the diagnostic work-up. Cross-sectional imaging is also important to further categorize the mass. Lung and bone metastases have been described and should be evaluated as part of the work-up. Histology may have either embryonal or botryoid features. In addition to chemotherapy and surgical resection, radiation therapy has been used in the management of BR. Endoscopic retrograde cholangiopancreatography may be required to address biliary obstruction.[52] There has been 1 case report of liver transplant for recurrent BR in an 8-year-old child.[54] Treatment complications include pancytopenia, sepsis, and peritonitis requiring broad-spectrum antibiotic coverage. Five-year OS is 60% to 70%.[53]

Hepatic angiosarcoma

Hepatic angiosarcoma (HAS) is a rare high-grade tumor of vascular endothelial cells that is believed to be the malignant transformation of infantile hepatic hemangioma (IHH).[55] Mean age of diagnosis is 3 years.[56] Patients may present with abdominal pain, abdominal swelling, feeding intolerance, or nausea.[17] Differentiating between a benign vascular liver tumor and a malignant vascular tumor with radiography may be difficult.[55] MRI may identify areas of necrosis and hemorrhage.[56] On histology, HAS consists of clusters or whorls of sarcomatous cells.[55] Because the cancer can develop from IHH, misdiagnosis as well as bleeding complications must be considered. Metastases to the lung, bone, lymph nodes, adrenal glands, and kidney have been described. Complete surgical resection is paramount but, given the large size of the tumor, this may be difficult. Although not standardized, chemotherapy is often part of the treatment plan. Successful liver transplant has been described in case report and series.[55,56] Prognosis is generally poor, with a median survival of 14 to 18 months and 5-year OS at 20% to 35%.[56] Given that HAS may develop from IHH, this unique subset of patients should have serial ultrasonography to monitor for malignant transformation.

Malignant rhabdoid tumors

Malignant rhabdoid tumor (MRT) is a rare and aggressive tumor initially thought to be a variant of Wilms tumor.[57] Its name is derives from the tumor's histologic resemblance to rhabdomyoblasts. The median age of presentation is 8 months and most patients present before the age of 2 years. Patients may present with nonspecific symptoms, including abdominal pain, early satiety, abdominal distension, or vomiting. Serum AFP level is usually normal. On imaging, rhabdoid tumors are large, heterogeneous, and may have cystic features as well as calcifications. Seventy percent of patients have metastatic disease at diagnosis, most commonly in the lungs and lymph nodes.[58] Rhabdoid tumors are cytologically discohesive, composed of round cells with large, irregularly, and eccentrically placed nuclei in abundant eosinophilic cytoplasm containing bundles of intermediate filaments that are cytokeratin and vimentin positive.[59] The tumor lacks muscle markers and demonstrates a loss of nuclear integrase interactor (INI) protein. Hepatoblastoma with small cell undifferentiated histology can mimic MRT but does not have INI mutation.[52] Treatment typically includes surgery and chemotherapy.[57] There was 1 pediatric liver transplant for MRT described in a case series by Trobaugh-Lotrario and colleagues,[59] and the child survived cancer free for at least 3 years posttransplant. Prognosis is poor, with a median survival of 2 months.[58]

Posttransplant care for malignant liver tumors

There is currently no standardized protocol for posttransplant immunosuppression for patients who were transplanted for malignant liver tumors, but, given that patients may have received chemotherapy before and after transplant, the authors recommend that this subset of patients receive a lower immunosuppression regimen. Transplant hepatologists are tasked to balance the risk of organ rejection, systemic infection, immunosuppression medication–related complications (ie, nephrotoxicity), posttransplant lymphoproliferative disease (PTLD), and other transplant-related conditions in a patient population that will also receive chemotherapy. Studies have previously suggested that patients with HB who receive liver transplants may have a lower risk for acute cellular rejection, thereby supporting the idea of reducing immunosuppression in this patient population.[60] Moreover, 1 case report described PTLD in a child after liver transplant for HB, again suggesting that a lower immunosuppression regimen should be considered.[61]

Patients with AFP-generating tumors need serial monitoring with serum AFP along with imaging to check for cancer recurrence. Persistent increase of AFP level postsurgery increases concern for residual disease. Patients with all other liver cancers should also have serial imaging to monitor for cancer recurrence. A multidisciplinary approach with members from pediatric transplant hepatology, pediatric transplant surgery, pediatric radiology, pathology, and pediatric oncology is imperative not only before liver transplant but also after transplant.

BENIGN TUMORS

Infantile Hepatic Hemangioma

IHH is the most common benign tumor of the liver in infancy.[41] IHH may be focal, multifocal, or diffuse. Children may present with abdominal mass and associated obstructive symptoms, such as vomiting and jaundice. A subset develop serious complications, such congestive heart failure, a consumptive coagulopathy with thrombocytopenia (Kasabach-Merritt syndrome), an abdominal compartment syndrome, and hypothyroidism from overproduction of type III iodothyronine deidonase.[62] Focal IHH, which is the hepatic analog of cutaneous rapidly involuting congenital hemangioma, typically involutes shortly after birth without any complications. Multifocal lesions involute in a similar pattern to cutaneous infantile hemangiomas, over a period of 6 to 10 years. Diffuse lesions tend to replace almost the entire liver parenchyma and are associated with complications.

Diagnosis is usually made based on a combination of clinical findings and imaging.[16] Ultrasonography, including prenatal imaging, shows a hypoechoic mass and Doppler shows a range of flow patterns. CT imaging shows a well-defined hypodense lesion that enhances with contrast from the periphery toward the center of the lesion. With MRI, T1-weighted images are hypointense unless hemorrhage is present, whereas T2-weighted images are hyperintense with centripetal contrast enhancement. Lesions can be complicated either by a central varix with arteriovenous shunt, necrosis, central thrombosis, or diffuse hemangiomatosis. In cases in which clinical findings or imaging are atypical, biopsy is recommended. Focal IHH is GLUT-1 (glucose transporter protein isoform 1) stain negative, whereas multifocal and diffuse IHH are GLUT-1 positive.[62]

Infantile lesions frequently regress but many patients need pharmacologic or surgical intervention.[41] In a large series of 55 patients, 13 (24%) required no intervention, whereas 24 (44%) used steroids or interferon-2a, and 18 (33%) required additional surgery or embolization. For patients who are symptomatic, an algorithm has been developed that incorporates steroids as first-line therapy.[63] Besides steroids and interferon-2α, the latter of which should not be used in children less than 1 year old given the risk of spastic diplegia, other drugs that are used include propranolol as well as chemotherapeutic agents such as vincristine and cyclophosphamide.[41,64] If pharmacologic therapy fails and the patient continues to be symptomatic, as occurs in nearly one-third of patients, then embolization can be considered for multifocal lesions, whereas transplant may be necessary for diffuse lesions.[65] Overall, diffuse lesions are the least responsive to medical therapy and most likely to need transplant. Although outcomes are generally favorable, screening abdominal ultrasonography is recommended for infants with 5 or more cutaneous infantile hemangiomas.[62] Patients with multifocal or diffuse IHH should have serial thyroid function checks and close cardiac follow-up until the IHH has regressed to monitor for congestive heart disease.

Mesenchymal Hamartoma

Mesenchymal hamartomas of the liver (MHL) are the second most common benign hepatic masses found in children, and typically present in the first 2 years of life.[66] Most masses are more than 10 cm at presentation but have been reported as large as 30 cm and are more commonly in the right lobe.[67] Consequently, most children present with abdominal swelling, although abdominal pain, anorexia, vomiting, diarrhea, and abnormal weight gain may occur.

Liver tests, including AFP, are typically normal, although increased levels of AFP have been reported and can be difficult to interpret in infants.[68] These tumors may be identified on prenatal or postnatal ultrasonography and findings are variable based on whether the mass is solid or cystic with septae.[16] CT and MRI can further identify variable elements, with lack of enhancement of cystic components and increased enhancement of solid components and septae after intravenous contrast is given. If necessary to further differentiate from other tumors (eg, embryonal sarcoma), ultrasonography-guided needle biopsy with multiple passes is preferred to fine needle aspiration.[52] MHL consists of spindle cells in a myxoid background, with occasional areas of extramedullary hematopoiesis, all in a disordered arrangement of mesenchyme, malformed bile ducts, and cords of normal-appearing hepatocytes.[16] It can be structurally porous, which allows fluid accumulation within its cystic spaces.

When identified in a fetus, intrauterine drainage of the cyst has been used.[69] Given the potential for spontaneous involution, watchful waiting may be considered if symptoms are minimal, as opposed to aspiration or surgical resection.[70] However, cyst drainage as well as marsupialization may be controversial given that malignant transformation to embryonal sarcoma, although rare, has been reported.[71] Liver transplant for unresectable MHL has been reported.[52]

Focal Nodular Hyperplasia

Focal nodular hyperplasia (FNH) is a well-circumscribed, nonneoplastic lesion characterized by benign-appearing hepatocytes in the presence of vascular anomalies and ductular proliferation, as well as prominent fibrous stroma that forms a stellate "scar."[72] FNH can occur in any age group, with a median age of 8.7 years, and approximately two-thirds of children with FNH are female.[73] Additional risk factors include history of malignancy as well as vascular malformations such as congenital absence of the portal vein and hemangiomas.

Most patients with FNH are asymptomatic. Among the 20% to 36% of children who do have symptoms, the most common presentation is a palpable mass with, or without, abdominal pain. Patients with prior malignancy are more likely to present without symptoms, presumably as a consequence of routine surveillance in this population. These patients are also more likely to present with multifocal FNH and the lesions are less likely to have central scars.[16]

Bloodwork, including AFP, is usually not informative, whereas imaging can yield characteristic findings.[16] Approximately one-quarter of cases have multifocal FNH, and these can range from 1 to 20 cm, with a mean of 6 cm. Ultrasonography, although not as specific as CT and MRI, shows a hyperechoic, homogeneous, and well-demarcated lesion. CT imaging shows a well-circumscribed, homogeneous lesion that is isodense to slightly hypodense to surrounding tissue and has a hypoattenuating central scar. With contrast, the mass enhances homogeneously and is hyperintense during the arterial phase and then becomes isointense during the venous and delayed phase. Similarly, MRI shows a stellate scar and masses are isointense to slightly hypointense lesions on T1-weighted images and slightly hyperintense lesions on T2-weighted images that become hyperintense in the arterial phase following administration of gadolinium. In the review by Lautz and colleagues,[73] a central scar was noted in only 60% of CT studies and 32% of MRI studies.

Atypical clinical, biochemical, or radiographic findings warrant lesion biopsy. FNH is characterized as bile duct proliferation and a central stellate scar containing blood vessels.[74] The glutamine synthetase (nitrogen metabolism enzyme) stain is commonly used to help differentiate FNH from other liver lesions.[52]

Management depends on confidence in the diagnosis, as well as the presence of symptoms. In a large series, nearly 60% of people had resection and the remainder were equally likely to have a biopsy with observation or observation alone.[73] Among those who had a resection, the most common indication was symptoms (48%), followed by an inability to rule out malignancy (24%), tumor growth (15%), and biopsy-proven malignancy (9%). These findings suggest that, despite the benign nature of FNH, children frequently require invasive procedures to confirm the diagnosis and/or manage symptoms.

Nodular Regenerative Hyperplasia

Nodular regenerative hyperplasia (NRH) represents a rare benign process that involves replacement of the normal hepatic architecture with regenerative nodules in the absence of fibrosis. Other names include idiopathic noncirrhotic portal hypertension, idiopathic portal hypertension, and hepatic portal sclerosis.[75] The disease is especially rare in children but may occur in the setting of other systemic diseases, such as thrombophilic conditions, vasculitis, myeloproliferative disorders, and other hematologic abnormalities. It has also been reported with the use of cytotoxic drugs and immunosuppression. De novo NRH has been described 2 pediatric patients after liver transplant.[76] In addition, there is a strong association between NRH and congenital portosystemic shunts. Patients are typically asymptomatic, although they may have clinically relevant sequelae of portal hypertension, including gastrointestinal bleeding.

NRH can be difficult to diagnose, with imaging that is largely nonspecific.[16] Because nodularity can be small and multifocal, ultrasonography may indicate only heterogeneous echotexture. Distinction from cirrhotic disease may be challenging, although elastography may be useful.[77] CT and T2-weighted MRI imaging typically show hypoattenuation or isoattenuation and do not enhance after contrast. Prognosis is generally favorable and management is directed toward monitoring for and treating portal hypertension.

Hepatic Adenoma

Although fairly common in young women and those using oral contraceptives, hepatic adenomas (HAs) are rare in children, accounting for 2% to 4% of all hepatic tumors in children.[16] Many conditions have been reported to predispose to HA, including glycogen storage disease (GSD) type 1 and 3, galactosemia, tyrosinemia, hyperthyroidism, familial adenomatosis polyposis, Turcot syndrome, Lynch syndrome, congenital portosystemic shunts, Fanconi anemia, use of anabolic steroids, polycystic ovarian syndrome, and diabetes. AFP level is normal in this tumor, and individuals with predisposing conditions should be monitored with serial AFP checks and ultrasounds. From a review of published cases, the overall likelihood of malignant transformation is reported as approximately 4% and yearly monitoring is recommended.[78,79] Risk also increases with size and it has rarely been reported as less than 8 cm in diameter.[79] However, individuals with GSD type I and III are at significantly increased risk of developing multiple HAs and are especially prone to malignant transformation to HCC.[80]

On imaging, these lesions are well circumscribed but can be distinguished from FNH given that HAs are typically heterogeneous with the presence of necrosis and hemorrhage, intratumoral fat, and/or calcifications.[16] In addition, these tumors do not have the characteristic central scar of FNH. On histology, HA is composed of benign-appearing hepatocytes, which may contain increased amounts of fat and glycogen, organized in sheets or cords. It is characterized by scattered thin-walled vascular channels within the mass and absence of portal and central veins, bile ducts, as well as connective tissue.

Observation, embolization, or ablation can be used for management of symptomatic HA. Masses can be resected provided at least 20% of functioning liver will remain. If necessary, transplant is indicated if the tumor cannot be resected, is at high risk of transformation, or the patient is symptomatic.[81,82]

SUMMARY

Although pediatric liver tumors are seen infrequently, their diagnosis and management often require not only a comprehensive understanding of the lesions but also a multidisciplinary approach in their management. Specific guidelines and recommendations have been implemented in recent years to guide treatment. Complicated cases, especially those that may require liver transplant, should be referred to centers with expertise in the lesions.

REFERENCES

1. Darbari A, Sabin KM, Shapiro CN, et al. Epidemiology of primary hepatic malignancies in U.S. children. Hepatology 2003;38(3):560–6.
2. Stocker J. Hepatic tumors in children. 2nd edition. Philadelphia: Lippincott Williams and Wilkins; 2001.
3. Weinberg AG, Finegold MJ. Primary hepatic tumors of childhood. Hum Pathol 1983;14(6):512–37.
4. Finegold MJ, Egler RA, Goss JA, et al. Liver tumors: pediatric population. Liver Transpl 2008;14(11):1545–56.
5. Pizzo P, Poplack D. Pediatric liver tumors. [Chapter: 28]. 6th edition. Philadelphia: Lippincott Williams and Wilkins; 2011.
6. Spector LG, Puumala SE, Carozza SE, et al. Cancer risk among children with very low birth weights. Pediatrics 2009;124(1):96–104.
7. Berland LL, Silverman SG, Gore RM, et al. Managing incidental findings on abdominal CT: white paper of the ACR incidental findings committee. J Am Coll Radiol 2010;7(10):754–73.
8. Suchy FJ, Sokol RJ, Balistreri WF. Liver disease in children. 3rd edition. New York: Cambridge University Press; 2007.
9. von Schweinitz D. Management of liver tumors in childhood. Semin Pediatr Surg 2006;15(1):17–24.
10. Huang SA, Tu HM, Harney JW, et al. Severe hypothyroidism caused by type 3 iodothyronine deiodinase in infantile hemangiomas. N Engl J Med 2000;343(3):185–9.
11. Mueller BU, Mulliken JB. The infant with a vascular tumor. Semin Perinatol 1999;23(4):332–40.
12. Isaacs H. Fetal and neonatal hepatic tumors. J Pediatr Surg 2007;42(11):1797–803.
13. De Ioris M, Brugieres L, Zimmermann A, et al. Hepatoblastoma with a low serum alpha-fetoprotein level at diagnosis: the SIOPEL group experience. Eur J Cancer 2008;44(4):545–50.
14. Meyers RL, Rowland JR, Krailo M, et al. Predictive power of pretreatment prognostic factors in children with hepatoblastoma: a report from the children's oncology group. Pediatr Blood Cancer 2009;53(6):1016–22.
15. Wu JT, Book L, Sudar K. Serum alpha fetoprotein (AFP) levels in normal infants. Pediatr Res 1981;15(1):50–2.
16. Chiorean L, Cui X-W, Tannapfel A, et al. Benign liver tumors in pediatric patients - review with emphasis on imaging features. World J Gastroenterol 2015;21(28):8541–61.
17. Aronson DC, Meyers RL. Malignant tumors of the liver in children. Semin Pediatr Surg 2016;25(5):265–75.
18. Linabery AM, Ross JA. Trends in childhood cancer incidence in the U.S. (1992-2004). Cancer 2008;112(2):416–32.
19. Spector LG, Birch J. The epidemiology of hepatoblastoma. Pediatr Blood Cancer 2012;59(5):776–9.
20. Secretan B, Straif K, Baan R, et al. A review of human carcinogens–Part E: tobacco, areca nut, alcohol, coal smoke, and salted fish. Lancet Oncol 2009;10(11):1033–4.

21. Buckley JD, Sather H, Ruccione K, et al. A case-control study of risk factors for hepatoblastoma. A report from the Childrens Cancer Study Group. Cancer 1989;64(5):1169–76.

22. Janitz AE, Ramachandran G, Tomlinson GE, et al. Maternal and paternal occupational exposures and hepatoblastoma: results from the HOPE study through the children's oncology group. J Expo Sci Environ Epidemiol 2017;27(4):359–64.

23. Czauderna P, Lopez-Terrada D, Hiyama E, et al. Hepatoblastoma state of the art: pathology, genetics, risk stratification, and chemotherapy. Curr Opin Pediatr 2014;26(1):19–28.

24. Takayasu H, Horie H, Hiyama E, et al. Frequent deletions and mutations of the beta-catenin gene are associated with overexpression of cyclin D1 and fibronectin and poorly differentiated histology in childhood hepatoblastoma. Clin Cancer Res 2001;7(4):901–8.

25. López-Terrada D, Alaggio R, de Dávila MT, et al. Towards an international pediatric liver tumor consensus classification: proceedings of the Los Angeles COG liver tumors symposium. Mod Pathol 2014;27(3):472–91.

26. Tanaka Y, Inoue T, Horie H. International pediatric liver cancer pathological classification: current trend. Int J Clin Oncol 2013;18(6):946–54.

27. Czauderna P, Haeberle B, Hiyama E, et al. The Children's Hepatic Tumors International Collaboration (CHIC): novel global rare tumor database yields new prognostic factors in hepatoblastoma and becomes a research model. Eur J Cancer 2016;52:92–101.

28. Haas JE, Feusner JH, Finegold MJ. Small cell undifferentiated histology in hepatoblastoma may be unfavorable. Cancer 2001;92(12):3130–4.

29. Maibach R, Roebuck D, Brugieres L, et al. Prognostic stratification for children with hepatoblastoma: the SIOPEL experience. Eur J Cancer 2012;48(10):1543–9.

30. Hishiki T. Current therapeutic strategies for childhood hepatic tumors: surgical and interventional treatments for hepatoblastoma. Int J Clin Oncol 2013;18(6): 962–8.

31. Haeberle B, Schweinitz DV. Treatment of hepatoblastoma in the German cooperative pediatric liver tumor studies. Front Biosci (Elite Ed) 2012;4:493–8.

32. Malogolowkin MH, Katzenstein HM, Krailo M, et al. Treatment of hepatoblastoma: the North American cooperative group experience. Front Biosci (Elite Ed) 2012;4: 1717–23.

33. Kremer N, Walther AE, Tiao GM. Management of hepatoblastoma: an update. Curr Opin Pediatr 2014;26(3):362–9.

34. Trobaugh-Lotrario AD, Meyers RL, O'Neill AF, et al. Unresectable hepatoblastoma: current perspectives. Hepat Med 2017;9:1–6.

35. Lovvorn HN, Ayers D, Zhao Z, et al. Defining hepatoblastoma responsiveness to induction therapy as measured by tumor volume and serum alpha-fetoprotein kinetics. J Pediatr Surg 2010;45(1):121–8 [discussion: 129].

36. Kueht M, Thompson P, Rana A, et al. Effects of an early referral system on liver transplantation for hepatoblastoma at Texas Children's Hospital. Pediatr Transplant 2016;20(4):515–22.

37. McAteer JP, Goldin AB, Healey PJ, et al. Surgical treatment of primary liver tumors in children: outcomes analysis of resection and transplantation in the SEER database. Pediatr Transplant 2013;17(8):744–50.

38. Ye J, Shu Q, Li M, et al. Percutaneous radiofrequency ablation for treatment of hepatoblastoma recurrence. Pediatr Radiol 2008;38(9):1021–3.

39. Zhang J, Xu F, Chen K, et al. An effective approach for treating unresectable hepatoblastoma in infants and children: pre-operative transcatheter arterial chemoembolization. Oncol Lett 2013;6(3):850–4.
40. Kelly D, Sharif K, Brown RM, et al. Hepatocellular carcinoma in children. Clin Liver Dis 2015;19(2):433–47.
41. Meyers RL. Tumors of the liver in children. Surg Oncol 2007;16(3):195–203.
42. Lau CSM, Mahendraraj K, Chamberlain RS. Hepatocellular carcinoma in the pediatric population: a population based clinical outcomes study involving 257 patients from the Surveillance, Epidemiology, and End Result (SEER) database (1973-2011). HPB Surg 2015;2015:670728.
43. Allan BJ, Wang B, Davis JS, et al. A review of 218 pediatric cases of hepatocellular carcinoma. J Pediatr Surg 2014;49(1):166–71 [discussion: 171].
44. Katzenstein HM, Krailo MD, Malogolowkin MH, et al. Hepatocellular carcinoma in children and adolescents: results from the Pediatric Oncology Group and the Children's Cancer Group intergroup study. J Clin Oncol 2002;20(12):2789–97.
45. Taouli B, Losada M, Holland A, et al. Magnetic resonance imaging of hepatocellular carcinoma. Gastroenterology 2004;127(5 Suppl 1):S144–52.
46. Czauderna P, Mackinlay G, Perilongo G, et al. Hepatocellular carcinoma in children: results of the first prospective study of the International Society of Pediatric Oncology group. J Clin Oncol 2002;20(12):2798–804.
47. Murawski M, Weeda VB, Maibach R, et al. Hepatocellular carcinoma in children: does modified platinum- and doxorubicin-based chemotherapy increase tumor resectability and change outcome? lessons learned from the SIOPEL 2 and 3 studies. J Clin Oncol 2016;34(10):1050–6.
48. Kim A, Widemann BC, Krailo M, et al. Phase 2 trial of sorafenib in children and young adults with refractory solid tumors: a report from the Children's Oncology Group. Pediatr Blood Cancer 2015;62(9):1562–6.
49. Kohorst MA, Warad DM, Matsumoto JM, et al. Management of pediatric hepatocellular carcinoma: a multimodal approach. Pediatr Transplant 2017;21(6). https://doi.org/10.1111/petr.13007.
50. Plant AS, Busuttil RW, Rana A, et al. A single-institution retrospective cases series of childhood undifferentiated embryonal liver sarcoma (UELS): success of combined therapy and the use of orthotopic liver transplant. J Pediatr Hematol Oncol 2013;35(6):451–5.
51. Shi Y, Rojas Y, Zhang W, et al. Characteristics and outcomes in children with undifferentiated embryonal sarcoma of the liver: a report from the National Cancer Database. Pediatr Blood Cancer 2017;64(4). https://doi.org/10.1002/pbc.26272.
52. Fernandez-Pineda I, Cabello-Laureano R. Differential diagnosis and management of liver tumors in infants. World J Hepatol 2014;6(7):486–95.
53. Spunt SL, Lobe TE, Pappo AS, et al. Aggressive surgery is unwarranted for biliary tract rhabdomyosarcoma. J Pediatr Surg 2000;35(2):309–16.
54. Shen C-H, Dong K-R, Tao Y-F, et al. Liver transplantation for biliary rhabdomyosarcoma with liver metastasis: report of one case. Transplant Proc 2017;49(1):185–7.
55. Xue M, Masand P, Thompson P, et al. Angiosarcoma successfully treated with liver transplantation and sirolimus. Pediatr Transplant 2014;18(4):E114–9.
56. Grassia KL, Peterman CM, Iacobas I, et al. Clinical case series of pediatric hepatic angiosarcoma. Pediatr Blood Cancer 2017;64(11). https://doi.org/10.1002/pbc.26627.
57. Nguyen H, Stelling A, Kuramoto A, et al. Malignant rhabdoid tumor of the liver: findings at US, CT, and MRI, with histopathologic correlation. Radiol Case Rep 2014;9(1):e00031.

58. Abe T, Oguma E, Nozawa K, et al. Malignant rhabdoid tumor of the liver: a case report with US and CT manifestation. Jpn J Radiol 2009;27(10):462–5.
59. Trobaugh-Lotrario AD, Finegold MJ, Feusner JH. Rhabdoid tumors of the liver: rare, aggressive, and poorly responsive to standard cytotoxic chemotherapy. Pediatr Blood Cancer 2011;57(3):423–8.
60. Ruth ND, Kelly D, Sharif K, et al. Rejection is less common in children undergoing liver transplantation for hepatoblastoma. Pediatr Transplant 2014;18(1):52–7.
61. Ng K, Rana A, Masand P, et al. Fatal central nervous system post-transplant lymphoproliferative disease in a patient who underwent liver transplantation for hepatoblastoma. J Pediatr Gastroenterol Nutr 2018;66(1):e21–3.
62. Gnarra M, Behr G, Kitajewski A, et al. History of the infantile hepatic hemangioma: from imaging to generating a differential diagnosis. World J Clin Pediatr 2016; 5(3):273–80.
63. Christison-Lagay ER, Burrows PE, Alomari A, et al. Hepatic hemangiomas: subtype classification and development of a clinical practice algorithm and registry. J Pediatr Surg 2007;42(1):62–7 [discussion: 67–8].
64. Wörle H, Maass E, Köhler B, et al. Interferon alpha-2a therapy in haemangiomas of infancy: spastic diplegia as a severe complication. Eur J Pediatr 1999;158(4): 344.
65. Kassarjian A, Zurakowski D, Dubois J, et al. Infantile hepatic hemangiomas: clinical and imaging findings and their correlation with therapy. AJR Am J Roentgenol 2004;182(3):785–95.
66. Stringer MD, Alizai NK. Mesenchymal hamartoma of the liver: a systematic review. J Pediatr Surg 2005;40(11):1681–90.
67. Kim SH, Kim WS, Cheon J-E, et al. Radiological spectrum of hepatic mesenchymal hamartoma in children. Korean J Radiol 2007;8(6):498–505.
68. Yen J-B, Kong M-S, Lin J-N. Hepatic mesenchymal hamartoma. J Paediatr Child Health 2003;39(8):632–4.
69. Tsao K, Hirose S, Sydorak R, et al. Fetal therapy for giant hepatic cysts. J Pediatr Surg 2002;37(10):E31.
70. Barnhart DC, Hirschl RB, Garver KA, et al. Conservative management of mesenchymal hamartoma of the liver. J Pediatr Surg 1997;32(10):1495–8.
71. Begueret H, Trouette H, Vielh P, et al. Hepatic undifferentiated embryonal sarcoma: malignant evolution of mesenchymal hamartoma? Study of one case with immunohistochemical and flow cytometric emphasis. J Hepatol 2001; 34(1):178–9.
72. International Working Party. Terminology of nodular hepatocellular lesions. Hepatology 1995;22(3):983–93.
73. Lautz T, Tantemsapya N, Dzakovic A, et al. Focal nodular hyperplasia in children: clinical features and current management practice. J Pediatr Surg 2010;45(9): 1797–803.
74. Ma IT, Rojas Y, Masand PM, et al. Focal nodular hyperplasia in children: an institutional experience with review of the literature. J Pediatr Surg 2015;50(3):382–7.
75. Schouten JNL, Garcia-Pagan JC, Valla DC, et al. Idiopathic noncirrhotic portal hypertension. Hepatology 2011;54(3):1071–81.
76. Devarbhavi H, Abraham S, Kamath PS. Significance of nodular regenerative hyperplasia occurring de novo following liver transplantation. Liver Transpl 2007; 13(11):1552–6.
77. Berzigotti A, Abraldes JG, Tandon P, et al. Ultrasonographic evaluation of liver surface and transient elastography in clinically doubtful cirrhosis. J Hepatol 2010;52(6):846–53.

78. Stoot JHMB, Coelen RJS, De Jong MC, et al. Malignant transformation of hepatocellular adenomas into hepatocellular carcinomas: a systematic review including more than 1600 adenoma cases. HPB (Oxford) 2010;12(8):509–22.
79. Ribeiro A, Burgart LJ, Nagorney DM, et al. Management of liver adenomatosis: results with a conservative surgical approach. Liver Transpl Surg 1998;4(5): 388–98.
80. Labrune P, Trioche P, Duvaltier I, et al. Hepatocellular adenomas in glycogen storage disease type I and III: a series of 43 patients and review of the literature. J Pediatr Gastroenterol Nutr 1997;24(3):276–9.
81. Wellen JR, Anderson CD, Doyle M, et al. The role of liver transplantation for hepatic adenomatosis in the pediatric population: case report and review of the literature. Pediatr Transplant 2010;14(3):E16–9.
82. Sundar Alagusundaramoorthy S, Vilchez V, Zanni A, et al. Role of transplantation in the treatment of benign solid tumors of the liver: a review of the united network of organ sharing data set. JAMA Surg 2015;150(4):337–42.

Acute Liver Failure
An Update

James E. Squires, MD, MS*, Patrick McKiernan, MD,
Robert H. Squires, MD

KEYWORDS

- Acute liver failure • Children • Acute liver failure management • Encephalopathy
- Diagnosis of acute liver failure

KEY POINTS

- Pediatric acute liver failure is a dynamic, life-threatening condition of disparate etiology.
- Management is dependent on intensive collaborative clinical care and support.
- Proper recognition and treatment of common complications of liver failure are critical to optimizing outcomes.
- Identifying underlying cause and implementing timely, appropriate treatment can be life-saving.

INTRODUCTION

Acute liver failure (ALF) is a dynamic clinical condition manifested by an abrupt onset of a liver-based coagulopathy and biochemical evidence of hepatocellular injury resulting from rapid deterioration in liver cell function. The Pediatric Acute Liver Failure (PALF) Study, funded by the National Institutes of Health and the National Institutes of Diabetes and Digestive and Kidney Diseases, identified clinical and biochemical study entry criteria (**Box 1**).

These criteria were not intended to define PALF, but rather to identify subjects with acute liver injury sufficiently severe to place the child at risk for progressive clinical deterioration that could result in liver transplantation or death. Beyond the PALF study, children meeting PALF study entry criteria should prompt referral, or at least contact with, a pediatric liver transplant center, as early referral is known to improve outcome.

The ALF phenotype can be precipitated by disparate etiologies that include drug-induced, metabolic and genetic, infectious, immune-mediated, hemodynamic, and oncologic injuries; however, a definitive diagnosis is not determined in up to 50% of

Disclosure Statement: Contributor to Up-to-Date (R.H. Squires). Nothing to disclose (P. McKiernan, J.E. Squires).
Department of Pediatric Gastroenterology and Hepatology, University of Pittsburgh School of Medicine, Children's Hospital of Pittsburgh, 4401 Penn Avenue, Pittsburgh, PA 15224, USA
* Corresponding author.
E-mail address: james.squires2@chp.edu

> **Box 1**
> **Pediatric Acute Liver Failure (PALF) study entry criteria**
>
> - No known evidence of chronic liver disease
> - International Normalized Ratio (INR), following parenteral administration of vitamin K, ≥ 1.5 with clinical hepatic encephalopathy (HE)
> - INR is ≥ 2.0 with or without HE
>
> *Data from* Squires RH Jr, Shneider BL, Bucuvalas J, et al. Acute liver failure in children: the first 348 patients in the pediatric acute liver failure study group. J Pediatr 2006;148(5):652–8.

cases. Proper management is dependent on intensive collaborative clinical care and support and, for a handful of conditions, specific therapy that can be life-saving. Outcomes in the pre–liver transplant era were limited to survival or death. Liver transplantation (LTx) interrupts the natural history of ALF and, consequently, this third outcome is most certainly composed of individuals who would have lived or would have died in the absence of LTx. Predicting patient outcome in the LTx era has been unfulfilling and better predictive models must be developed for proper stewardship of the limited resource of organ availability.

GENERAL MANAGEMENT AND COMPLICATIONS
General

Once a patient meets PALF study entry criteria, general management strategies should be undertaken regardless of etiology. Early transfer to a pediatric liver transplant center before development of clinical encephalopathy is associated with improved outcomes.[1] A general algorithm for patients meeting PALF study entry criteria is presented in **Fig. 1**.

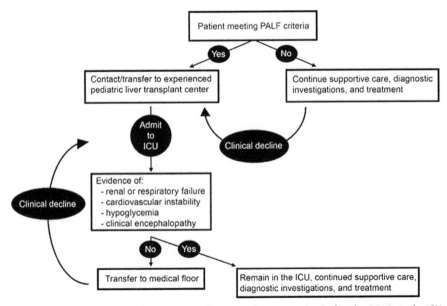

Fig. 1. A general algorithm for patients who meet the entry criteria for the PALF study. ICU, intensive care unit.

The initial history should include critical points preceding the development of PALF, while remaining focused on age-specific differential diagnoses. Physical examination is critical to assess for evidence of HE, ascites, edema, disease chronicity, heart murmur, or gallop (**Box 2**).

A plan for laboratory and clinical assessments should be initiated immediately and occur at least twice per day initially, then adjusted based on trends and interventions. The presence and degree of HE is critical in determining appropriate management (**Table 1**).

In the presence of cardiovascular instability, fluid or colloid resuscitation should occur. Once the child is stable, or if shock was not evident on presentation, total fluids should be restricted to between 90% and 100% maintenance fluids. This can be difficult to accomplish, as intravenous medications and blood product administration must be counted within the total daily volume. Accurate measurement of daily intake and output is critical. Overhydration can precipitate pulmonary edema, ascites, and cerebral edema, whereas underhydration can precipitate hepatorenal syndrome, acute tubular necrosis, worsening encephalopathy, and hypotension. A central catheter is needed for most children, and monitoring central venous pressure in the intensive care unit can assist in assessing the critically ill child. A comprehensive overview of common complications and general diagnostic and management strategies is presented (**Table 2**).

Hepatic Encephalopathy

HE is difficult to assess and may not be clinically apparent, particularly in infants and young children (**Table 3**).[26] An altered metal status due to severe illness, metabolic decompensation, electrolyte abnormality, cardiovascular instability, or fear may confound assessment of HE.[27] Pathogenesis extends beyond an elevated ammonia to include systemic inflammation and neuroinflammation.[28]

Coagulopathy

The INR is elevated in ALF and is a marker for severe hepatocellular dysfunction. However, a prolonged INR is not a measure of bleeding risk in patients with ALF.[29] Patients

---

Box 2
Medical history and physical examination in PALF

Important historical points:
- Onset of jaundice
- Perceived changes in mental status, such as confusion, slurred speech, agitation
- Constitution symptoms, such as nausea, vomiting, diarrhea, fever, rash
- Careful medication history, including over-the-counter medications and medications in the house
- Travel, exposure to farm animals
- Previous history of seizures, developmental delay, liver disease
- Family history of infant deaths, Wilson disease, autoimmune disease

Physical findings that suggest an underlying chronic liver disease would include the following:
- Prominent superficial abdominal vessels secondary to severe portal hypertension
- Digital clubbing
- Palmar erythema
- Xanthoma

Neurologic assessments should be frequent and, ideally, assessed by the same individual to identify subtle differences and progression.
- If able, having the child write his or her name on paper for a family member to assess the quality and subsequently to assess deterioration in handwriting over time, which can be seen with evolving encephalopathy.

Table 1
Laboratory testing and clinical assessments in pediatric acute liver failure

		Initial Testing	
Liver function	PT/INR Bilirubin (total and fractionated) Total protein and albumin Ammonia Glucose	Liver injury	ALT AST GGT Ferritin
Multisystem assessment	BMP + calcium, magnesium, phosphorus CBC + platelets and differential Amylase and lipase Blood gases (mixed, venous, or arterial)		

Frequency of testing accounting for HE

Interval	HE grade 0–I	HE grade II	HE grade III–IV
Q 30 min			Neurologic checks
Q 60 min		Neurologic checks	Vital signs
Q 2 h	Neurologic checks		
Q 4 h		vital signs	Dextrostik[b]
Q 6 h	Vital signs		BMP, magnesium, ammonia, CBC[c]
Q 8 h	Dextrostik	Dextrostik,[a] BMP, magnesium, ammonia, CBC	
Q 12 h	Dextrostik, BMP, magnesium, ammonia, CBC, liver function and injury	Liver function and injury	Liver function and injury

Abbreviations: ALT, alanine aminotransferase; AST, aspartate aminotransferase; BMP, basic metabolic panel; CBC, complete blood count; GGT, gamma glutamyl transferase; HE, hepatic encephalopathy; INR, international normalized ratio; PALF, pediatric acute liver failure; PT, prothrombin time; Q, every.
[a] No hypoglycemia in the past 48 hours.
[b] When there are acute changes in mental status. When hypoglycemia is identified, obtain serum blood sugar to ensure glucose is greater than 100 mg/dL and is stable within the normal range.
[c] When severe ascites and/or hypoalbuminemia.

Table 2
General diagnostic and management strategies of common complications in pediatric acute liver failure

Complication	Diagnosis	Management
Fluid and electrolytes		
Hyper/hypoglycemia	Routine blood monitoring/ dextrostik	• Maintain glucose levels between 90 and 120 mg/dL • Both hyperglycemia and hypoglycemia are associated with complications[2] • Protracted and profound hypoglycemia may be suggestive of an underlying metabolic defect • The glucose infusion rate may need to be 10–15 mg/kg per min and glucose concentrations in the IV fluids required to maintain proper glucose levels may need to be above 20% dextrose
Hyper/hyponatremia	Routine blood monitoring	• Maintain sodium requirements of 2–3 mEq/kg per day • Treat hyponatremia when patient is symptomatic or Na <120 mEq/L or fluid restriction not possible • Hypernatremia (145–155 mmol/L) may improve intracranial hypertension, but only temporarily and sustained hypernatremia should be avoided[3]
Hypophosphatemia	Routine blood monitoring	• Hypophosphatemia is common and should be treated to keep serum level more than 3 mg/dL[4]
HE and hyperammonemia	Physical examination, EEG, CT[a]	Clinical management • Elevate head to 30° • Dim and quiet room with no sudden noises or unnecessary chatter • Place pads on bed rails to prevent injury from sudden movements • Minimize tracheal suctioning if intubated Medical management • Reduce protein intake to 1 mg/kg • Lactulose 0.5 mL/kg per dose up to 30 mL/dose; adjust to produce 2–4 stools per day; acid environment converts ammonia produced by the gut from NH3 to NH4+ thus decreasing intestinal absorption[5] • Rifaximin to alter intestinal microbiome and decrease NH3 production; efficacy is comparable to lactulose in adults,[6] but very sparse data in children • There are conflicting studies on the efficacy of L-ornithine-L-aspartate in adults,[7,8] but has not been studied satisfactorily in children Exacerbating factors include sepsis, shock or hypotension, gastrointestinal bleeding, renal failure, electrolyte imbalance[9]

(continued on next page)

Table 2
(continued)

Complication	Diagnosis	Management

Cerebral edema	• CT: effacement of Sylvain fissures, sulci, and basil cisterns, loss of gray and white matter differentiation
	• Ultrasonography of optic nerve sheath diameter[10,b]
	• Ammonia >200 mmol/L is risk factor[6]
	• Clinically: rapid HE progression, abnormal pupillary responses, sustained or paroxysmal hypertension
		ICP monitoring considered in
		• Patients with stage III or IV coma
		• Require mechanical ventilation
		• EEG with slowing
		• ↑↑ ammonia
		• CT scan with features of edema
		• Hemorrhage is most feared complication[11]
		Overall goals[12]:
		• Clinical stability or improvement
		• ICP pressure <20 mm Hg
		• Maintain cerebral perfusion pressure >50 mm Hg for children <4 y, >55 mm Hg for children 4–10 y, and >60 mm Hg for children >10 y
		Specific therapies:
		• Hypothermia (core body temperature 32°–33°) was reported to improve outcome in small case series, but was not found to confer benefit in 2 randomized trials[13,14]
		• Indomethacin has been studied for its anti-inflammatory properties,[15] but concerns regarding bleeding risk and renal toxicity have likely precluded its acceptance as a reasonable treatment option
		• Forced hyperventilation to reduce P_{CO_2} below 34 mm Hg; brief (eg, 20 min) bursts of forced hyperventilation may be most effective, as extended hypocapnia may place the patient at risk for hypoxia[16]
		• Hyperosmolar therapy[17]
		  ○ Mannitol 0.5–1.0 g/kg. Can be given via a peripheral vein. Can produce a brisk diuresis, so careful monitoring of cardiovascular status is needed. No additional benefit is serum osmolality >320 mOsm/kg.
		  ○ Hypertonic saline (2.0% to 23.4%) to maintain serum sodium between 145 and 155 meq/L. Transtentorial herniation has been reversed with 23.4% may extend the window for liver transplantation.[18]

Coagulopathy	↑↑ INR ↓ Factor V and VII ↓ Fibrinogen	• Fresh frozen plasma (FFP) and or platelets for active bleeding or an invasive procedure • Avoid FFP and platelets to just correct the INR or improve platelet count in the absence of bleeding, as both are associated with transfusion-related lung injury and fluid overload[19] • Cryoprecipitate for low fibrinogen levels (eg, <100 mg/dL) • Recombinant factor VII has been used to correct the INR before placement of an intracranial monitor. It is very expensive and there is a risk of thrombosis.[20]
Kidney injury	RIFLE criteria ↓ Creatinine clearance ↓ Urine output	• Continuous renal replacement therapy[21]

Nutritional support[22–25]	Patients with PALF are likely catabolic and will required more calories than basal needs	• Enteral feeding is preferred over TPN
		• Oral feeding should not be interrupted if safe; nasogastric or naso-jejunal feeds should be attempted before starting TPN
		• TPN may be necessary to provide maximal calories with minimal volume if fluid overload is an issue and/or if ensuring euglycemia is not possible with enteral feeding
		• If TPN started,
		  ○ No protein restriction unless hyperammonemia
		  ○ If hyperammonemia present, protein should be restricted to 1 g protein/kg per day
		  ○ Lipids can be started unless suspected disorder of fatty acid oxidation or mitochondrial disease

Infections	Positive culture	Suspect infection if
		  ○ Onset of spontaneous bleeding
		  ○ Spontaneous hypothermia
		  ○ Worsening status of other organs (eg, pulmonary, cardiovascular, renal)
		  ○ Worsening mental status or progression of cerebral edema
		  ○ Elevation on WBC, neutrophils, or appearance of immature WBCs
		If clinical or biochemical changes occur, blood cultures and tracheal cultures, if intubated, should be obtained and broad-spectrum antibiotics started until cultures return negative

Abbreviations: ↑, increase in; ↓, decrease in; CT, computerized tomography; EEG, electroencephalogram; HE, hepatic encephalopathy; ICP, intracranial pressure; INR, international normalized ratio; IV, intravenous; PALF, pediatric acute liver failure; RIFLE, risk, injury, failure, loss, end-stage; TPN, total parenteral nutrition; WBC, white blood cell.

[a] Avoid contrast if evidence of renal injury.

[b] Greater than 6.1 mm is a potentially novel approach studied in pediatric traumatic brain injury, but not in PALF.

Table 3
Hepatic encephalopathy in pediatric acute liver failure

Stage		Clinical	Reflexes	Neurologic Signs	EEG Changes
0		None	Normal	None	Normal
I	Infant/child	Inconsolable, crying, inattention to task, parents describe child as "not acting like self"	Normal or hyperreflexia	Difficult or impossible to assess	Normal or diffuse slowing to theta rhythm, triphasic waves
	Adolescent/young adult	Confused, mood changes, altered sleep habits, forgetful	Normal	Tremor, apraxia, impaired handwriting	
II	Infant/child	Inconsolable, crying, inattention to task, parents describe child as "not acting like self"	Normal or hyperreflexia	Difficult or impossible to assess	Abnormal, generalized slowing, triphasic waves
	Adolescent/young adult	Drowsy, inappropriate behavior, decreased inhibitions	Hyperreflexia	Dysarthria, ataxia	
III	Infant/child	Somnolence, stupor, combativeness	Hyperreflexia	Difficult or impossible to assess	Abnormal, generalized slowing, triphasic waves
	Adolescent/young adult	Stuporous, obeys simple commands	Hyperreflexia, (+) Babinski	Rigidity	
IV	Infant/child	Comatose, arouses with painful stimuli (IVa) or no response (IVb)	Absent	Decerebrate or decorticate	Abnormal, very slow, delta activity
	Adolescent/young adult	Comatose, arouses with painful stimuli (IVa) or no response	Absent	Decerebrate or decorticate	

Abbreviation: EEG, electroencephalography.
Adapted from Squires RH Jr. Acute liver failure in children. Semin Liver Dis 2008;28(2):157; with permission.

with ALF appear to have a comparable decrease in both procoagulant and anticoagulant factors.[30] As a result, the overall coagulation profile, as measured by thromboelastography, typically reflects normal hemostasis.[31] However, the coagulation profile can be dynamic in ALF. Although most individuals have normal hemostasis despite a prolonged INR, some may have manifestation of a hypercoagulable state (eg, portal vein thrombosis) or hypocoagulable (eg, active bleeding episodes).[32]

Renal

As most children with ALF were healthy before presentation, renal insufficiency is a result of acute kidney injury (AKI). Settling on a consensus definition of AKI has been problematic. More recently, the *R*isk of renal failure; *I*njury to the kidney; *F*ailure of kidney function; with outcomes of *L*oss of kidney function and *E*nd-stage kidney disease (RIFLE classification) appears to be able to characterize AKI in critically ill children.[33] The RIFLE classification used estimated creatinine clearance and/or urine output to determine Risk, Injury, and Failure.[34]

The etiology of AKI in PALF includes the following:

- Acetaminophen toxicity
- Nephrotoxic medications
- Infection
- Hypovolemia

Hepatorenal syndrome (HRS) rarely, if ever, occurs in the setting of PALF. HRS can be seen in those with acute on chronic changes, such as a patient with established cirrhosis and ascites receiving aggressive diuretic therapy. This results in a contracted central blood volume resulting in reduced renal blood flow with treatment directed to expand the blood volume.[35] Expanding blood volume in PALF, in the absence of shock or hypotension, may precipitate worsening HE, cerebral edema, increased intracranial pressure, and fluid overload.

Secondary Infections

Secondary bacterial infections are not commonly reported at the time of presentation in PALF and routine administration of intravenous antibiotics are not customarily initiated on admission. A retrospective study in adults with ALF did not support antibacterial prophylaxis.[36] However, sepsis in children is more common after 2 weeks of hospitalization.[37] The clinical signs of sepsis can be subtle and often do not include an elevated temperature (see "Infections" section in **Table 2**).

Aplastic Anemia

Hepatitis-associated aplastic anemia (HAAA) is rare and presents following PALF or acute severe hepatitis of indeterminate cause. The clinical phenotype often includes serum aminotransferase values more than 3 times the upper limit of normal but often reaching well over 1000 IU/L and bilirubin levels that are more than 5 mg/dL but also reaching over 20 gm/dL at times. The etiology remains unknown, although associated viral infections have been noted. Pancytopenia develops in the weeks to months following the initial liver injury.[38] A liver biopsy without viral inclusions, but containing a marked inflammatory infiltrate with a predominance of CD8+ cytotoxic T cells, may identify an individual at risk for developing HAAA.[39] If a liver transplant interrupted the clinical course of PALF, HAAA can develop following liver transplantation.

The diagnosis is suspected by gradual diminishment of the white blood cell count, neutrophil count, platelet count, and hemoglobin accompanied by a low reticulocyte count. A bone marrow will confirm the diagnosis.

Treatment ideally uses an allogeneic bone marrow transplant from an HLA-matched sibling. Immunosuppressive therapy with antithymocyte globulin and cyclosporine is often required.[38]

Liver Support Therapy

Various iterations of extracorporeal liver support systems have been investigated in children with ALF to determine if they might have a meaningful improvement in clinical outcome. Unfortunately, virtually all of them that include albumin dialysis, plasma exchange, bioartificial liver support systems (human hepatoblastoma cells), extracorporeal liver assist device (human-based cells), HepatAssist (porcine cell-based), and molecular absorbent recirculating system (MARS) have fallen short of the mark or have been underpowered to assess benefit. Therefore, they cannot be recommended.[40]

Plasmapheresis

Plasmapheresis or plasma exchange (PE) has been used successfully in a variety of conditions, such as myasthenia gravis, Guillain-Barre, and cryoglobulinemia. Case reports and case series have suggested PE can serve as a bridge to LTx by improving coagulation and other biochemical parameters. In a study of 243 PE procedures in 49 children, coagulation parameters improved, but it had no effect on neurologic complications and only 3 of 49 recovered with their native liver.[41] In patients with Wilson disease presenting with ALF and hemolytic anemia, PE may serve to remove toxic levels of copper and stabilize the hemolytic process before LTx.[42] A recent multicenter, randomized controlled trial compared 90 participants who received standard medical therapy with 90 who received standard medical therapy plus 3 days of PE. Those who received PE experienced improved transplant-free survival, decreased frequency of systemic inflammatory response syndrome, and sequential organ failure assessment scores compared with the control group.[43] Similar studies should be performed in children.

Molecular absorbent recirculating system

Over the past 15 years, efforts to establish the relevance of this liver support system in the management of ALF have been largely unsuccessful. A recent study suggested MARS may serve to bridge patients with severe liver trauma to spontaneous recovery.[44] There is a paucity of data using MARS in children, but a recent cohort of 20 children with ALF who were MARS-treated were compared with 20 who did not receive MARS, and although the heterogeneous patient cohort precluded a statistical analysis for benefit, biochemical parameters, such as ammonia, bilirubin, and creatinine, improved and it appeared to be safe.[45] Adequately powered studies are essential to determine if children receive a meaningful benefit from MARS.

ETIOLOGY, MECHANISM OF INJURY, CLINICAL CHARACTERISTICS, DIAGNOSTIC TESTING, TREATMENT, AND PROGNOSIS

Over the course of 10 years, the PALF Study Group enrolled more than 1000 participants in North America and England. Specific diagnoses within broad diagnostic categories, such as metabolic, infectious, drug-related, and immune-mediated liver injury differ with age and geographic location. Historically, PALF in developing nations was predominantly due to viral hepatitis, as single or dual infections; however, recent publications reflect an increasing number of metabolic/genetic, immune-mediated, and drug/herbal/toxin-related causes of PALF.[46]

A diagnosis is not established for many children with PALF. This is due to a variety of reasons that include an incomplete differential diagnosis, inadequate diagnostic testing, or clinical progression that precludes further diagnostic testing. The clinical course of PALF can be rapid, dynamic, and unpredictable. The interval between presentation and a clinical outcome, such as liver transplant, death, or spontaneous recovery, can be as short as a few hours or days for some children. Thus, there is an urgency to establishment a specific diagnosis, as timely therapeutic intervention can affect clinical outcome.

Drug-Induced Liver Injury

Acetaminophen toxicity

Acetaminophen (APAP) is one of the most frequently used medications in the United States and is the most common identified cause of ALF in children[47,48] (**Table 4**). If taken as directed (maximum dose 75 mg/kg per day for children, 4 g/d for adults), APAP is well generally well tolerated; however, a well-designed study in healthy adults taking 4 g/d of APAP found elevations in alanine aminotransferase (ALT) of more than 3 times the upper limit of normal when taken for 4 or more days, with the serum APAP level in the therapeutic range.[49]

Non-acetaminophen drug-induced or toxin-induced liver injury

Although APAP toxicity is the most common cause for drug-induced liver injury (DILI) associated with PALF, many other medications, toxins, and herbal remedies have been identified as etiologic[58–62] (**Table 5**). An excellent resource for DILI is the LiverTox Web site: https://livertox.nlm.nih.gov/.

Metabolic/Genetic Diseases

As a disease category, metabolic conditions account for approximately 10% of all cases of PALF and 18% of PALF cases among children younger than 3 years (**Table 6**).[63] Tyrosinemia, galactosemia, urea cycle disorders, mitochondrial hepatopathies, and respiratory chain defects are common in younger patients.[64] In older children, Wilson disease is the most common metabolic defect; however, mitochondrial disorders, respiratory chain defects, and partial ornithine transcarbamylase deficiency also can present in older patients.

Viral Hepatitis

In North America, a viral cause for PALF is uncommon, with the notable exceptions of herpes simplex virus and enterovirus in children younger than 90 days.[63,82] There are many reasons for this that include vaccines for hepatitis A and B, safe potable water, hygienic requirements for food processing, and a sound sanitary system. In countries or regions in which these prevention practices are not available, then infectious diseases, particularly hepatitis A, B, and E, are the most common cause of ALF (**Table 7**).

Other Viruses

A variety of other viruses have been reported to cause PALF, but their ubiquitous nature and confounding exposure to potentially hepatotoxic medications makes it difficult to invoke a cause-and-effect of the identified virus at the time of clinical presentation. Human herpes virus-6 is typically a self-limited infection associated with exanthem subitum and a mononucleosis-type syndrome,[96,99] but has been identified in liver tissue of patients with ALF.[100] Influenza virus was reported to be a cause of ALF, but all recovered with their native liver, had chronic exposure to acetaminophen, and some had a biochemical phenotype similar to acetaminophen toxicity.[101] Parvovirus B19, another ubiquitous virus, can cause mild elevations of serum aminotransferase levels when children present with Fifth disease.[102] However, parvovirus

Table 4
Acetaminophen and acute liver failure: non-acetaminophen drug-induced or toxin-induced liver injury

Etiology	Mechanism of Injury	Clinical Characteristics	Diagnosis	Treatment	Prognosis

APAP	• Hepatic glutathione depletion following acute APAP toxicity allows highly reactive APAP derivatives to exact hepatocellular injury.[50]	• Most common identifiable cause of PALF
		• Ingestion ≥ 100 mg/kg is considered potentially toxic
		• Most common among white, adolescent girls
		• Extremely ↑↑↑ AST and ALT
		• Modest ↑ bilirubin
		• Centrilobular hepatic necrosis on liver biopsy
		• Acute and chronic exposure can cause PALF[51,52]
			• Relies heavily on a detailed history (not all patients will report a single toxic ingestion or chronic APAP ingestion)
			• APAP levels
			  ○ Levels obtained before 4 h are not sufficiently reliable to predict APAP hepatotoxicity unless the level is very low or undetectable[53]
			  ○ Level can be <10 mg/L in a third of patients with either an acute toxic ingestion or chronic exposure[54]
			  ○ APAP adducts
			    ■ Generated from binding of electrophilic APAP by-products to intracellular proteins
			    ■ Have been identified in most, but not all, patients with PALF due to acute APAP toxicity
			    ■ Present in a small percentage of those with an indeterminate diagnosis suggesting a possible role of APAP adducts in the diagnosis of APAP toxicity[55,56]
				• NAC
				• Initial NAC bolus (between 50 and 150 mg/kg) infused over 15–60 min followed by either a continuous or intermittent infusion over the next 20–48 h[57]
					Full recovery occurs in more than 90% of cases, but liver transplantation can be life-saving for those with clinical deterioration despite NAC therapy[54]

Abbreviations: ↑, increase; ALT, alanine aminotransferase; APAP, acetaminophen; AST, aspartate aminotransferase; NAC, N-acetylcysteine; PALF, pediatric acute liver failure.

Table 5
Non-acetaminophen drug-induced or toxin-induced liver injury

Classification	Drug/Toxin	Interval Between Exposure and Manifestations	Clinical Features
Analgesic	Halothane	1–30 d	Fever, jaundice
Antibiotic	Isoniazid	0–14 mo	Fatigue, anorexia, malaise, then jaundice
	Rifampin	Weeks	Jaundice, severe hepatitis
	Pyrazinamide	4–8 wk	Fatigue, anorexia, malaise, then jaundice
	Amoxicillin/clavulanic acid	Days–2 mo	DRESS, severe hepatitis, cholestasis
	Tetracycline	4–6 d into therapy	Nausea, vomiting, abdominal pain, mild jaundice
	Minocycline	Days–2 mo	DRESS, severe hepatitis
		Months to a year	Autoimmune hepatitis
	Macrolide	1–3 wk	Nausea, abdominal pain, jaundice, fever
	Sulfonomide	Days–1 mo	Fever, rash, eosinophilia, jaundice
	Ketoconazole	1–6 mo	Acute hepatitis
	Itraconazole	1–6 mo	Fatigue, jaundice, severe hepatitis
Antiepileptic	Phenytoin	2–8 wk	Hepatitis, cholestasis, atypical lymphocytes, lymphadenopathy
	Carbamazepine	1–8 wk	DRESS, severe hepatitis
	Lamotrigine	1–8 wk	DRESS, mild to moderate hepatitis, cholestasis
	Felbamate	1–6 mo	Severe hepatitis, cholestasis
	Valproate	Months to years	hyperammonemia
		1–6 mo	Jaundice, severe hepatitis
Recreational drugs	Marijuana	Days	Acute severe hepatitis
	Cocaine	Hours to a few days	Acute hepatic necrosis
	Amphetamine	3–14 d	Acute severe hepatitis
Herbal medications	Amanita phalloides	6–40 h	Nausea, vomiting, then liver and renal failure
	Germander	2–18 wk	Nausea, vomiting, fatigue, severe hepatocellular injury
	Kava	2–24 wk	Nausea, fatigue, severe hepatocellular injury, cholestasis

Abbreviation: DRESS, drug rash with eosinophilia and systemic symptoms.

Table 6
Metabolic diseases and acute liver failure

Etiology	Mechanism of Injury	Clinical Characteristics	Diagnosis	Treatment	Prognosis
Wilson disease	• Due to mutations of the *ATP7B* gene, which prevent copper incorporation into ceruloplasmin and biliary excretion of copper	• Hepatic disease may present from age 3 to 60 y, but the peak incidence is between 6 and 20 y • ALF may be accompanied by a history of school deterioration or speech abnormality • ↓ Alkaline phosphatase • Nonimmune hemolytic anemia • Liver biopsy with steatosis/fibrosis	• Pathogenic mutations in *ATP7B* • Increased urinary copper excretion • Kayser- Fleischer rings • ↑↑ Hepatic copper	• Trientene or penicillamine and zinc • Monitor Wilson disease score[65] • LTx if Wilson disease score ≥11 or encephalopathy	• Lifelong chelation therapy required
Tyrosinemia	• Defect in FAH, the final enzymatic step in the tyrosine degradation pathway[66]	• Present within the first few weeks of life with hepatomegaly, and a profound coagulopathy • ↑ bilirubin • Modest ↑ ALT and AST • *Escherichia coli* sepsis may be presenting feature • ↑↑ Risk of HCC • Risk is lowered with early treatment[67]	• Urine test for succinylacetone is diagnostic • NBS is available for tyrosinemia in most states • Diagnostic testing should be performed if the clinical phenotype is consistent with tyrosinemia regardless of the results of the NBS	• Nitisinone (NTBC, Orfadin), treatment is lifelong • Low tyrosine diet • LTx is performed for treatment failure with NTBC or clinical concern for HCC regardless of whether the patient is receiving NTBC	• Ongoing monitoring for development of HCC, even if NTBC was initiated

Galactosemia	• GALT deficiency	• Hepatosplenomegaly, coagulopathy • ↑↑ Bilirubin • *E coli* sepsis may be presenting feature • Modest ↑ ALT and AST	• NBS testing using dried blood spots includes assessment of GALT level[68] ○ Red blood cell transfusion before obtaining the test will void the usefulness of the test • + Urine reducing substances	• A galactose-restricted diet (eg, lactose free) is the lifelong therapy • Dietary restrictions appear to become lax into adulthood, but the consequences are not clear[69]	• Mild intellectual impairment is common
Urea cycle defects (UCD)	• OTCD is the most common UCD to present with PALF • Citrullinemia type 1 has also been described[70]	• Typical presentation of a metabolic crisis with poor feeding, altered mental status ± seizures, and ↑↑ serum NH3 • One-third of patients with UCD will also have a ↑ ALT, AST and INR that meets entry criteria for PALF[71] • Bilirubin usually normal • PALF can be transient or recurrent	• Quantitative serum/plasma amino acids will reveal patterns of elevation and deficiency that can lead to a suspected diagnosis • Urinary orotic acid and amino acid analysis • Single gene mutation analysis when a specific diagnosis is strongly suspected from results of the previously mentioned tests • Multigene panel that includes the 8 genes generating UCD enzymes • Enzyme activity in liver, fibroblasts, or red blood cells[72]	• Dialysis to remove NH3 • NH3 scavengers (eg, sodium phenylacetate, sodium benzoate) • Low-protein diet supplemented with amino acids, preferably administered enterally; but may require TPN • LTx will cure some UCDs (eg, CPS1, OTCD, argininosuccinate synthetase), as these enzymes are found almost exclusively in the liver; arginosuccinate lyase and arginase 1 are expressed outside the liver and more careful post-LTx monitoring is needed[73]	• Most common identifiable cause of PALF

(continued on next page)

Table 6
(continued)

Etiology	Mechanism of Injury	Clinical Characteristics	Diagnosis	Treatment	Prognosis
Fatty acid oxidation defects[74]	• ≥20 individual defects are recognized • ALF described in LCHAD, ACAD9, MCAD, CACT deficiency	• Hepatomegaly, ↑ ALT and AST, and modest ↑ NH3 occur in ≥ 80% of cases • ↑Bilirubin in up to one-third • Neurologic, cardiac, and muscular symptoms are frequent	• Blood acylcarnitine profile and urinary organic analysis at the time of metabolic instability • ↑ plasma-free fatty acids/3-hydroxybutyrate ratio • Mutation detection using multigene panel • Fibroblast palmitate and myristate oxidation studies	• Treatment with intravenous carbohydrate • Avoiding fasting and use of a carbohydrate-containing emergency regimen during intercurrent illnesses • In long-chain defects, dietary long-chain fat should be restricted	• PALF recovers spontaneously with supportive care • Neurologic sequalae from hypoglycemia are common
NBAS deficiency[75]	• Normal function in retrograde transport between endoplasmic reticulum and the Golgi apparatus • Role in PALF not fully understood	• Infantile liver failure precipitated by febrile illness • Mild jaundice • Recurrent PALF	• Pathogenic mutations in *NBAS* • Liver biopsy shows steatosis	• Aggressive supportive care • Prompt antipyresis • Use of intravenous lipid during acute episodes • LTx appears to prevent recurrent episodes	• Episodes may be fatal but recovery usually occurs within days if normalization of liver function • Recurrent PALF, may become less severe with age
Hepatocerebellar neuropathy syndrome[76]	• Due to deficiency of SCYL1, which has a role in maintaining Golgi integrity	• Recurrent bouts of PALF provoked by fever starting in infancy	• MRI shows cerebellar vermis atrophy • Pathogenic mutations in *SCYL1*	• Aggressive supportive care • Prompt antipyresis • LTx has not been described	• Spontaneous recovery occurs, but progressive fibrosis and PHTN develop • Episodes decrease with age and are rare after age 10 • Delayed motor milestones are common and eventually progressive cerebellar dysfunction and motor myopathy develop

Disease	Pathogenesis	Clinical Features	Genetics	Management	Outcome
Infantile liver failure syndrome type 1[77]	• Mutations in *LARS*, which encodes a transfer RNA synthase	• Multisystem disorder with low birth weight, anemia, and seizures • PALF with fever in infancy • ↓↓ albumin • Liver biopsy with microvesicular steatosis • Microcytic anemia	• Pathogenic mutations in *LARS*	• Aggressive supportive care • Prompt antipyresis • High-protein diet during acute episodes • LTx has not been described	• Spontaneous clinical and biochemical recovery occurs over 3–4 wk • Chronic liver disease develops in some cases • Episodes decrease with age, but intermittent encephalopathy and seizures unrelated to liver dysfunction persist
Wolcot-Rallison syndrome[78]	• Due to mutations in *EIF2AK3*	• Neonatal diabetes and skeletal dysplasia • Up to 80% develop recurrent liver failure, often associated with febrile illness, from infancy	• Pathogenic mutations in *EIF2AK3*	• Aggressive supportive care • LTx has prevented recurrent episodes and has been combined with pancreas	• Up to 80% develop recurrent liver failure, often associated with febrile illness, from infancy • Most episodes are self-limiting but cumulative mortality in childhood remains high

(continued on next page)

Table 6
(continued)

Etiology	Mechanism of Injury	Clinical Characteristics	Diagnosis	Treatment	Prognosis

Bile acid (BA) synthetic disorders[79]	• Due to defect in any of the 14 enzymes of BA synthesis
	• Liver injury is a consequence of decreased primary BAs that are critical for BA-dependent bile flow, combined with the production of atypical, hepatotoxic metabolites
	• Liver failure is reported in
	  ○ Delta 4-3-oxosteroid 5α-reductase deficiency
	  ○ Oxysterol 7α-hydroxylase deficiencies
		• Low gamma glutamyl transferase neonatal cholestasis
		• Fat-soluble deficiency
		• Low plasma BAs
			• Pathogenic mutations in select BA synthesis enzymes
			• Urinary fast atom bombardment spectroscopy
				• Cholic and/or chenodeoxycholic acid supplementation
				• LTx if supplementation fails
					• Excellent outcomes have been reported with initiation of early supplementation
					• LTx provides a metabolic cure

Hereditary fructose intolerance	• Deficiency of fructose-1-phosphate aldolase resulting in the accumulation of fructose-1 phosphate	• Symptoms occur with the introduction of sucrose or fructose into the diet and include vomiting, failure to thrive, and jaundice with hepatomegaly • Classically occurring following weaning, the widespread availability of fructose-containing feeds means that presentation can occur in early infancy • In older children and adults there is a history of avoiding fruit and sweets	• Pathogenic mutations in *ALDOB*	• Avoidance of dietary fructose	• Removal of dietary fructose results in rapid improvement, although hepatomegaly and abnormal transaminases may persist

Mitochondrial hepatopathy[80]	• Dysfunction of the electron transport chain resulting in cellular ATP deficiency, impaired fat oxidation and the generation of toxic free radicals	• Highly variable but multisystem disease is usual
		• ALF is most commonly caused by mtDNA depletion syndromes
		• Elevated lactate is sensitive but non-specific
		• Liver biopsy often shows microvesicular steatosis
			• Tissue measurements of respiratory chain activity and mtDNA levels
			• Pathogenic mutations causing mtDNA depletion have been described in 10 genes to date, of which at least 4 result in liver disease
			   ○ DGUOK
			   ○ POLG
			   ○ MPV17
			   ○ Twinkle
				• Aggressive supportive care
				• Once considered a general contraindication to LTx, recent experience suggests a potential role of LTx in management.[81]
					• Multisystem disease progresses in most cases

(continued on next page)

Table 6
(continued)

Etiology	Mechanism of Injury	Clinical Characteristics	Diagnosis	Treatment	Prognosis
Alpers syndrome	• mtDNA depletion disorder due to mutations in *POLG*	• Characterized by degenerative brain and liver disease in the first decade that may be precipitated by Valproate treatment • Seizures, which are focal and refractory, usually precede liver disease • EEG may show characteristic pattern	• Pathogenic mutations in *POLG*	• Stop valproate • Intravenous carnitine and NAC if valproate associated	

Abbreviations: ↑, increase; ACAD9, Acyl-CoA dehydrogenase family member 9; ALT, alanine aminotransferase; AST, aspartate aminotransferase; CACT, Carnitine-acylcarnitine translocase; CPS1, carbamoylphosphate synthetase; DGUOK, deoxyguanosine kinase; EEG, electroencephalogram; FAH, fumarylacetoacetase; GALT, galactose-1-phosphate uridyl transferase; HCC, hepatocellular carcinoma; LCHAD, Long-chain 3-hydroxyacyl-CoA dehydrogenase; LTx, Liver transplant; MCAD, Medium-chain acyl-CoA dehydrogenase deficiency; MRI, magnetic resonance imaging; mtDNA, mitochondrial DNA; NAC, N-acetylcysteine; NBAS, neuroblastoma amplified sequence; NBS, newborn screen; OTCD, ornithine transcarbamylase deficiency; PALF, pediatric acute liver failure; PHTN, portal hypertension; POLG, polymerase gamma; TPN, total parenteral nutrition.

Table 7
Viral infection and acute liver failure

Etiology	Clinical Characteristics	Diagnosis	Treatment/Prognosis
Herpes simplex virus[83–85]	• Most common cause of neonatal ALF • Transmission from asymptomatic mother to infant likely occurs at or shortly after birth • Symptoms generally begin in first week of life • Can occur in older children (ie, history of immunosuppression and/or sexual activity) • ↑↑ Transaminases	• PCR in the serum • HSV serologies may not be present early in the disease • Culture of vesicle, blood, liver tissue • IHC stain of the liver	• Acyclovir (should be started immediately in all newborns presenting with ALF; it can be stopped if the HSV PCR returns negative) • LTx has been successful
Enterovirus[82]	• Affects all age groups • In older children, nausea, vomiting, and/or diarrhea are common • Occasionally, more serious conditions include flaccid paralysis or cardiomyopathy • Second most common cause of neonatal ALF	• PCR for enterovirus, Coxsackie virus, echovirus • Liver tissue culture	• Supportive care • LTx has been performed • If the infant survives ALF, complete recovery without sequelae occurs in most cases
Epstein-Barr virus[86–88]	• ↑ ALT and AST • ± Cholestasis • ALF is rare • EBV can trigger HLH (see below)	• Serology helpful, but not diagnostic • PCR for EBV ± IHC increases likelihood	• Supportive care • Corticosteroids have been used for EBV-ALF
Hepatitis A virus[89]	• ALF occurs in 1% of primary infections • Incidence dramatically decreased with HAV vaccine	• HAV IgM	• Supportive care • LTx has been performed
Hepatitis B virus[48,90]	• 1% of adults with ALF, only 0.3% of children • Incidence decreased with HBV vaccine	• HBV DNA • + HBV surface antigen • + HBV surface antibody • HBV e-antigen and antibody • HBV core antibody	• Children born to HBV+ mothers should receive HBV vaccine and HBIG • Although no studies in children, entecavir or tenofovir is recommended[91,92] • LTx has been performed

(continued on next page)

Table 7
(continued)

Etiology	Clinical Characteristics	Diagnosis	Treatment/Prognosis
Hepatitis E virus[93]	• Common cause of ALF in developing countries • Can cause ALF in pregnant women	• HEV IgM • HEV IgG + viral RNA	• Ribavirin with or without pegylated interferon[94,95] but guidelines are not established.
Cytomegalovirus[96]	• ALF more common in immunosuppressed and infant populations	• PCR + serology suggesting recent infection • Liver biopsy with CMV inclusions	• Supportive care, spontaneous resolution can occur • Reduce immunosuppression medications if possible • Ganciclovir or valganciclovir has been used[97]
Adenovirus[98]	• Common in immunosuppressed patients	• Blood PCR • Liver tissue: culture, viral inclusions, IHC	• Cidofovir

Abbreviations: ALF, acute liver failure; CMV, cytomegalovirus; EBV, Epstein-Barr virus; HAV, Hepatitis A virus; HBIG, Hepatitis B immune globulin; HBV, Hepatitis B virus; HEV, Hepatitis E virus; HLH, hemophagocytic lymphohistiocytosis; HSV, herpes simplex virus; Ig, immunoglobulin; IHC, immunohistochemistry; LTx, liver transplantation; PCR, polymerase chain reaction.

DNA can be present in liver tissue for months following infection, raising questions about causality when found in patients with ALF.[102] A study of adult patients found no evidence that parvovirus was associated with ALF.[103]

Immune-Mediated

Immune mechanisms have been shown to play a critical role in the pathogenesis of many liver injuries in children. Immune injury can occur secondary to autoinflammation and injury (classical autoimmune hepatitis and hemophagocytic lymphohistiocytosis) or by an allogeneic immune response of maternal antibodies to antigens associated with neonatal liver cells (gestational alloimmune liver disease) **(Table 8)**. Importantly, autoantibodies (auto-AB), such as antinuclear antibody, smooth muscle antibody, and liver-kidney microsomal antibody (LMK), are associated with but not exclusive to autoimmune hepatitis. In the setting of PALF, serum auto-AB can be present among disease categories that include indeterminate, autoimmune hepatitis, and other known diagnoses (particularly Wilson disease).[104] Auto-AB detected in the serum of PALF patients can be transient and reflect their release from the inflammatory milieu in the context of severe hepatocellular injury.[105] Thus, it is important to recognize differences that may exist between classic autoimmune hepatitis (AIH), which can cause ALF, and auto-AB–positive PALF.

Cardiovascular

Shock/ischemia
Ischemic hepatitis, resulting from conditions such as hypoplastic left heart, interruption of the aortic arch, and cardiomyopathy, may initially manifest as severe liver injury or ALF.[110–112] Serum aminotransferase levels are often well over 1000 IU/L associated with acute hepatic necrosis. LTx is rarely used as an intervention, as complete hepatic recovery can occur if satisfactory blood flow to the liver can be established.

Budd-Chiari syndrome
Budd-Chiari syndrome is a rare cause of PALF. Obstruction of hepatic venous outflow either from hepatic vein thrombi, intravascular web within the inferior vena cava (IVC) cephalad from the hepatic veins, or a tumor results in the clinical manifestation of hepatomegaly, ascites, and evidence of hepatocellular injury. The cause for hepatic vein thrombosis is often not determined in children, although coagulation disorders (eg, antithrombin III deficiency, protein C or S deficiency, Factor V Leiden mutations) and myeloproliferative conditions associated with Janus kinase 2 mutations should be investigated.[113,114]

Diagnosis
- Ultrasound of the liver with Doppler
- Computerized axial tomography with angiography
- Angiography of the IVC to assess for intravascular web and patency of hepatic veins

Treatment
- Anticoagulation, even if the INR is prolonged.[115]
- Angioplasty of hepatic veins
- Transhepatic portosystemic shunt
- Liver transplant

Oncologic

Congenital leukemia as well acute lymphoblastic leukemia in older children can present with ALF.[116] Physical examination revealing splenomegaly and lymphadenopathy,

Table 8
Immune-mediated disease and acute liver failure

Etiology	Mechanism of Injury	Clinical Characteristics	Diagnosis	Treatment	Prognosis
Autoimmune hepatitis	• Exact etiology unclear • Suspect that auto-antigenic peptide, with particular cytokine milieu results in Th1 cell stimulation of T lymphocytes and macrophages and Th2 stimulation of auto-AB • Possible role of regulatory T cell and Th17 dysfunction	• + abdominal pain, fatigue, arthralgia • Often other autoimmune diseases • ALF can be presenting feature • ↑↑ AST and ALT • ↑/− bilirubin • ↑↑ IgG • + Auto-AB	• + Auto-AB • ↑↑ IgG • Liver histology compatible with AIH (interface hepatitis, plasma cell infiltrate, fibrosis) • Absence of viral hepatitis	• Steroids in acute setting • Long-term management often with Imuran, 6-MP, mycophenolate mofetil • Second-line agents such as budesonide, tacrolimus, rituximab, infliximab have been used	• Variable prognosis • Infectious complications can occur due to treatment • Long-term immunosuppression therapy is needed • LTx has been performed
Auto-AB–positive PALF[48]	• Unclear, likely multiple etiologies	• Can be similar to AIH	• + Auto-AB • Liver histology with hepatic necrosis	• Steroids have been used successfully in some but not all	• Infectious complications can occur due to treatment • LKM-positive patients are more likely to receive LTx • LTx has been performed • Most patients can be weaned completely off immunosuppression without disease recurrence
Gestational alloimmune liver disease (a.k.a.	• Alloimmune disease where to-be-determined fetal antigen crosses the ○ Liver	• Abnormal iron deposition in ○ Liver	• Extrahepatic siderosis in salivary gland (lip biopsy) or other organ (MRI)	• Exchange transfusion with IVIG	• Spectrum of disease, but in its most severe from is

neonatal hemochromatosis[106]	placenta, induces maternal antibody production that returns to the fetal circulation and devastates the fetal liver • High recurrence rate (~80%) in subsequent pregnancies	o Heart o Brain o Salivary glands • Leading cause of neonatal ALF • Present in first days of life • ↑↑ INR, ↑ bilirubin • Normal AST and ALT	• + MAC stain in liver biopsy is sensitive, but not entirely specific	• Antenatal treatment with IV immunoglobulins beginning at 14–18 wk of gestation can prevent recurrence in subsequent pregnancies	universally fatal without prompt therapy or LTx • LTx has been performed
Hemophagocytic lymphohistiocytosis (HLH)[107,108]	• Disorder of immune overactivation • Primary/familial type associated with PRF1, FHL2, FHL3, syntaxin 11 mutations • Secondary type most commonly associated with EBV infection • Other conditions associated include malignancy, metabolic d/o, and autoimmune disease	• Fever, hepatosplenomegaly, and cytopenia associated with a robust hyperinflammatory state • ↑ sIL-2r • ↑ ferritin	Must meet 5 of the following 8 criteria[109]: • Fever • Splenomegaly • Cytopenia affecting ≥ 2 lineages o Hemoglobin <9 o Platelet count <100 × 10⁹/L o Absolute neutrophil count <1 × 10⁹/L • Hypertriglyceridemia and/or hypofibrinogenemia o Triglycerides ≥ 265 mg/dL o Fibrinogen ≤150 mg/dL • Hemophagocytosis in bone marrow, spleen, or lymph nodes • Low or absent NK cell activity • Ferritin ≥500 µg/L • sCD25 (sIL2Rα) ≥2400 U/ml	• Immunosuppression o Corticosteroids o Etoposide o IVIG o Cyclosporine o Antithymocyte globulin • ± Bone marrow or hematopoietic stem cell transplant • LTx should be avoided, but has been successfully reported • Antiviral therapy for example, acyclovir/ valganciclovir) combined with rituximab has been used in EBV-related HLH	

Abbreviations: ↑, increase; ↓, decrease; +, positive; −, negative; AIH, autoimmune hepatitis; ALF, acute liver failure; ALT, alanine aminotransferase; AST, aspartate aminotransferase; d/o, disorder; EBV, Epstein-Barr virus; Ig, immunoglobulins; IVIG, intravenous immunoglobulins; LKM, liver-kidney microsomal antibody; LTx, liver transplant; MAC, membrane attack complex; NK, natural killer; PALF, pediatric acute liver failure; sIL-2r, soluble interleukin 2 receptor.

abdominal ultrasonography with evidence of enlarged abdominal lymph nodes, and abnormalities noted on the peripheral blood smear would suggest examination of the bone marrow should be performed as soon as possible. Metastatic, but previously undiagnosed, tumors such as adenocarcinoma also have been reported in children.[117]

Indeterminate

An indeterminate diagnosis (IN) is one of exclusion, although oftentimes the diagnostic evaluation is either interrupted by death, liver transplant, or spontaneous recovery. Therefore, the IN cohort is likely the most heterogenous final diagnosis among all others. An IN diagnosis can occur in all age groups, but appears to be highest among children between 1 to 10 years of age.[63] Clinical features associated with an IN diagnosis include a higher total bilirubin, but comparable levels of aminotransferase elevation and encephalopathy grade compared to those with an established diagnosis. However, those with an IN diagnosis are much more likely to receive a liver transplant that those with an established diagnosis.

Recent studies have hypothesized an underlying immune dysregulation as a mechanism of injury associated with an IN diagnosis.[118,119] Children with an IN diagnosis often have clinical features similar to other hyperinflammatory conditions such as macrophage activation syndrome and HLH. However, the hyperinflammatory milieu does not appear to be a genetic disorder of the immune or inflammatory response, as episodes of ALF do not recur after spontaneous recovery with the native liver.

Treatment

- Supportive therapy.
- Anecdotal reports and small case series report a benefit from corticosteroids, but given the severe complications associated with steroid treatment in ALF, further study is needed before a recommendation can be made.
- LTx.

PROGNOSIS

There are no satisfactory tools or models to predict outcome in PALF. Efforts to construct such a model are hampered by LTx. Most models include both death and LT into a single outcome. However, these 2 outcomes are not the same, as the LTx cohort includes patients who would have lived or would have died had LTx not interrupted the natural course of ALF. Existing models such as King's College Hospital Criteria and the Liver Injury Unit score that combined outcomes were unable to be validated when the outcomes of death and LTx separated.[120,121] Examination of dynamic inflammatory networks do appear to segregate outcomes of death and survival, whereas those who received an LTx had an inflammatory network that appeared to have features seen in those who died and those who survived.[122,123] Using a growth mixture model that included clinical data (INR, encephalopathy, total bilirubin) collected over 7 days, 5 different trajectories were generated with differing likelihoods for death or survival.[124] Other models using the trajectory of data collected over time suggest dynamic models hold some promise.[125,126]

OUTCOME

Most patients who meet PALF entry criteria are alive with their native liver at 21 days after enrollment. Very rarely, recurrent episodes of ALF are noted and have been associated with disorders of long-chain fatty acid oxidation, dihydrolipoamide dehydrogenase (E3) deficiency, Wolcott-Rallison syndrome, as well as children with mutations in the *LARS* (leucyl-tRNA synthase) gene[127] and *NBAS* (neuroblastoma amplified sequence) gene.[128] The frequency of LTx has decreased since 2000, and currently is performed in approximately 38% of patients. Outcome following LTx for both patient and graft survival has improved, but remains lower than patients receiving LTx for chronic cholestatic diseases. For those patients who survive with their native liver or received an LTx, neurocognitive testing has identified deficits in executive functions, fatigue, motor skills, attention, and health-related quality of life.[129] The frequency of death among those who met entry criteria for the PALF study has remained between 3% and 5%.

REFERENCES

1. Devictor D, Desplanques L, Debray D, et al. Emergency liver transplantation for fulminant liver failure in infants and children. Hepatology 1992;16:1156–62.
2. Srinivasan A, Venkataraman S, Hansdak SG, et al. Hyperglycaemia as an indicator of concurrent acute pancreatitis in fulminant hepatic failure associated with hepatitis B infection. Singapore Med J 2005;46(5):236–7.
3. Gonda DD, Meltzer HS, Crawford JR, et al. Complications associated with prolonged hypertonic saline therapy in children with elevated intracranial pressure. Pediatr Crit Care Med 2013;14(6):610–20.
4. Baquerizo A, Anselmo D, Shackleton C, et al. Phosphorus as an early predictive factor in patients with acute liver failure. Transplantation 2003;75(12):2007–14.
5. Gluud LL, Vilstrup H, Morgan MY. Nonabsorbable disaccharides for hepatic encephalopathy: a systematic review and meta-analysis. Hepatology 2016;64(3):908–22.
6. Wijdicks EF. Hepatic encephalopathy. N Engl J Med 2016;375(17):1660–70.
7. Acharya SK, Bhatia V, Sreenivas V, et al. Efficacy of L-ornithine L-aspartate in acute liver failure: a double-blind, randomized, placebo-controlled study. Gastroenterology 2009;136(7):2159–68.
8. Sidhu SS, Sharma BC, Goyal O, et al. L-ornithine L-aspartate in bouts of overt hepatic encephalopathy. Hepatology 2017. https://doi.org/10.1002/hep.29410.
9. Kodali S, McGuire BM. Diagnosis and management of hepatic encephalopathy in fulminant hepatic failure. Clin Liver Dis 2015;19(3):565–76.
10. Young AM, Guilfoyle MR, Donnelly J, et al. Correlating optic nerve sheath diameter with opening intracranial pressure in pediatric traumatic brain injury. Pediatr Res 2017;81(3):443–7.
11. Maloney PR, Mallory GW, Atkinson JL, et al. Intracranial pressure monitoring in acute liver failure: institutional case series. Neurocrit Care 2016;25(1):86–93.
12. Stevens RD, Shoykhet M, Cadena R. Emergency neurological life support: intracranial hypertension and herniation. Neurocrit Care 2015;23(Suppl 2):S76–82.
13. Bernal W, Murphy N, Brown S, et al. A multicentre randomized controlled trial of moderate hypothermia to prevent intracranial hypertension in acute liver failure. J Hepatol 2016;65(2):273–9.
14. Karvellas CJ, Todd Stravitz R, Battenhouse H, et al. Therapeutic hypothermia in acute liver failure: a multicenter retrospective cohort analysis. Liver Transpl 2015;21(1):4–12.
15. Tofteng F, Larsen FS. The effect of indomethacin on intracranial pressure, cerebral perfusion and extracellular lactate and glutamate concentrations in patients with fulminant hepatic failure. J Cereb Blood Flow Metab 2004;24(7):798–804.

16. Coles JP, Minhas PS, Fryer TD, et al. Effect of hyperventilation on cerebral blood flow in traumatic head injury: clinical relevance and monitoring correlates. Crit Care Med 2002;30(9):1950–9.

17. Francony G, Fauvage B, Falcon D, et al. Equimolar doses of mannitol and hypertonic saline in the treatment of increased intracranial pressure. Crit Care Med 2008;36(3):795–800.

18. Koenig MA, Bryan M, Lewin JL 3rd, et al. Reversal of transtentorial herniation with hypertonic saline. Neurology 2008;70(13):1023–9.

19. Argo CK, Balogun RA. Blood products, volume control, and renal support in the coagulopathy of liver disease. Clin Liver Dis 2009;13(1):73–85.

20. Krisl JC, Meadows HE, Greenberg CS, et al. Clinical usefulness of recombinant activated factor VII in patients with liver failure undergoing invasive procedures. Ann Pharmacother 2011;45(11):1433–8.

21. Cardoso FS, Gottfried M, Tujios S, et al. Continuous renal replacement therapy is associated with reduced serum ammonia levels and mortality in acute liver failure. Hepatology 2017. https://doi.org/10.1002/hep.29488.

22. Lutfi R, Abulebda K, Nitu ME, et al. Intensive care management of pediatric acute liver failure. J Pediatr Gastroenterol Nutr 2017;64(5):660–70.

23. European Association for the Study of the Liver, easloffice@easloffice.eu, Clinical practice guidelines panel, Wendon J, Cordoba J, Dhawan A, et al. EASL clinical practical guidelines on the management of acute (fulminant) liver failure. J Hepatol 2017;66(5):1047–81.

24. Plauth M, Schuetz T, Working group for developing the guidelines for parenteral nutrition of The German Association for Nutritional M. Hepatology - guidelines on parenteral nutrition [Chapter 16]. Ger Med Sci 2009;7:Doc12.

25. Kerwin AJ, Nussbaum MS. Adjuvant nutrition management of patients with liver failure, including transplant. Surg Clin North Am 2011;91(3):565–78.

26. Ng VL, Li R, Loomes KM, et al. Outcomes of children with and without hepatic encephalopathy from the pediatric acute liver failure study group. J Pediatr Gastroenterol Nutr 2016;63(3):357–64.

27. Squires RH Jr. Acute liver failure in children. Semin Liver Dis 2008;28(2):153–66.

28. Butterworth RF. The liver-brain axis in liver failure: neuroinflammation and encephalopathy. Nat Rev Gastroenterol Hepatol 2013;10(9):522–8.

29. Kawada PS, Bruce A, Massicotte P, et al. Coagulopathy in children with liver disease. J Pediatr Gastroenterol Nutr 2017;65(6):603–7.

30. Lisman T, Stravitz RT. Rebalanced hemostasis in patients with acute liver failure. Semin Thromb Hemost 2015;41(5):468–73.

31. Stravitz RT, Lisman T, Luketic VA, et al. Minimal effects of acute liver injury/acute liver failure on hemostasis as assessed by thromboelastography. J Hepatol 2012;56(1):129–36.

32. Barton CA. Treatment of coagulopathy related to hepatic insufficiency. Crit Care Med 2016;44(10):1927–33.

33. Schneider J, Khemani R, Grushkin C, et al. Serum creatinine as stratified in the RIFLE score for acute kidney injury is associated with mortality and length of stay for children in the pediatric intensive care unit. Crit Care Med 2010;38(3):933–9.

34. Plotz FB, Bouma AB, van Wijk JA, et al. Pediatric acute kidney injury in the ICU: an independent evaluation of pRIFLE criteria. Intensive Care Med 2008;34(9):1713–7.

35. Leventhal TM, Liu KD. What a nephrologist needs to know about acute liver failure. Adv Chronic Kidney Dis 2015;22(5):376–81.

36. Karvellas CJ, Cavazos J, Battenhouse H, et al. Effects of antimicrobial prophylaxis and blood stream infections in patients with acute liver failure: a retrospective cohort study. Clin Gastroenterol Hepatol 2014;12(11):1942–9.e1.
37. Godbole G, Shanmugam N, Dhawan A, et al. Infectious complications in pediatric acute liver failure. J Pediatr Gastroenterol Nutr 2011;53(3):320–5.
38. Rauff B, Idrees M, Shah SA, et al. Hepatitis associated aplastic anemia: a review. Virol J 2011;8:87.
39. Patel KR, Bertuch A, Sasa GS, et al. Features of hepatitis in hepatitis-associated aplastic anemia: clinical and histopathologic study. J Pediatr Gastroenterol Nutr 2017;64(1):e7–12.
40. Jain V, Dhawan A. Extracorporeal liver support systems in paediatric liver failure. J Pediatr Gastroenterol Nutr 2017;64(6):855–63.
41. Singer AL, Olthoff KM, Kim H, et al. Role of plasmapheresis in the management of acute hepatic failure in children. Ann Surg 2001;234(3):418–24.
42. Kiss JE, Berman D, Van Thiel D. Effective removal of copper by plasma exchange in fulminant Wilson's disease. Transfusion 1998;38(4):327–31.
43. Larsen FS, Schmidt LE, Bernsmeier C, et al. High-volume plasma exchange in patients with acute liver failure: an open randomised controlled trial. J Hepatol 2016;64(1):69–78.
44. Hanish SI, Stein DM, Scalea JR, et al. Molecular adsorbent recirculating system effectively replaces hepatic function in severe acute liver failure. Ann Surg 2017; 266(4):677–84.
45. Lexmond WS, Van Dael CM, Scheenstra R, et al. Experience with molecular adsorbent recirculating system treatment in 20 children listed for high-urgency liver transplantation. Liver Transpl 2015;21(3):369–80.
46. Alam S, Khanna R, Sood V, et al. Response to profile and outcome of first 109 cases of paediatric acute liver failure at a specialized paediatric liver unit in India: methodological issues. Liver Int 2017;37(11):1741.
47. Kaufman DW, Kelly JP, Rosenberg L, et al. Recent patterns of medication use in the ambulatory adult population of the United States: the Slone survey. JAMA 2002;287(3):337–44.
48. Narkewicz MR, Dell Olio D, Karpen SJ, et al. Pattern of diagnostic evaluation for the causes of pediatric acute liver failure: an opportunity for quality improvement. J Pediatr 2009;155(6):801–6.e1.
49. Watkins PB, Kaplowitz N, Slattery JT, et al. Aminotransferase elevations in healthy adults receiving 4 grams of acetaminophen daily: a randomized controlled trial. JAMA 2006;296(1):87–93.
50. Rumack BH, Bateman DN. Acetaminophen and acetylcysteine dose and duration: past, present and future. Clin Toxicol (Phila) 2012;50(2):91–8.
51. Heubi JE, Barbacci MB, Zimmerman HJ. Therapeutic misadventures with acetaminophen: hepatoxicity after multiple doses in children. J Pediatr 1998;132(1):22–7.
52. Alonso EM, Sokol RJ, Hart J, et al. Fulminant hepatitis associated with centrilobular hepatic necrosis in young children. J Pediatr 1995;127:888–94.
53. Seifert SA, Kirschner RI, Martin TG, et al. Acetaminophen concentrations prior to 4 hours of ingestion: impact on diagnostic decision-making and treatment. Clin Toxicol (Phila) 2015;53(7):618–23.
54. Leonis MA, Alonso EM, Im K, et al. Chronic acetaminophen exposure in pediatric acute liver failure. Pediatrics 2013;131(3):e740–6.
55. Alonso EM, James LP, Zhang S, et al. Acetaminophen adducts detected in serum of pediatric patients with acute liver failure. J Pediatr Gastroenterol Nutr 2015;61(1):102–7.

56. Bond GR. Acetaminophen protein adducts in children with acute liver failure of indeterminate cause. Pediatrics 2007;119(2):418–9 [author reply: 19–20].

57. Wong A, Graudins A. N-acetylcysteine regimens for paracetamol overdose: time for a change? Emerg Med Australas 2016;28(6):749–51.

58. Murray KF, Hadzic N, Wirth S, et al. Drug-related hepatotoxicity and acute liver failure. J Pediatr Gastroenterol Nutr 2008;47(4):395–405.

59. Reuben A, Koch DG, Lee WM. Drug-induced acute liver failure: results of a U.S. multicenter, prospective study. Hepatology 2010;52(6):2065–76.

60. Santi L, Maggioli C, Mastroroberto M, et al. Acute liver failure caused by amanita phalloides poisoning. Int J Hepatol 2012;2012:487480.

61. Fontana RJ. Acute liver failure due to drugs. Semin Liver Dis 2008;28(2):175–87.

62. Devarbhavi H, Patil M, Reddy VV, et al. Drug-induced acute liver failure in children and adults: results of a single-centre study of 128 patients. Liver Int 2017. https://doi.org/10.1111/liv.13662.

63. Squires RH Jr, Shneider BL, Bucuvalas J, et al. Acute liver failure in children: the first 348 patients in the pediatric acute liver failure study group. J Pediatr 2006; 148(5):652–8.

64. Hegarty R, Hadzic N, Gissen P, et al. Inherited metabolic disorders presenting as acute liver failure in newborns and young children: King's College Hospital experience. Eur J Pediatr 2015;174(10):1387–92.

65. Dhawan A, Taylor RM, Cheeseman P, et al. Wilson's disease in children: 37-year experience and revised King's score for liver transplantation. Liver Transpl 2005; 11(4):441–8.

66. de Laet C, Dionisi-Vici C, Leonard JV, et al. Recommendations for the management of tyrosinaemia type 1. Orphanet J Rare Dis 2013;8:8.

67. Bartlett DC, Lloyd C, McKiernan PJ, et al. Early nitisinone treatment reduces the need for liver transplantation in children with tyrosinaemia type 1 and improves post-transplant renal function. J Inherit Metab Dis 2014;37(5):745–52.

68. Pasquali M, Yu C, Coffee B. Laboratory diagnosis of galactosemia: a technical standard and guideline of the American College of Medical Genetics and Genomics (ACMG). Genet Med 2017. https://doi.org/10.1038/gim.2017.172.

69. Adam S, Akroyd R, Bernabei S, et al. How strict is galactose restriction in adults with galactosaemia? International practice. Mol Genet Metab 2015; 115(1):23–6.

70. Faghfoury H, Baruteau J, de Baulny HO, et al. Transient fulminant liver failure as an initial presentation in citrullinemia type I. Mol Genet Metab 2011;102(4): 413–7.

71. Gallagher RC, Lam C, Wong D, et al. Significant hepatic involvement in patients with ornithine transcarbamylase deficiency. J Pediatr 2014;164(4): 720–5.e6.

72. Ah Mew N, Simpson KL, Gropman AL, et al. Urea cycle disorders overview. In: Adam MP, Ardinger HH, Pagon RA, et al, editors. GeneReviews((R)). Seattle (WA): University of Washington, Seattle; 1993.

73. Squires RH, Ng V, Romero R, et al. Evaluation of the pediatric patient for liver transplantation: 2014 practice guideline by the American Association for the Study of Liver Diseases, American Society of Transplantation and the North American Society for Pediatric Gastroenterology, Hepatology and Nutrition. Hepatology 2014;60(1):362–98.

74. Baruteau J, Sachs P, Broue P, et al. Clinical and biological features at diagnosis in mitochondrial fatty acid beta-oxidation defects: a French pediatric study of 187 patients. J Inherit Metab Dis 2013;36(5):795–803.

75. Staufner C, Haack TB, Kopke MG, et al. Recurrent acute liver failure due to NBAS deficiency: phenotypic spectrum, disease mechanisms, and therapeutic concepts. J Inherit Metab Dis 2016;39(1):3–16.
76. Schmidt WM, Rutledge SL, Schule R, et al. Disruptive SCYL1 mutations underlie a syndrome characterized by recurrent episodes of liver failure, peripheral neuropathy, cerebellar atrophy, and ataxia. Am J Hum Genet 2015;97(6):855–61.
77. Casey JP, Slattery S, Cotter M, et al. Clinical and genetic characterisation of infantile liver failure syndrome type 1, due to recessive mutations in LARS. J Inherit Metab Dis 2015;38(6):1085–92.
78. Habeb AM, Al-Magamsi MS, Eid IM, et al. Incidence, genetics, and clinical phenotype of permanent neonatal diabetes mellitus in northwest Saudi Arabia. Pediatr Diabetes 2012;13(6):499–505.
79. Clayton PT. Disorders of bile acid synthesis. J Inherit Metab Dis 2011;34(3):593–604.
80. Rahman S. Gastrointestinal and hepatic manifestations of mitochondrial disorders. J Inherit Metab Dis 2013;36(4):659–73.
81. McKiernan P, Ball S, Santra S, et al. Incidence of primary mitochondrial disease in children younger than 2 years presenting with acute liver failure. J Pediatr Gastroenterol Nutr 2016;63(6):592–7.
82. Sundaram SS, Alonso EM, Narkewicz MR, et al. Characterization and outcomes of young infants with acute liver failure. J Pediatr 2011;159(5):813–8.e1.
83. Corey L, Wald A. Maternal and neonatal herpes simplex virus infections. N Engl J Med 2009;361(14):1376–85.
84. Levitsky J, Duddempudi AT, Lakeman FD, et al. Detection and diagnosis of herpes simplex virus infection in adults with acute liver failure. Liver Transpl 2008;14(10):1498–504.
85. Norvell JP, Blei AT, Jovanovic BD, et al. Herpes simplex virus hepatitis: an analysis of the published literature and institutional cases. Liver Transpl 2007;13(10):1428–34.
86. Shkalim-Zemer V, Shahar-Nissan K, Ashkenazi-Hoffnung L, et al. Cholestatic hepatitis induced by Epstein-Barr virus in a pediatric population. Clin Pediatr (Phila) 2015;54(12):1153–7.
87. Stefanou C, Tzortzi C, Georgiou F, et al. Combining an antiviral with rituximab in EBV-related haemophagocytic lymphohistiocytosis led to rapid viral clearance; and a comprehensive review. BMJ Case Rep 2016;2016:1–6.
88. Kunitomi A, Kimura H, Ito Y, et al. Unrelated bone marrow transplantation induced long-term remission in a patient with life-threatening Epstein-Barr virus-associated hemophagocytic lymphohistiocytosis. J Clin Exp Hematop 2011;51(1):57–61.
89. Lee HW, Chang DY, Moon HJ, et al. Clinical factors and viral load influencing severity of acute hepatitis A. PLoS One 2015;10(6):e0130728.
90. Manka P, Verheyen J, Gerken G, et al. Liver failure due to acute viral hepatitis (A-E). Visc Med 2016;32(2):80–5.
91. Terrault NA, Bzowej NH, Chang KM, et al. AASLD guidelines for treatment of chronic hepatitis B. Hepatology 2016;63(1):261–83.
92. European Association for the Study of the Liver. EASL clinical practice guidelines: management of chronic hepatitis B virus infection. J Hepatol 2012;57(1):167–85.
93. Bhatia V, Singhal A, Panda SK, et al. A 20-year single-center experience with acute liver failure during pregnancy: is the prognosis really worse? Hepatology 2008;48(5):1577–85.

94. Hajji H, Gerolami R, Solas C, et al. Chronic hepatitis E resolution in a human immunodeficiency virus (HIV)-infected patient treated with ribavirin. Int J Antimicrob Agents 2013;41(6):595–7.

95. Dalton HR, Keane FE, Bendall R, et al. Treatment of chronic hepatitis E in a patient with HIV infection. Ann Intern Med 2011;155(7):479–80.

96. Tsunoda T, Inui A, Iwasawa K, et al. Acute liver dysfunction not resulting from hepatitis virus in immunocompetent children. Pediatr Int 2017. https://doi.org/10.1111/ped.13249.

97. Hasosah MY, Kutbi SY, Al-Amri AW, et al. Perinatal cytomegalovirus hepatitis in Saudi infants: a case series. Saudi J Gastroenterol 2012;18(3):208–13.

98. Schaberg KB, Kambham N, Sibley RK, et al. Adenovirus hepatitis: clinicopathologic analysis of 12 consecutive cases from a single institution. Am J Surg Pathol 2017;41(6):810–9.

99. Harma M, Hockerstedt K, Lautenschlager I. Human herpesvirus-6 and acute liver failure. Transplantation 2003;76(3):536–9.

100. Chevret L, Boutolleau D, Halimi-Idri N, et al. Human herpesvirus-6 infection: a prospective study evaluating HHV-6 DNA levels in liver from children with acute liver failure. J Med Virol 2008;80(6):1051–7.

101. Whitworth JR, Mack CL, O'Connor JA, et al. Acute hepatitis and liver failure associated with influenza A infection in children. J Pediatr Gastroenterol Nutr 2006;43(4):536–8.

102. Young NS, Brown KE. Parvovirus B19. N Engl J Med 2004;350(6):586–97.

103. Lee WM, Brown KE, Young NS, et al. Brief report: no evidence for parvovirus B19 or hepatitis E virus as a cause of acute liver failure. Dig Dis Sci 2006;51(10):1712–5.

104. Narkewicz MR, Horslen S, Belle SH, et al. Prevalence and significance of autoantibodies in children with acute liver failure. J Pediatr Gastroenterol Nutr 2017;64(2):210–7.

105. Bernal W, Ma Y, Smith HM, et al. The significance of autoantibodies and immunoglobulins in acute liver failure: a cohort study. J Hepatol 2007;47(5):664–70.

106. Taylor SA, Whitington PF. Neonatal acute liver failure. Liver Transpl 2016;22(5):677–85.

107. Lin M, Park S, Hayden A, et al. Clinical utility of soluble interleukin-2 receptor in hemophagocytic syndromes: a systematic scoping review. Ann Hematol 2017;96(8):1241–51.

108. Al-Samkari H, Berliner N. Hemophagocytic lymphohistiocytosis. Annu Rev Pathol 2017. https://doi.org/10.1146/annurev-pathol-020117-043625.

109. Henter JI, Horne A, Arico M, et al. HLH-2004: diagnostic and therapeutic guidelines for hemophagocytic lymphohistiocytosis. Pediatr Blood Cancer 2007;48(2):124–31.

110. Verhoeven NM, Wallot M, Huck JH, et al. A newborn with severe liver failure, cardiomyopathy and transaldolase deficiency. J Inherit Metab Dis 2005;28(2):169–79.

111. Ichihashi K, Matsui A, Yanagisawa M, et al. Hepatic cell necrosis with congenital heart disease in the newborn. Acta Paediatr Jpn 1991;33(1):87–92.

112. Tapper EB, Sengupta N, Bonder A. The incidence and outcomes of ischemic hepatitis: a systematic review with meta-analysis. Am J Med 2015;128(12):1314–21.

113. Parekh J, Matei VM, Canas-Coto A, et al. Budd-Chiari syndrome causing acute liver failure: a multicenter case series. Liver Transpl 2017;23(2):135–42.

114. O'Grady JG. Budd-Chiari syndrome and acute liver failure: a complex condition requiring a rapid response. Liver Transpl 2017;23(2):133–4.

115. Seijo S, Plessier A, Hoekstra J, et al. Good long-term outcome of Budd-Chiari syndrome with a step-wise management. Hepatology 2013;57(5):1962–8.
116. Litten JB, Rodriguez MM, Maniaci V. Acute lymphoblastic leukemia presenting in fulminant hepatic failure. Pediatr Blood Cancer 2006;47(6):842–5.
117. Hussain SZ, Jaiswal A, Bader AA, et al. Fatal acute liver failure in a child with metastatic gastric adenocarcinoma. J Pediatr Gastroenterol Nutr 2006;43(1): 116–8.
118. Alonso EM, Horslen SP, Behrens EM, et al. Pediatric acute liver failure of undetermined cause: a research workshop. Hepatology 2017;65(3):1026–37.
119. Bucuvalas J, Filipovich L, Yazigi N, et al. Immunophenotype predicts outcome in pediatric acute liver failure. J Pediatr Gastroenterol Nutr 2013;56(3):311–5.
120. Lu BR, Zhang S, Narkewicz MR, et al. Evaluation of the liver injury unit scoring system to predict survival in a multinational study of pediatric acute liver failure. J Pediatr 2013;162(5):1010–6.e4.
121. Sundaram V, Shneider BL, Dhawan A, et al. King's College Hospital criteria for non-acetaminophen induced acute liver failure in an international cohort of children. J Pediatr 2013;162(2):319–23.
122. Azhar N, Ziraldo C, Barclay D, et al. Analysis of serum inflammatory mediators identifies unique dynamic networks associated with death and spontaneous survival in pediatric acute liver failure. PLoS One 2013;8(11):e78202.
123. Zamora R, Vodovotz Y, Mi Q, et al. Data-driven modeling for precision medicine in pediatric acute liver failure. Mol Med 2016;22:821–9.
124. Li R, Belle SH, Horslen S, et al. Clinical course among cases of acute liver failure of indeterminate diagnosis. J Pediatr 2016;171:163–70.e1-3.
125. Rajanayagam J, Frank E, Shepherd RW, et al. Artificial neural network is highly predictive of outcome in paediatric acute liver failure. Pediatr Transplant 2013; 17(6):535–42.
126. Kumar R, Shalimar, Sharma H, et al. Prospective derivation and validation of early dynamic model for predicting outcome in patients with acute liver failure. Gut 2012;61(7):1068–75.
127. Casey JP, McGettigan P, Lynam-Lennon N, et al. Identification of a mutation in LARS as a novel cause of infantile hepatopathy. Mol Genet Metab 2012;106(3): 351–8.
128. Haack TB, Staufner C, Kopke MG, et al. Biallelic mutations in NBAS cause recurrent acute liver failure with onset in infancy. Am J Hum Genet 2015;97(1):163–9.
129. Sorensen LG, Neighbors K, Zhang S, et al. Neuropsychological functioning and health-related quality of life: pediatric acute liver failure study group results. J Pediatr Gastroenterol Nutr 2015;60(1):75–83.

Liver Transplantation in Children

Yen H. Pham, MD[a], Tamir Miloh, MD[b],*

KEYWORDS

- Pediatric liver transplant • Immunosuppression • Split liver • Living donor
- Liver failure

KEY POINTS

- Liver transplantation (LT) is a lifesaving procedure in children with acute or chronic liver disease, hepatic tumors, and some genetic metabolic diseases.
- A multidisciplinary team is required to address the clinical needs of patients and assure optimal outcome.
- Because of scarcity of donors and better size matching between graft and recipients, most of the pediatric LTs in recent practice consist of variant techniques instead of whole LTs. The outcomes are similar to those following whole LTs.
- Advances in surgical techniques, postoperative management, and immunosuppressive treatment have allowed LT to be an effective treatment modality for patients with liver failure. LT for children has excellent short- and long-term patient and graft survival.

INTRODUCTION

Since the first successful pediatric liver transplant (LT) by Dr Starzl in 1967 in a patient with biliary atresia (BA), LT is now preformed in approximately 600 children a year in the United States and there are more than 15,000 pediatric recipients (Scientific Registry of Transplant Recipients [SRTR] data). Pediatric transplants account for about 7% to 8% of total number of LTs performed in the United States. Improvement in pretransplant management, patient selection, surgical techniques, organ preservation, immunosuppression, and posttransplant follow-up has led to outstanding results in patient and graft survival and quality of life (QOL). LT has become the standard of care for children with end-stage liver disease, acute or chronic, selected liver tumors; and metabolic disorders. The indications for LT in children are different than in adults, with BA remaining the most common cause. Many children are transplanted at a

Disclosure Statement: The authors have nothing to disclose.
[a] Pediatric Gastroenterology, Hepatology, and Nutrition, Baylor College of Medicine, Texas Children's Hospital, 18200 Katy Freeway, Suite 250, Houston, TX 77094, USA; [b] Pediatric Gastroenterology, Hepatology, and Nutrition, Baylor College of Medicine, Texas Children's Hospital, 6701 Fannin Street, Houston, TX 77030, USA
* Corresponding author.
E-mail address: tamiloh@texaschildrens.org

young age, necessitating the use of technical variants with improving success. The scarcity of cadaveric donors has led to using living donor grafts that are currently approximately 15% of transplants.[1] In 2002, the Pediatric End-Stage Liver Disease (PELD) for patients younger than 12 years and Model of End-Stage Liver Disease (MELD) for patients older than 12 years were implemented to allocate organs according to clinical need.

There are LT recipients who survive beyond 20 years after transplant. Tailoring the immunosuppressant to the individual patient is pertinent, on one hand, for prevention of acute cellular, chronic, and antibody-mediated rejection and, on the other hand, for avoiding significant morbidities such as infection, posttransplant lymphoproliferative disease (PTLD), and medication side effects.[2] Patients need close monitoring of liver enzymes, function, immunosuppressant levels, and viral polymerase chain reactions. Adherence with lifelong medication is challenging, in particular with adolescents. Nonadherence is associated with rejection and graft loss and should be addressed with every visit. The true ceiling for patient survival and graft longevity in pediatric LT recipients remains unknown. Some centers perform surveillance liver biopsies and have found increased hepatitis and fibrosis despite normal transaminases.[3] A unique aspect is that some children may develop operational tolerance and may be weaned off immunosuppressant.[4]

INDICATIONS FOR LIVER TRANSPLANT

LT in children should increase life expectancy and/or QOL. The indications for LT in children may be end-stage liver disease with significant synthetic dysfunction (acute or chronic), intractable portal hypertension, refractory ascites, coagulopathy, encephalopathy, variceal bleed, recurrent life-threatening episodes of cholangitis, spontaneous bacterial peritonitis, refractory pruritus, deforming xanthomas, failure to thrive despite maximal nutritional support, unresectable hepatic tumors, and certain metabolic diseases. The common disease processes leading to LT evaluation are listed in **Table 1**. The SRTR data show that the most common indication for pediatric LT is BA across all ages. This could be due to a late diagnosis, failed Kasai portoenterostomy, recurrent cholangitis, and progressive portal hypertension. The indications for LT change with the recipient's age. In the young population the common indications for LT are BA, metabolic disease, acute liver failure, and cholestasis. In the age group of 1 to 5 years, malignant liver tumors become the 4th indication for LT. In the population aged 11 to 17 years, noncholestatic cirrhosis is the most common cause for LT, followed by acute liver failure, metabolic disease, BA and cholestatic cirrhosis.

Indications for LT may change overtime. With earlier screening, diagnosis, and Kasai portoenterostomy, BA may decrease as the indication for LT. Only 16% of children with BA survive up to 2 years with their native liver if the total serum bilirubin measured 3 months following Kasai procedure is greater than 6 mg/dL, compared with 84% for those with a total bilirubin less than 2 mg/dL.[5] Parenteral nutrition-associated liver disease has decreased as an indication for LT, likely due to improved chronic total parenteral nutrition management and intestinal rehabilitation.[6] Metabolic diseases can lead to cirrhosis and be a risk factor for liver tumors (α-1 antitripsin deficiency, tyrosinemia, and Wilson disease) or acute liver failure. There are other metabolic diseases in which an LT replaces the defective enzyme and decreased associated morbidity (urea cycle defects, organic acidemias, and Crigler–Najjar syndrome type I). In some metabolic diseases the LT does not correct the enzyme deficiency in other organs beside the liver but is expected to improve QOL and decrease extrahepatic complications. There are some diseases in which an LT is needed to prevent progression of extrahepatic disease, such as primary hyperoxaluria type 1 and organic acidemias. There are a few

Table 1
Indications for liver transplantation in children

Cholestatic Conditions	• Biliary atresia • Sclerosing cholangitis • Parenteral nutrition-associated cholestasis • Alagille syndrome • Progressive familial intrahepatic cholestasis • Langerhans cell histiocytosis
Hepatitis	• Hepatitis B • Hepatitis C • Autoimmune hepatitis
Metabolic Disease	• Alpha 1 antitrypsin deficiency • Cystic fibrosis • Crigler–Najjar syndrome • Urea cycle defects • Organic academia • Maple syrup urine disease • Tyrosinemia • Wilson disease • Primary hyperoxaluria • Glycogen storages disorders • Hemophilia • Familial hypercholesterolemia • Certain mitochondrial disorders
Tumors	• Hepatoblastoma • Hemangioendothelioma • Hepatocellular carcinoma • Sarcoma
Other	• Cryptogenic cirrhosis • Gestational alloimmune liver disease • Budd–Chiari syndrome • Congenial hepatic fibrosis • Caroli disease • Drug induced • Hepatopulmonary syndrome
Acute Liver Failure	

metabolic and genetic diseases that, with improved LT outcome, have become an indication for LT as have better outcomes than conservative care. These include maple syrup urine disease and a few mitochondrial disorders.[7] In certain circumstances, a combined liver kidney (hyperoxaluria, methyl malonic acidemia) or combined liver lung (in cystic fibrosis [CF]) transplant is required. With a growing obesity epidemic, nonalcoholic fatty liver disease is becoming one of the leading causes of LT in adults and young adolescents.[8] LT can be beneficial in selected patients with secondary hemophagocytic lymphohistiocytosis.[9]

Current contraindications to LT in children are the following:

1. Nonresectable extrahepatic malignant tumor;
2. Multisystem organ failure with concomitant end-stage organ failure that cannot be corrected by a combined transplant;
3. Uncontrolled sepsis;
4. Irreversible serious neurologic damage; and
5. Uncorrectable life-limiting defects in critical organs such as heart, lungs, and kidneys.

There may be a few relative contraindications such as lack of social support; however, this is an ethical dilemma in pediatrics, and occasionally social work and child protective services can be involved.

ALLOCATION

Liver candidates younger than 18 years at the time of registration may be assigned any of the following:

- Pediatric status 1A
- Pediatric status 1B
- Calculated MELD or PELD score
- Exception MELD or PELD score
- Inactive status (status 7)

Status 1A is assigned to children with conditions such as fulminant liver failure without preexisting liver disease, defined as the onset of hepatic encephalopathy within 56 days of the first signs and symptoms of liver disease and has at least one of the following criteria: ventilator dependent, dialysis, or international normalized ratio (INR) greater than 2; primary nonfunction of a transplanted liver within 7 days of transplant; hepatic artery thrombosis (HAT) in a transplanted liver within 14 days of transplant; or acute decompensated Wilson disease.

Status 1B is assigned to children with the conditions such as hepatoblastoma without evidence of metastatic disease, organic acidemia or urea cycle defect (after 30 days of transplant with PELD score of 30), and chronic liver disease with a calculated PELD/MELD score greater than 25 and at least one of the following criteria: mechanical ventilator, gastrointestinal bleeding requiring greater than 30 mL/kg of red blood cell within previous 24 hours, dialysis, or Glasgow coma score less than 10 within 48 hours.

The PELD scoring system was applied since 2002. It is a formula developed to provide a numerical assessment of the risk of death in patients younger than 12 years: 0.436 (Age <1 yr.) – 0.687 x Loge (albumin g/dL) + 0.480 x Loge (total bilirubin mg/dL) + 1.857 x Loge (INR) +0.667 (Growth failure <−2 Std. Deviations present). However, the PELD score has been criticized and found not to predict well mortality on the wait list.[10] Other suggested scores such as the pCLIF-SOFA scores were suggested to better prognosticate the 28-day mortality.[11] Candidates who are at least 12 years old receive the following initial MELD score: 0.957 x Loge(creatinine mg/dL) + 0. 378 x Loge (bilirubin mg/dL) + 1.120 x Loge (INR) + 0.643. For candidates with an initial MELD score greater than11, the MELD Na score is recalculated as follows: MELD = MELD(i) + 1.32*(137-Na) – [0.033*MELD(i)*(137-Na)]. Sodium values less than 125 mmol/L will be set to 125.

Candidates meeting specific standardized MELD/PELD exceptions can be found on the OPTN Website and include patients with CF, hepatocellular carcinoma (HCC), cholangiocarcinoma, hepatopulmonary syndrome, portopulmonary hypertension, and hyperoxaluria. As both calculated PELD and MELD often do not reflect the risk of mortality on the wait list, nonstandard exceptions appeals are requested in 44% of children. Common conditions for appeal include failure to thrive, intractable ascites, pathologic bone fractures, refractory pruritus, and hemorrhage due to complications associated with portal hypertension. For children aged 2 to 18 years at listing, exception denial increased the risk of waitlist and post-LT mortality.[12] There is widespread regional variations in exception acceptance and disparity in use of exceptions by race that is not explained by clinical disease severity, diagnosis, geography, or other demographic factors.[13] United Network for Organ Sharing is currently moving from a regional review board to a national review board to assess nonstandard exceptions.

Once an organ becomes available, the allocation priority is based on the pediatric versus adult recipient, age of donor, geographic location of the donor and recipient (within donor service area, region, or nationally), and recipient–donor blood type match (identical vs compatible). There is a difference in pediatric organ allocation policies across the world. Some countries such as Brazil would triple the calculated PELD score to prioritize children. In the United States there are 20 to 30 children who die on the wait list every year, of which close to 50% received no offers. Pediatric prioritization in the allocation and development of improved risk stratification systems is required to reduce wait-list mortality among children.[14]

LIVER TRANSPLANT EVALUATION

Referral to LT depends on the child's clinical circumstances: emergent in acute liver failure or acute decompensation, urgent in progressive disease, or anticipatory. The timing of referral may depend on disease progression. In some metabolic diseases, early referral may offer the benefit of avoiding multisystemic complications and irreversible organ damage.[15] The primary goal of the evaluation process is to identify appropriate candidates for LT and establish a peritransplantation plan. Children have distinct diseases, clinical susceptibilities, physiologic responses, as well as neurocognitive and neurodevelopmental features that distinguish them from adults and differ within the pediatric age group. The multidisciplinary members of the pediatric LT team include transplant surgeon, hepatologist/gastroenterologist with expertise in pediatric liver disease, transplant coordinator, social worker, dietician, transplant pharmacist, and financial counselor. In selected patients, other disciplinarians are involved, including infectious disease specialist, transplant immunology, critical care specialist, anesthesiologist, psychologist/neuropsychologist/child development specialist, psychiatrist, child life specialist, cardiologist, nephrologist, neurologist, genetic/metabolic specialist, oncologist, pulmonologist, radiologist (diagnostic or interventional), dentist, ethics specialist, or other subspecialists.

The goal of the evaluation process is to confirm the indication for transplantation, discuss alternative treatments, exclude contraindications; discuss complications associated with end-stage liver disease (ascites, pruritus, portal hypertension, malnutrition, vitamin deficiencies, and delayed growth), and optimize pretransplant medical therapy and immunizations (as live vaccines are relatively contraindicated post-LT). Completion of all age-appropriate vaccinations, for the child and family members, should occur before transplantation on an accelerated schedule. Inactivated influenza vaccination should be given to patients and their family members. Previous exposure to Epstein-Barr virus (EBV) and cytomegalovirus (CMV) is assessed, because it effects the risk of PTLD and duration of CMV prophylaxis posttransplant. Serologies for vaccine preventable disease are done. Aggressive nutritional support for children awaiting LT should be initiated to optimize outcomes. Nasogastric tube feedings and parenteral nutrition may be needed in some circumstances because nutrition status is strongly associated with peritransplant survival.[16] Nutritional assessment includes vitamins and trace elements and often supplements are warranted. Neurocognitive testing should be performed in children awaiting LT to identify areas warranting early intervention to minimize later cognitive difficulties. Other important components include obtaining prior records; assessing disease severity and urgency for LT; considering appropriateness of a live donor option; establishing a trusting relationship among the child, family, and transplant team; ensuring finances are available; and developing a management and communication plan with the local managing physician.

During the evaluation process, it is pertinent to evaluate the liver and kidney function. Serum creatinine alone should not be used to assess renal function; either cystatin C or the revised Schwartz Formula should be used to estimate the glomerular filtration rate in children with chronic liver disease.[15] Children undergo a chest X-ray, ultrasound Doppler, electrocardiogram, and echocardiogram. In selected case, computed tomography or MRI may be required. Informed consent from parents includes discussing indication, contraindications, alternative for transplant, organ availability and option of living donor, increased risk donors, right to refuse transplant, and posttransplant complications. There should be a set plan on what to do when an organ becomes available and need to transport to the hospital.

Following are a few disease-specific considerations: children with hepatoblastoma should be evaluated pre-LT to rule out extrahepatic disease. Children at risk of HCC (cirrhosis or metabolic disease) with elevated or rising alpha-fetoprotein should be screened for HCC. As the Milan criteria may not be applicable to children, transplantation for HCC must be individualized and should be considered in the absence of radiological evidence of extrahepatic disease or gross vascular invasion, irrespective of size of the lesion or number of lesions. Alagille syndrome may carry a risk structural cardiac and renal disease and cerebral vascular malformations.[17] LT in FIC1 disease can be associated with worsening extrahepatic manifestations (diarrhea) and steatohepatitis.[18] Screening transcutaneous oxygen saturation with the patient in the upright position should be performed in all patients with possible portosystemic shunting. Patients with portal hypertension and end-stage liver disease may develop hepatopulmonary syndrome (HPS) and portopulmonary hypertension (PPHN). If the right ventricular systolic pressure is greater than 50 mm Hg by 2-dimensional echo, a right-heart cardiac catheterization is necessary to establish the diagnosis of PPHN. Children with HPS and mild PPHN should be prioritized on the wait list. In patients with CF, pulmonary function tests, including forced expiratory volume in 1 second and forced vital capacity, should be performed.[15] In some cases, multiorgan transplant should be considered.

SURGICAL TECHNIQUES AND VARIANT TRANSPLANTS

Because of the natural history of their liver diseases, the most children are very young (younger than 1 year) at the time of listing for transplantation. The number of pediatric candidates exceeds the number of small-sized pediatric donors of similar weight who need full-size LT to be performed. The result has been high mortality on the cadaveric waiting list, up to 25% in some North American centers.[19]

Because of scarcity of donors and better size matching between graft and recipients, most of the pediatric LTs in recent practice consist of variant techniques instead of whole LTs. The first variant techniques for LT consisted of graft reduction of cadaveric livers, which aimed to improve size matching. Early data from large series show that life expectancy of children who receive a cut-down LT is similar to that after full-size LT.[20,21]

Later techniques including living related donor and split transplant have the added benefit of increasing the donor pool.[21] These techniques require precise knowledge of the internal anatomy of the liver, which is divided into lobes and segments that have their own separated vascular and biliary network. The split technique allows a cadaveric liver to be divided into 2 functional segments, thus increasing the total number of organs available for transplant. The larger right lobe is typically transplanted into an adult recipient and the left lateral segment or left lobe transplanted into a child.[22] The first split was made in 1988 by Pichlmayr and colleagues,[23] and early report by Broelsch[24] (30 transplants in 25 children and 5 adults) showed inferior patient and graft survival rates compared with conventional transplants; however, progressive technical improvements began to achieve results similar to those of standard transplantations.[25] More recent meta-analysis continues to suggest that pediatric whole LT is associated with better outcomes than technical variant LT. The 1-, 3-, and 5-year patient survival rates and 1- and 3-year graft survival rates were higher in whole LT than technical variant LT. There was no significant difference in 5-year graft survival rate between the 2 groups. The incidence of portal vein thrombosis and biliary complications were significantly lower in the whole LT group, whereas the incidence of HAT was comparable between the 2 groups.[26] Because variant techniques will remain absolutely necessary in pediatric LT, continued efforts to minimize surgical complications is essential to improve outcomes.

In living donor LT, the donor undergoes removal of the left lateral segment, which represents between 15% and 20% of the total liver mass, or the full left lobe, which represents 30% to 35%, depending on the weight of the potential recipient. The remaining liver mass quickly regenerates without functional sequelae.[27,28] Raia in Sao Paulo performed the first living related donor transplant (LRDT) in 1988 on a patient who, unfortunately, did not survive the procedure.[29] Strong in Brisbane performed the first successful LRDT a year later, and Broelsch and Tanaka in Chicago and Kyoto, respectively, popularized the techniques soon after.[30,31] Their series is the largest one published so far, with 600 receptors younger than 18 years (850 including adults).[32,33] Multiple other large series demonstrate comparable long-term results between LRDT and cadaveric hepatic transplantation.[34–36]

With regard to recipient complications, biliary complications are the most frequent (14%–15%); arterial thrombosis has been much reduced using microsurgical techniques, so much so that the group from Kyoto reported an incidence of only 3.3%; portal thrombosis occurred in 7.5% and suprahepatic vein stenosis in 3.7% of cases from the same series. Vascular complications are more frequent in younger children.[36] For the donor, the potential risks of mortality and morbidity would be that of a left lateral segmentectomy or full left hepatectomy in a young, healthy patient with a normal liver. This is around 0.5% in cases donating the right hepatic lobe and less than 0.1% in cases donating left lobe.[34]

MEDICATIONS

Controlling host cellular responses and minimizing infection are key in reducing morbidity and mortality associated with LT. Success in pediatric solid organ transplantation has resulted in large part from control of T-cell–mediated acute rejection episodes. The incidence of acute cellular rejection and chronic rejection in pediatric LTs has been reported to be as high as 49.7% and 9%, respectively.[2] The use of increasingly potent T-cell–directed immunosuppressants has led to a reduction in graft loss from acute cellular rejection.[37]

Most immunosuppression protocols from pediatric LT programs include calcineurin inhibitors (CNI) (tacrolimus or cyclosporine), corticosteroids, and mycophenolate mofetil (MMF). Typically, patients are placed on 2 or more immunosuppressants postoperatively as induction. Most of these children then continue on tacrolimus monotherapy lifelong. Tacrolimus (Prograf) has become the preferred CNI due to reduction in steroid-resistant acute rejection, improved graft survival, and reduced rates of nephrotoxicity compared with cyclosporine. These immunosuppressants are very effective but are not without significant physiologic consequences. In order to ensure their immunomodulating effect while minimizing toxicity, drug levels and dosing have to be monitored closely. Dosages and target therapeutic drug levels vary depending on the time since transplantation and should be personalized to the individual patient. Some children may require more immunosuppression (ie, children with autoimmune hepatitis may require 2 immunosuppressants) and some may require intentional dose reduction (ie, after EBV seroconversion). Care must be taken in balancing risk of overimmunosuppression (side effects, infection, PTLD, etc.) and underimmunosuppression (rejection).

Commonly used immunosuppressive agents, dosing, side effects, and administration considerations in pediatric LT are outlined in **Table 2**.[38]

OUTCOME AND COMPLICATIONS

Advances in surgical techniques, postoperative care, and immunosuppressive treatment have allowed LT to be an effective treatment modality for patients with liver failure. Recent outcomes of pediatric LT are good. According to recent US Organ Procurement and Transplantation Network and Studies in Pediatric Liver Transplantation (SPLIT), patient survival rates at 1 and 5 years after a pediatric LT are now 91% to 91.4% and 84% to 86.5%.[2,39,40]

HAT remains a significant cause of graft loss after a LT in children, with incidence ranging from 5.7% to 8.4%.[41] Microsurgical techniques with an operational microscope have been used in hepatic arterial anastomosis reconstruction to lower the risk of HAT.[42]

Portal vein thrombosis, another significant complication in pediatric LT, reportedly affects approximately 5% to 10% of pediatric recipients. The diameter of the portal vein tends to decrease because of a reduced flow in children with portal hypertension. In addition, in patients with BA, the inflammation can extend to the portal vein.[43] Optimizing the graft weight to body weight ratios (GWBWR) and technical skills while avoiding redundancy, kinking, or stretching can help to prevent portal vein thrombosis. Doppler ultrasound is routinely performed after reperfusion to ensure vascular flow before closing the abdomen.

The SPLIT group reported the overall incidence of early biliary complications were more frequent in segmental LTs (21.8%) than in whole LTs (5.8%).[41] Kanmatz et al. recommends Roux-en-Y hepaticojejunostomy as the first choice for left lateral segment LT.

SPLIT registry data indicate that infection contributed to nearly half of all patients (46%), typically through multisystem organ failure or cardiopulmonary failure. Malignancy accounted for an additional 5.1%. Rejection contributed directly or indirectly, by necessitating retransplantation to only 4.7%. Infants were at highest risk to develop infection and at lowest risk to experience rejection.

Sepsis/infection, multisystem organ failure, and PTLD, as complications of immunosuppression, accounted for 41% of late deaths in pediatric LT. Chronic rejection accounted for rare deaths but was the dominant cause, along with acute rejection, for graft loss, accounting for half of the cases.[40,41] The morbidity from posttransplant lymphoproliferative disease was reduced by early detection of EBV infection, decreasing the dosage of immunosuppressive medication and continuing intravenous ganciclovir.

Large pediatric series demonstrate better survival rates in patients with less than 25 PELD points, GWBWR less than 3%, and weighing more than 7 kg. Important transplant predictors of graft survival include weight, renal function, modern era, warm

Table 2
Commonly used immunosuppressive agents, dosing, and side effects in pediatric liver transplantation

Medication	Dose	Side Effects
Tacrolimus	0.15–0.2 mg/kg/d po divided q12 h	Alopecia, pruritus, photosensitivity, constipation, diarrhea, nausea, vomiting, anemia, leukocytosis, thrombocytopenia, headache, insomnia, paresthesia, tremor, seizure, leukoencephalopathy (rare), nephrotoxicity, hypertension, cardiomyopathy, prolonged QT interval,, diabetes mellitus, hypercholesterolemia, lymphoproliferative disease, hypomagnesaemia, hyperkalemia, hypophosphatemia
Cyclosporine	15 mg/kg/d po divided q12 h for 2 wk posttransplant, then 4–12 mg/kg/d po divided bid	Nephrotoxicity, hypertension, edema, arrhythmia, hirsutism, gingival hyperplasia, gynecomastia, diarrhea, leukopenia, hypomagnesaemia, hyperkalemia, hyperuricemia hyperglycemia, hyperlipidemia, tremor, paresthesia, leg cramps, weakness, encephalopathy, progressive multifocal leukoencephalopathy, seizure
Sirolimus	Loading dose: 3 mg/m^2 on day 1 Maintenance dose: 1 mg/m^2/d divided q12 h or given daily	Hyperlipidemia, proteinuria, myelosuppression, pneumonitis, hypersensitivity reactions, hepatic artery thrombosis, poor wound healing, mouth ulcers, acne, edema, anemia, thrombocytopenia, arthralgia, headache, increased serum creatinine, fever, pain, progressive multifocal leukoencephalopathy
Mycophenolate mofetil	10–15 mg/kg/dose po BID (max 1 g/dose)	Diarrhea, abdominal pain, constipation, nausea, teratogenic, neutropenia, anemia, thrombocytopenia, constipation, nausea, hypertension, edema, opportunistic infections, hyperglycemia, hypocalcemia, hypokalemia, hypomagnesaemia, hypercholesterolemia, pleural effusion, lymphoma, progressive multifocal leukoencephalopathy
Corticosteroids	Induction with high-dose methylprednisolone IV 20 mg/kg/dose (max 1 g) Taper over 5 d to maintenance prednisone or prednisolone (approximately 0.2–0.3 mg/kg/dose po daily)	Hypertension, impaired wound healing, gastrointestinal ulcers, diabetes mellitus, fluid retention, adrenal insufficiency, depression, mood swings, insomnia, cataracts, weight gain, osteopenia, pancreatitis, cosmetic (acne, cushing, striae), decreased growth
Basiliximab	Wt <35 kg: 10 mg IV ×2 Wt ≥35 kg: 20 mg IV ×2 First dose given within 2 h of transplant, second dose on day 4	Hypersensitivity reaction, abdominal pain, vomiting, asthenia, dizziness, insomnia, edema, hypertension, anemia, dysuria, cough, dyspnea, fever

(continued on next page)

Table 2 (continued)		
Medication	Dose	Side Effects
Antithymocyte globulin (rabbit)	1.5 mg/kg/d administered by IV infusion for 7–14 d	Cytokine-release storm, serum sickness, thrombocytopenia, leukopenia, neutropenia, hypertension, peripheral edema, post-transplant lymphoproliferative disease, hyperkalemia

From Miloh T, Barton A, Wheeler J, et al. Immunosuppression in pediatric liver transplant recipients: unique aspects. Liver Transpl 2017;23(2):244–56; with permission.

ischemia time, and time between primary transplantation and re-pLTx. Renal function, mechanical ventilation, and underlying cause of liver disease affect patient survival.[42,44]

LONG-TERM MANAGEMENT

Advancements in surgical techniques, organ procurement, pre- and postoperative management, and immunosuppression have led to outstanding strides in pediatric LT. As more and more recipients enter into adulthood, more attention is paid to the potential harm of chronic immunosuppressive therapy itself, with side effects including renal insufficiency, cardiovascular disease, diabetes mellitus, PTLD, and osteopenia. Opportunistic infection and PTLD account for 30% of late mortality in pediatric LT recipients.[40,45,46]

As a result of the concern for potential side effect morbidities, there is a rise in interest in immunosuppression minimization and withdrawal. It is estimated that 20% to 25% of pediatric LT recipients will be operationally tolerant without immunosuppression.[4,47]

Abnormal liver enzymes are common among long-term pediatric LT survivors, with up to one-third having abnormal transaminases, and nearly half have abnormal gamma-glutamyltransferases 5 years post-LT.[48] Furthermore, chronic hepatitis, liver fibrosis, or both have been described in 40% to 50% of otherwise asymptomatic 5-year survivors with normal liver function tests, supporting the need for protocol biopsies and further investigation.[3,49–52]

ADHERENCE AND TRANSITION

The long-term outcomes after LT strongly depend on adherence with medical regimen and lifelong intake of immunosuppression and close medical follow-up. The definition of adherence is compliance with agreed upon therapy; therefore the child and family are active members. The most common cause of late graft loss is chronic and late rejection.[40] Nonadherence (NA) was estimated to occur in 35% to 50% of adolescents and is the most common cause of late acute rejection in children who receive an LT.[53] NA is associated with graft loss, increased expenditures on care, and ultimately death.[54,55] As children get older, the medication intake responsibility shifts from caregiver (usually parent) to child. By 9 years of age, 30% of children are expected to be responsible for taking their medication, which is a vulnerable time for NA.[53] Pediatric LT recipients' medical and psychosocial needs change over time as they transition from childhood to adolescence and early adulthood.[56]

It may be challenging to identify NA. Subjective methods such as patient reports are unreliable; pill counts, refills, and electronic monitoring impose additional burden on the patient. Increased medication level variability index greater than 2.5 in children was associated with increased risk of rejection[57] and may be used to predict NA. It is crucial to better identify high-risk populations, improve detection methods, and plan earlier interventions. The most reported barrier to adherence was forgetfulness and vomiting (70%), followed by bad taste and interruptions in routine (60%), anxiety, depression, and posttraumatic stress disorder.[58] The medication regimen should be clear and simplified as possible. A systematic review of immunosuppressant adherence interventions in transplant recipients revealed only a few successful interventions, including counseling, increased clinic visits, mobile devices with automated reminders, and telemonitoring.[59] It is important to address adolescent psychosocial health issues with the patients and their families and provide counseling on smoking, illicit drug use, alcohol use, birth control, and sexually transmitted disease. Female LT patients who are of child-bearing age on MMF should use methods of birth control due to the known teratogenicity of this immunosuppressive agent. Adolescents may lose insurance coverage into adulthood, which may restrict care. Addressing these topics early and repeatedly is important in improving adherence and thereby maximizing long-term outcome.

As patients mature into young adulthood, a process of transition has to take place to allow safe and effective transfer of care from a pediatric facility to the care of adult providers. In the absence of a transfer process, patients may experience anxiety, confusion, distress, inability to manage the requirements of the new setting, increased risk of NA, rejection, and even mortality.[60] There are various potential barriers to transitioning and ultimately transferring care. These barriers arise at the level of the patient, parent/family, and the pediatric and adult provider. In adult settings, patients are expected to display behaviors consistent with self-management for instance, independently discussing one's illness and concerns with the treatment team, scheduling and attending appointments, and so on. However, when patients endorse more responsibility for their care too early, clinical outcomes are worse, indicating that indiscriminate promotion of self-management by adolescents may not be advisable.[61] Assessment of adolescent executive function skills may help guide the development of individualized transition readiness guidelines to promote successful gains in self-management abilities as well as eventual transfer to adult medical services. There are a few transition readiness tolls available, and the process can start as early as 11 to 12 years of age, such as The Readiness for Transition Questionnaire.[62] A 2014 technical review by the Agency for Healthcare Research and Quality emphasized the importance of transition programs, transition coordinator, a special clinic for young adults in transition, and provision of educational materials.[63] A multidisciplinary approach aiming at fostering adherence should be used. Parents should be supported to move from a "managerial" to a "supervisory" role during transition to help young people engage independently with the health care team.

REFERENCES

1. Mogul DB, Luo X, Bowring MG, et al. Fifteen-year trends in pediatric liver transplants: split, whole deceased, and living donor grafts. J Pediatr 2018;196: 148–53.e2.

2. Ng VL, Alonso EM, Bucuvalas JC, et al. Health status of children alive 10 years after pediatric liver transplantation performed in the US and Canada: report of

the studies of pediatric liver transplantation experience. J Pediatr 2012;160(5): 820–6.e3.

3. Scheenstra R, Peeters PM, Verkade HJ, et al. Graft fibrosis after pediatric liver transplantation: ten years of follow-up. Hepatology 2009;49(3):880–6.

4. Feng S, Ekong UD, Lobritto SJ, et al. Complete immunosuppression withdrawal and subsequent allograft function among pediatric recipients of parental living donor liver transplants. JAMA 2012;307(3):283–93.

5. Shneider BL, Brown MB, Haber B, et al. A multicenter study of the outcome of biliary atresia in the United States, 1997 to 2000. J Pediatr 2006;148(4):467–74.

6. Nandivada P, Fell GL, Gura KM, et al. Lipid emulsions in the treatment and prevention of parenteral nutrition-associated liver disease in infants and children. Am J Clin Nutr 2016;103(2):629S–34S.

7. Mazariegos G, Shneider B, Burton B, et al. Liver transplantation for pediatric metabolic disease. Mol Genet Metab 2014;111(4):418–27.

8. Alkhouri N, Hanouneh IA, Zein NN, et al. Liver transplantation for nonalcoholic steatohepatitis in young patients. Transpl Int 2016;29(4):418–24.

9. Amir AZ, Ling SC, Naqvi A, et al. Liver transplantation for children with acute liver failure associated with secondary hemophagocytic lymphohistiocytosis. Liver Transpl 2016;22(9):1245–53.

10. Shneider BL, Neimark E, Frankenberg T, et al. Critical analysis of the pediatric end-stage liver disease scoring system: a single center experience. Liver Transpl 2005;11(7):788–95.

11. Bolia R, Srivastava A, Yachha SK, et al. Pediatric CLIF-SOFA score is the best predictor of 28-day mortality in children with decompensated chronic liver disease. J Hepatol 2018;68(3):449–55.

12. Braun HJ, Perito ER, Dodge JL, et al. Nonstandard exception requests impact outcomes for pediatric liver transplant candidates. Am J Transplant 2016; 16(11):3181–91.

13. Hsu EK, Shaffer M, Bradford M, et al. Heterogeneity and disparities in the use of exception scores in pediatric liver allocation. Am J Transplant 2015;15(2):436–44.

14. Hsu EK, Shaffer ML, Gao L, et al. Analysis of liver offers to pediatric candidates on the transplant wait list. Gastroenterology 2017;153(4):988–95.

15. Squires RH, Ng V, Romero R, et al. Evaluation of the pediatric patient for liver transplantation: 2014 practice guideline by the American Association for the Study of Liver Diseases, American Society of Transplantation and the North American Society for Pediatric Gastroenterology, Hepatology and Nutrition. Hepatology 2014;60(1):362–98.

16. Carter-Kent C, Radhakrishnan K, Feldstein AE. Increasing calories, decreasing morbidity and mortality: is improved nutrition the answer to better outcomes in patients with biliary atresia? Hepatology 2007;46(5):1329–31.

17. Carpenter CD, Linscott LL, Leach JL, et al. Spectrum of cerebral arterial and venous abnormalities in Alagille syndrome. Pediatr Radiol 2018;48(4):602–8.

18. Squires JE. Protecting the allograft following liver transplantation for PFIC1. Pediatr Transplant 2016;20(7):882–3.

19. Busuttil RW, Colonna JO 2nd, Hiatt JR, et al. The first 100 liver transplants at UCLA. Ann Surg 1987;206(4):387–402.

20. Otte JB, de Ville de Goyet J, Reding R, et al. Pediatric liver transplantation: from the full-size liver graft to reduced, split, and living related liver transplantation. Pediatr Surg Int 1998;13(5–6):308–18.

21. Otte JB, de Ville de Goyet J, Sokal E, et al. Size reduction of the donor liver is a safe way to alleviate the shortage of size-matched organs in pediatric liver transplantation. Ann Surg 1990;211(2):146–57.

22. Otte JB, de Ville de Goyet J, Alberti D, et al. The concept and technique of the split liver in clinical transplantation. Surgery 1990;107(6):605–12.

23. Pichlmayr R, Ringe B, Gubernatis G, et al. Transplantation of a donor liver to 2 recipients (splitting transplantation)–a new method in the further development of segmental liver transplantation. Langenbecks Arch Chir 1988;373(2):127–30 [in German].

24. Broelsch CE, Emond JC, Whitington PF, et al. Application of reduced-size liver transplants as split grafts, auxiliary orthotopic grafts, and living related segmental transplants. Ann Surg 1990;212(3):368–75 [discussion: 375–7].

25. Rogiers X, Malagó M, Gawad K, et al. In situ splitting of cadaveric livers. The ultimate expansion of a limited donor pool. Ann Surg 1996;224(3):331–9 [discussion: 339–41].

26. Ye H, Zhao Q, Wang Y, et al. Outcomes of technical variant liver transplantation versus whole liver transplantation for pediatric patients: a meta-analysis. PLoS One 2015;10(9):e0138202.

27. Iwatsuki S, Shaw BW Jr, Starzl TE. Experience with 150 liver resections. Ann Surg 1983;197(3):247–53.

28. Nagao T, Inoue S, Mizuta T, et al. One hundred hepatic resections. Indications and operative results. Ann Surg 1985;202(1):42–9.

29. Raia S, Nery JR, Mies S. Liver transplantation from live donors. Lancet 1989; 2(8661):497.

30. Singer PA, Siegler M, Lantos JD, et al. The ethical assessment of innovative therapies: liver transplantation using living donors. Theor Med 1990;11(2):87–94.

31. Strong RW, Lynch SV, Ong TH, et al. Successful liver transplantation from a living donor to her son. N Engl J Med 1990;322(21):1505–7.

32. Kiuchi T, Inomata Y, Uemoto S, et al. Living-donor liver transplantation in Kyoto, 1997. Clin Transplant 1997;191–8.

33. Tanaka K, Ogura Y, Kiuchi T, et al. Living donor liver transplantation: Eastern experiences. HPB (Oxford) 2004;6(2):88–94.

34. Burgos L, Hernández F, Barrena S, et al. Variant techniques for liver transplantation in pediatric programs. Eur J Pediatr Surg 2008;18(6):372–4.

35. Otte JB. Paediatric liver transplantation–a review based on 20 years of personal experience. Transpl Int 2004;17(10):562–73.

36. Tanaka K, Uemoto S, Tokunaga Y, et al. Surgical techniques and innovations in living related liver transplantation. Ann Surg 1993;217(1):82–91.

37. Meier-Kriesche HU, Schold JD, Kaplan B. Long-term renal allograft survival: have we made significant progress or is it time to rethink our analytic and therapeutic strategies? Am J Transplant 2004;4(8):1289–95.

38. Miloh T, Barton A, Wheeler J, et al. Immunosuppression in pediatric liver transplant recipients: unique aspects. Liver Transpl 2017;23(2):244–56.

39. McDiarmid SV, Anand R, Martz K, et al. A multivariate analysis of pre-, peri-, and post-transplant factors affecting outcome after pediatric liver transplantation. Ann Surg 2011;254(1):145–54.

40. Soltys KA, Mazariegos GV, Squires RH, et al. Late graft loss or death in pediatric liver transplantation: an analysis of the SPLIT database. Am J Transplant 2007; 7(9):2165–71.

41. Diamond IR, Fecteau A, Millis JM, et al. Impact of graft type on outcome in pediatric liver transplantation: a report from Studies of Pediatric Liver Transplantation (SPLIT). Ann Surg 2007;246(2):301–10.

42. Kanmaz T, Yankol Y, Mecit N, et al. Pediatric liver transplant: a single-center study of 100 consecutive patients. Exp Clin Transplant 2014;12(1):41–5.

43. Takahashi Y, Nishimoto Y, Matsuura T, et al. Surgical complications after living donor liver transplantation in patients with biliary atresia: a relatively high incidence of portal vein complications. Pediatr Surg Int 2009;25(9):745–51.

44. Venick RS, Farmer DG, Soto JR, et al. One thousand pediatric liver transplants during thirty years: lessons learned. J Am Coll Surg 2018;226(4):355–66.

45. Mohammad S, Hormaza L, Neighbors K, et al. Health status in young adults two decades after pediatric liver transplantation. Am J Transplant 2012;12(6):1486–95.

46. Duffy JP, Kao K, Ko CY, et al. Long-term patient outcome and quality of life after liver transplantation: analysis of 20-year survivors. Ann Surg 2010;252(4):652–61.

47. Porrett P, Shaked A. The failure of immunosuppression withdrawal: patient benefit is not detectable, inducible, or reproducible. Liver Transpl 2011;17(Suppl 3):S66–8.

48. Ng VL, Fecteau A, Shepherd R, et al. Outcomes of 5-year survivors of pediatric liver transplantation: report on 461 children from a north american multicenter registry. Pediatrics 2008;122(6):e1128–35.

49. Ekong UD, Melin-Aldana H, Seshadri R, et al. Graft histology characteristics in long-term survivors of pediatric liver transplantation. Liver Transpl 2008;14(11):1582–7.

50. Evans HM, Kelly DA, McKiernan PJ, et al. Progressive histological damage in liver allografts following pediatric liver transplantation. Hepatology 2006;43(5):1109–17.

51. Fouquet V, Alves A, Branchereau S, et al. Long-term outcome of pediatric liver transplantation for biliary atresia: a 10-year follow-up in a single center. Liver Transpl 2005;11(2):152–60.

52. Herzog D, Soglio DB, Fournet JC, et al. Interface hepatitis is associated with a high incidence of late graft fibrosis in a group of tightly monitored pediatric orthotopic liver transplantation patients. Liver Transpl 2008;14(7):946–55.

53. McDiarmid SV. Adolescence: challenges and responses. Liver Transpl 2013;19(Suppl 2):S35–9.

54. Fredericks EM, Lopez MJ, Magee JC, et al. Psychological functioning, nonadherence and health outcomes after pediatric liver transplantation. Am J Transplant 2007;7(8):1974–83.

55. Shemesh E, Shneider BL, Savitzky JK, et al. Medication adherence in pediatric and adolescent liver transplant recipients. Pediatrics 2004;113(4):825–32.

56. Alonso EM, Neighbors K, Barton FB, et al. Health-related quality of life and family function following pediatric liver transplantation. Liver Transpl 2008;14(4):460–8.

57. Shemesh E, Bucuvalas JC, Anand R, et al. The medication level variability index (MLVI) predicts poor liver transplant outcomes: a prospective multi-site study. Am J Transplant 2017;17(10):2668–78.

58. Shemesh E. Non-adherence to medications following pediatric liver transplantation. Pediatr Transplant 2004;8(6):600–5.

59. Duncan S, Annunziato RA, Dunphy C, et al. A systematic review of immunosuppressant adherence interventions in transplant recipients: decoding the streetlight effect. Pediatr Transplant 2018;22(1).

60. Annunziato RA, Emre S, Shneider B, et al. Adherence and medical outcomes in pediatric liver transplant recipients who transition to adult services. Pediatr Transplant 2007;11(6):608–14.
61. Annunziato RA, Bucuvalas JC, Yin W, et al. Self-management measurement and prediction of clinical outcomes in pediatric transplant. J Pediatr 2018;193: 128–33.e2.
62. Fredericks EM. Transition readiness assessment: the importance of the adolescent perspective. Pediatr Transplant 2017;21(3).
63. Davis AM, Brown RF, Taylor JL, et al. Transition care for children with special health care needs. Pediatrics 2014;134(5):900–8.

Moving?

Make sure your subscription moves with you!

To notify us of your new address, find your **Clinics Account Number** (located on your mailing label above your name), and contact customer service at:

Email: journalscustomerservice-usa@elsevier.com

800-654-2452 (subscribers in the U.S. & Canada)
314-447-8871 (subscribers outside of the U.S. & Canada)

Fax number: 314-447-8029

Elsevier Health Sciences Division
Subscription Customer Service
3251 Riverport Lane
Maryland Heights, MO 63043

*To ensure uninterrupted delivery of your subscription, please notify us at least 4 weeks in advance of move.